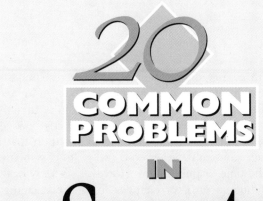

20 COMMON PROBLEMS IN

Sports Medicine

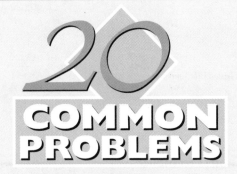

Sports Medicine

EDITOR

JAMES C. PUFFER, M.D.

Professor and Chief
Division of Sports Medicine
Department of Family Medicine
UCLA School of Medicine
Los Angeles, California

SERIES EDITOR

BARRY D. WEISS, M.D.

Professor of Clinical Family and Community Medicine
University of Arizona College of Medicine, Tucson, Arizona

McGraw-Hill

Medical Publishing Division

New York   Chicago   San Francisco   Lisbon   London   Madrid   Mexico City
Milan   New Delhi   San Juan   Seoul   Singapore   Sydney   Toronto

McGraw-Hill

A Division of The McGraw·Hill Companies

20 COMMON PROBLEMS IN SPORTS MEDICINE

Copyright © 2002 by The **McGraw-Hill Companies**, Inc. All rights reserved. Printed in the United States of America. Except as permitted under the United States Copyright Act of 1976, no part of this publication may be reproduced or distributed in any form or by any means, or stored in a data base or retrieval system, without the prior written permission of the publisher.

1234567890 DOCDOC 0987654321

ISBN 0-07-052720-2

This book was set in Garamond by Better Graphics, Inc.
The editors were Andrea Seils, Susan Noujaim, and Nicky Panton.
The production supervisor was Richard Ruzycka.
The cover designer was Marsha Cohen/Parallelogram.
The index was prepared by Geraldine Beckford.

R.R. Donnelley and Sons Company was printer and binder.

This book is printed on acid-free paper.

Library of Congress Cataloging-in-Publication Data

20 common problems in sports medicine / editor, James Puffer.
    p. ; cm.
   Includes bibliographical references and index.
   ISBN 0-07-052720-2
    1. Sports medicine. 2. Sports injuries. I. Title: Twenty common problems in sports medicine. II. Puffer, James
   [DNLM: 1. Athletic Injuries--diagnosis. 2. Athletic Injuries--therapy. 3. Pain--therapy. QT 261 Z999 2002]
   RC1210 .A15 2002
   617.1′027--dc21

                                        2001018050

INTERNATIONAL EDITION ISBN 112465-9
Copyright © 2002. Exclusive rights by The McGraw-Hill Companies, Inc., for manufacture and export. This book cannot be reexported from the country to which it is consigned by McGraw-Hill. The International Edition is not available in North America.

We dedicate this book in memory of
Harry L. Galanty, M.D.
Loving husband and father, devoted son,
respected colleague and friend.

Contents

Contributors

ANTERIOR KNEE PAIN
(CHAPTER 7)
Harry L. Galanty, M.D. (deceased)
Formerly Assistant Professor of Orthopedics
  and Pediatrics
Texas Tech University
Health Sciences Center
Lubbock, Texas

APOPHYSITIS
(CHAPTER 17)
Paul R. Stricker, M.D.
Physician
Department of Orthopaedic Surgery
Scripps Clinic
La Jolla, California

Cheryl Wasilewski, P.T.
Physical Therapist
Vanderbilt University Sports Medicine
Nashville, Tennessee

CONCUSSION
(CHAPTER 15)
John McShane, M.D.
Clinical Assistant Professor of Family Medicine
  and Director, Sports Medicine Fellowship Program
Jefferson Medical College
Thomas Jefferson University Hospital
Philadelphia, Pennsylvania

Eugene Hong, M.D.
Clinical Assistant Professor
Family Medicine and Sports Medicine
Department of Family Medicine
Jefferson Medical College
Thomas Jefferson University Hospital
Philadelphia, Pennsylvania

Jennifer M. Naticchia, M.D.
Clinical Instructor & Assistant Director of Sports Medicine
Family Medicine and Sports Medicine
Department of Family Medicine
Jefferson Medical College
Thomas Jefferson University Hospital
Philadelphia, Pennsylvania

**DEVELOPMENTAL AND
MATURATIONAL ISSUES**
(CHAPTER 16)
Sally S. Harris, M.D.
Physician
Departments of Pediatrics and Sports Medicine
Palo Alto Medical Foundation
Palo Alto, California

ELBOW PAIN
(CHAPTER 3)
Robert G. Hosey, M.D.
Assistant Professor of Family Practice/Sports Medicine
University of Kentucky
Chandler Medical Center
Lexington, Kentucky

**EXERCISE-INDUCED
BRONCHOSPASM**
(CHAPTER 13)
Andrew W. Nichols, M.D.
Director of Sports Medicine and Associate Professor
Department of Family Practice and Community Health
John A. Burns School of Medicine
University of Hawaii at Manoa
Honolulu, Hawaii

FOOT PAIN
(CHAPTER 11)
Todd D. Larson, M.D.
Staff Physician
Saint Joseph Medical Clinic
Tacoma, Washington

FRACTURES IN PEDIATRIC ATHLETES
(CHAPTER 18)
Suzanne S. Hecht, M.D.
Assistant Professor
UCLA Departments of Family Medicine and Orthopedics
Division of Sports Medicine
Los Angeles, California

Joseph P. Luftman, M.D.
Clinical Instructor
UCLA Department of Family Medicine
Clinical Faculty, Kaiser Sunset Family Practice Residency
　Program and Division of Sports Medicine
Los Angeles, California

HEAT ILLNESS
(CHAPTER 14)
Daniel V. Vigil, M.D.
Sports Medicine Director and Faculty Physician
Family Practice Residency Program
Kaiser Permanente—Los Angeles
Los Angeles, California
and
Clinical Instructor
UCLA School of Medicine
University of California, Los Angeles
Los Angeles, California

HIP PAIN
(CHAPTER 6)
Jeffrey A. Housner, M.D.
Clinical Assistant Professor of Family Practice
University of Michigan
Department of Family Practice Center
Ann Arbor, Michigan

LEG PAIN
(CHAPTER 9)
John P. DiFiori, M.D.
Associate Professor and Assistant Team Physician
Department of Family Medicine and Intercollegiate Athletics
UCLA Division of Sports Medicine
University of California, Los Angeles
Los Angeles, California

LOW BACK PAIN
(CHAPTER 19)
David J. Shaskey, M.D.
Staff Physician
Sports Medicine and Rheumatology
Wasatch Internal Medicine
Salt Lake City, Utah

MENSTRUAL DYSFUNCTION
(CHAPTER 12)
Kimberly A. Fulton, M.D.
Primary Care Sports Medicine Fellow
The Cleveland Clinic
Cleveland, Ohio

Aurelia Nattiv, M.D.
Associate Professor
UCLA Department of Family Medicine
Division of Sports Medicine
and
Department of Orthopaedic Surgery
UCLA School of Medicine
Los Angeles, California

SHOULDER DISLOCATION
(CHAPTER 2)
James Dunlap, M.D.
Associate Professor, Program Director, and Chair
Department of Family Medicine—Las Vegas
University of Nevada School of Medicine
Las Vegas, Nevada

SHOULDER PAIN
(CHAPTER 1)
James J. Kinderknecht, M.D.
Assistant Professor of Family Medicine
　and Community Medicine
Department of Family and Community Medicine
University of Missouri—Columbia
Columbia, Missouri

STRESS FRACTURES
(CHAPTER 20)
Thomas D. Armsey, M.D.
Assistant Professor
Department of Family Practice and Orthopaedics
University of Kentucky College of Medicine
Lexington, Kentucky

THE ACUTELY INJURED KNEE
(CHAPTER 8)
Bryan W. Smith, M.D.
Clinical Assistant Professor of Pediatrics and Orthopaedics
University of North Carolina School of Medicine
Chapel Hill, North Carolina

THE ACUTELY INJURED WRIST
(CHAPTER 4)
Philip H. Cohen, M.D.
Assistant Team Physician
Rutgers University
Piscataway, New Jersey

Bassil Aish, M.D.
Director of Clinical Research
Beach Physicians and Surgeons Medical Group
and
Team Physician
Golden West College
Huntington Beach, California

THE INJURED ANKLE
(CHAPTER 10)
Edward J. Reisman, M.D.
Specialty Consultant, Primary Care Physician
Group Health Permanente
Corporate Center, Spokane Division
Spokane, Washington

THE INJURED FINGER
(CHAPTER 5)
Dennis Y. Wen, M.D.
Assistant Professor of Clinical Family Medicine
University of Missouri—Columbia
Columbia, Missouri

Preface

This book is the latest in McGraw-Hill's *20 Common Problems* series, which is a collection of books devoted to the most common problems confronted by primary care providers in the ambulatory setting. This book deals specifically with the most common problems seen in sports medicine. It is to the credit of series editor Barry Weiss, M.D. that a decision was made to include sports medicine in this series. Musculoskeletal problems rank second only to upper respiratory complaints as the most frequent problems seen by primary care providers. Unfortunately, little attention is paid to these common problems in the training of medical professionals. With that thought in mind, this book has been written in a manner similar to the books that have preceded it. Specifically, each chapter focuses on a problem in sports medicine, and concentrates on the most important information that the clinician needs to know to adequately diagnose and manage each problem. Since the primary care provider sees patients of all ages who participate in recreational and competitive activities, we have included both the medical and musculoskeletal problems that are encountered by the clinician on a frequent basis. Particular attention has been paid to identifying those problems that can be managed by the primary care provider and differentiating them from those that should be referred for more specialized care. The book has been written to complement the clinical skills of a broad cohort of clinicians from multi-

ple disciplines who practice in the primary care setting, as well as to serve as a useful resource to medical students, nurses and residents who are training to eventually practice in the primary care setting.

What are the 20 Most Common Problems in Sports Medicine?

Little data exist to document the most common problems in sport medicine seen by primary care providers. Therefore, we have relied upon our collective experience of treating sports medicine problems in the UCLA Family Health Center and the UCLA Comprehensive Sports Medicine Center in order to develop our compilation. The first serves as our training and faculty practice site for our residency training program in Family Practice, and the second serves as the training site for the faculty and fellows of our sports medicine fellowship for primary care physicians. Our selection of the *20 most common problems* has been somewhat arbitrary, but we feel that it accurately reflects the typical problems seen by the practicing clinician in the primary care setting. As you will see, we have organized the book into five discrete parts. *Part I* deals with problems of the upper extremity and includes shoulder pain, shoulder dislocation, elbow pain, the acutely injured wrist, and the injured finger. *Part II* deals with problems of the lower extremity and concentrates on hip pain, anterior knee pain, the acutely injured knee, leg pain, the sprained ankle, and foot pain. *Part III* focuses on medical problems and includes menstrual dysfunction, exercise-induced bronchospasm, heat illness, and concussion. *Part IV* addresses pediatric problems, including developmental aspects of children participating in athletic activity, apophysitis, and fractures. The final section, *Part V*, deals with the problems of low back pain and stress fractures.

About the Authors

We have had the great pleasure to train 28 fellows in sports medicine at our institution. Twenty-four of these fellows have finished our program and serve as team physicians and practice primarily in academic settings throughout the country. Twenty-two of these fellows serve as the primary authors for the chapters in this book. These include Chap. 4, co-authored by Philip H. Cohen and Bassil Aish, and Chap. 18, co-authored by Suzanne S. Hecht and Joseph P. Luftman. Aurelia Nattiv co-authored Chap. 12 with one of our former residents, and John McShane co-authored Chap. 15 with two colleagues from his training program. Since each of the authors has received their training in the same program, each chapter has a degree of uniformity in its approach to each specific problem. In a sense, it represents the approach that we take at UCLA in solving musculoskeletal and medical problems in the active patient. But more importantly, each chapter is flavored by the unique experience that each author has acquired

since completing their training. It is for these reasons that we have enjoyed the process of putting this book together; we have viewed this as a special opportunity to share our training and expertise with the many learners who will hopefully enjoy reading and using this book.

A Special Note

Unfortunately, during the writing of this text, we lost one of our dear friends and colleagues, Harry L. Galanty. Harry finished his chapter during the end of a long illness that took him prematurely from his wonderful family and us. So, it was with considerable sorrow that we dedicated this book to his memory, but it was with renewed energy that we dedicated ourselves to make the book the best that we could, so as to appropriately honor his life and his commitment to his patients, residents, and students.

Acknowledgments

Before closing, I would like to acknowledge some special people whose help was critical in completing this project. Barry D. Weiss, series editor, was particularly helpful in the initial review of the chapters and offered many useful suggestions that strengthened the overall presentation of the topics. Marty Quan, our residency program director, diligently read each chapter and served as an important resource who helped make certain that each chapter was written in a manner which would be easily grasped by readers with varying levels of experience and expertise. Susan Noujaim, senior developmental editor at McGraw-Hill, has been incredibly patient in assisting us with this task and was indispensable throughout every phase of the project. Finally, a special thanks to our administrative assistant, Mark Demars, who has done everything from retyping manuscripts to politely reminding authors of their missed deadlines!

James C. Puffer, M.D.

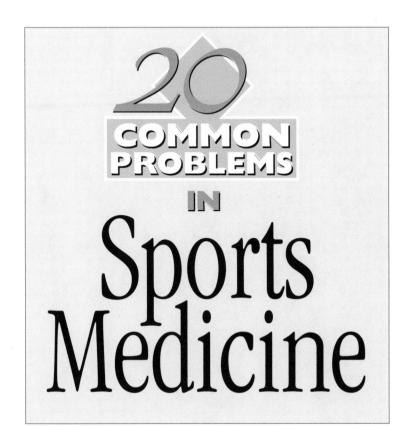

20 COMMON PROBLEMS IN Sports Medicine

Upper Extremity
Problems

James J. Kinderknecht

Shoulder Pain

Introduction

Shoulder pain is an extremely common problem in sports medicine, and pain in the shoulder can be one of the most challenging to diagnose and treat. Shoulder function is governed by the complex interplay of a number of anatomic and biomechanic factors, and therefore, to evaluate, diagnose, and treat the painful shoulder, a thorough understanding of shoulder anatomy and biomechanics is essential.

Shoulder pain can be divided into disorders related to the bony structures, soft tissues, and nerves. The soft tissues include the tendons, bursae, and the glenoid labrum. The onset of pain can be an acute, traumatic event or the result of repetitive activities. It is commonly associated with sports activities, occupational activities, as well as activities of daily living involving patients of all ages. The chapter focuses on shoulder pain in sports. Shoulder dislocations are discussed in Chap. 2.

Anatomy

Bone

The shoulder is comprised of several joints. The glenohumeral joint, acromioclavicular joint, sternoclavicular joint, and the scapulothoracic articulation are all critical in facilitating normal motion of the shoulder. The bony anatomy consists of the humerus, scapula, clavicle, and the sternum. The scapula includes the glenoid, acromion, coracoid, and the scapular body.

Musculature

The soft tissue anatomy is comprised of the musculature, ligaments, labrum, and neural structures. The rotator cuff is a key muscular structure. It is the dynamic stabilizer of the glenohumeral joint and is made up of the supraspinatus, infraspinatus, subscapularis, and teres minor muscles.[1] The subscapularis is an internal rotator of the joint. External rotation is provided by the infraspinatus and teres minor. The supraspinatus is an abductor of the shoulder. The pectoralis major, deltoid, latissimus dorsi, and biceps are primary movers of the shoulder and also assist with stabilization to enable normal joint function. The rhomboids (major and minor), trapezius, levator scapulae, and serratus anterior stabilize the scapula.

Ligaments

The glenohumeral ligaments are the static stabilizers of the glenohumeral joint (Fig. 1-1). The superior glenohumeral, middle glenohumeral, and inferior glenohumeral ligaments all constrain the joint. The inferior ligament contributes most to the restraint of anterior translation of the head of the humerus within the glenoid fossa, especially when the shoulder is abducted and externally rotated. The acromioclavicular ligament and the coracoclavicular ligaments stabilize the acromioclavicular joint. The labrum is also a stabilizer of the glenohumeral joint, providing an anchor site for the glenohumeral ligaments and a "bumper" along the glenoid rim.

The coracoacromial arch consists of the coracoid process, acromion, and coracoacromial ligament. This arch, along with the acromioclavicular joint, defines the subacromial space containing the subacromial bursa, the supraspinatus tendon, and the tendon of the long head of the biceps (Fig. 1-2, on p. 6). Understanding this anatomy is vital when considering impingement of the shoulder.

Figure 1-1

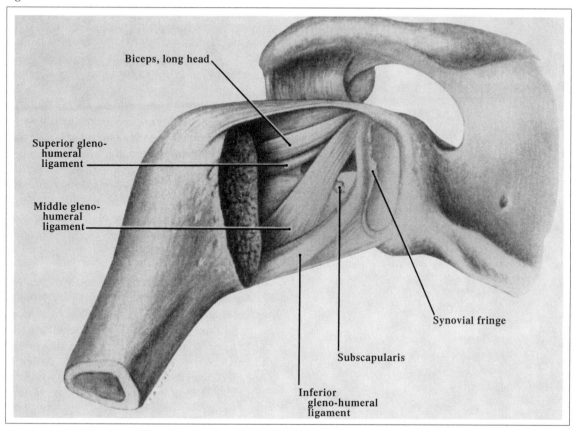

The glenohumeral ligaments. *(Reproduced with permission from Pettrone FA: Athletic Injuries of the Shoulder. New York: McGraw-Hill; 1995).*

Clinical Evaluation

History

The ability to obtain an appropriate and detailed history is critical in evaluating shoulder pain. The questions that are the most helpful in reaching a diagnosis are included in Table 1-1.

Determining the mechanism of injury is helpful. Shoulder pain may be the result of a traumatic event or it may be more insidious in onset.

Common traumatic mechanisms include a fall with the shoulder contacting the ground, direct blows with another person, or a fall on an outstretched hand. The insidious onset of pain is frequently related to doing repetitive, overhead activities. Overhead motion is essential in several different sports. Pain at night with difficulty sleeping is an extremely common complaint in the setting of impingement syndrome.

The pain may be anterior, lateral, or posterior and, therefore, the location of the pain may not be a very helpful symptom. However, it is common for the patient to complain of pain radiating

Figure 1-2

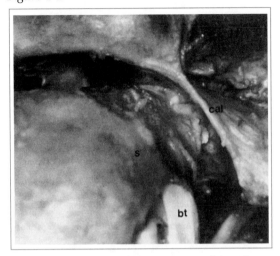

The biceps tendon and upper 20 percent of the subscapularis, shown to lie under the coracoacromial ligament. *(Reproduced with permission from Pettrone FA: Athletic Injuries of the Shoulder. New York: McGraw-Hill; 1995).*

Table 1-1

History of Shoulder Pain

What is the duration of the symptoms?

Was the shoulder pain preceded by a traumatic event?

Was there an activity that brought on the shoulder pain?

What activities aggravate the pain?

What activities improve the pain?

Where is the pain located?

Are there symptoms of instability (does the arm go dead)?

Does the pain get worse at night?

Does the shoulder feel weak?

Is there painful popping of the shoulder?

Is the shoulder stiff?

What shoulder activities are involved in the patient's occupation?

What recreational/sports activities does the patient participate?

Have you had previous shoulder problems?

to the lateral upper arm near the deltoid muscle insertion on the humerus. It is important to remember that this is a common site for referred pain, and to not be directed away from pathology that originates in the shoulder.

Weakness of the shoulder can be difficult to interpret as it can be due to pain or may be the result of a tendon tear. Stiffness of the shoulder is also a complaint seen in several disorders.

It is not unusual for patients to have pain and dysfunction for several months before presenting to the physician. If during this time the patient restricts activities to what is not painful, adhesive capsulitis can develop. Daily activities such as pulling out a wallet, putting on a shirt or coat, putting on a bra, or reaching overhead may be nearly impossible to perform in the setting of adhesive capsulitis.

Mechanical symptoms, such as the sensation of popping, are usually not very helpful. Numerous conditions of the shoulder may have popping and this sensation may not be pathologic. Painful popping is typically more concerning and can occur with various disorders. Activities associated with the athlete's specific sport or training are extremely important to review. These activities are often responsible for the development of overuse injuries. Symptoms of overuse can result in the alteration of normal throwing mechanics and this can lead to exacerbation of symptoms. A common history for these injuries is one in which the patient has performed a sudden increase in overhead motions, seen in sports like tennis, swimming, baseball, weight lifting, or volleyball.

The differential diagnosis should be well established after the history is obtained. A comprehensive list is included in Table 1-2.

Physical Examination

The physical examination of the shoulder should be approached systematically. This systematic examination consists of inspection, palpation, range of motion, muscle testing, stability, and

Table 1-2

Causes of Shoulder Pain

Problem	Presentation	Laboratory/Radiographic Findings	Treatment
Impingement	Positive impingement signs, painful motion, night pain	Radiographs may be normal or may show outlet obstruction (spurs, type 2 or type 3 acromion), aided with lidocaine injection	NSAIDs, rehabilitation, subacromial steroid injection, subacromial decompression
Rotator cuff tear	Weakness, atrophy; end result of chronic impingement, frequently precipitated by injury	Radiographs may show decreased subacromial space, osteophytes; MRI shows tears	Rehabilitation, especially in older patients; surgery in younger patients
Biceps tendon rupture	Bulge in the distal humerus ("Popeye" muscle), usually precipitated by injury; weakness in the supinators (20% loss), weakness in the elbow flexors (8% loss)	Radiographs normal or same as in impingement	NSAIDs, rehabilitation, repair in younger patients for both strength and cosmesis (competitive body builders)
Acute calcific tendinitis	Severe acute shoulder pain, very painful, restricted motion, tenderness on greater tuberosity	Radiographs show calcific deposits	NSAIDs and analgesics, rehabilitation and analgesics, steroid injection (usually), arthroscopic decompression (sometimes)
Adhesive capsulitis (frozen shoulder)	Loss of active and passive range of motion, pain at extremes of patient's motion; usually secondary to pain from a previous shoulder problem	Same as in impingement, tears	NSAIDs, rehabilitation modalities; if no improvement after 18 months, manipulation under anesthesia; most patients respond to a dedicated rehabilitation program
AC arthritis	Pain, swelling at AC joint, usually associated with impingement	AC joint narrowing, hypertrophy, spurs	Ice, NSAIDs, steroid injections in AC joint (difficult injection); resect distal clavicle if conservative treatment does not work
Glenohumeral arthritis	Chronic pain, loss of motion, crepitus, disuse atrophy	Joint space narrowing, changes in humeral head	NSAIDs, physical therapy, total shoulder arthroplasty in advanced cases
Septic arthritis	Acute painful limited motion, fever, chills	Elevated white blood cell count, erythrocyte sedimentation rate, synovial fluid white blood cell count >100,000 per mm^3 (10.0 × 10^9 per L), positive culture and Gram stain; early radiographs normal, later radiographs show erosive changes	Intravenous antibiotics, surgical irrigation
Rheumatoid arthritis	Usually multiple, small-joint, symmetric	Radiograph shows joint space narrowing, osteoporosis; rheumatoid factor, erythrocyte sedimentation rate	NSAIDs, DMARDs, steroid injection
Gout	Podagra, monoarthritis	Serum uric acid, crystals in joint fluid	Colchicine, NSAIDs, allopurinol (Purinol, Zyloprim), probenecid (Benemid, Benuryl)
Lyme disease	Tick bite, erythema migrans	Lyme titer, characteristic rash	Antibiotics
Lupus erythematosus	Multiple joints affected	Antinuclear antibody, erythrocyte sedimentation rate	NSAIDs, antimetabolites
Spondylo-arthropathy	Sacroiliac joint	HLA B27	NSAIDS
Avascular necrosis	Predisposing factors such as steroid use, trauma, alcoholism; frequently idiopathic; painful motion	Early radiographs normal; later radiographs show humeral head flattening; proceeds to degenerative arthritis	NSAIDs, physical therapy, hemi- or total shoulder arthroplasty
Cervical radiculopathy	Radiating pain below shoulder or to upper back, decreased and painful range of motion in neck, positive Spurling's test,* neurologic changes in arms, normal shoulder examination	Radiographs show degenerative changes in cervical spine; MRI may show compressive radiculopathy	NSAIDs, physical therapy, traction, surgical decompression
Tumor	Mass, history of smoking	Chest radiograph may show Pancoast's tumor	Surgery, chemotherapy
Thoracic outlet	Decreased pulses with provocative maneuvers	May require angiography	Surgery

*Radicular pain reproduced with head compression.
ABBREVIATIONS: NSAIDs, nonsteroidal antiinflammatory drugs; AC, acromioclavicular; DMARDs, disease-modifying antirheumatic drugs (including immunosupressants); MRI, magnetic resonance imaging.
SOURCE: Reproduced with permission from Fongemie AE, Buss DD, Rolnick JJ: Management of shoulder impingement and rotator cuff tears. *American Family Physician* 57:672, 1998.

assessing neurologic function. Additionally, examination of the cervical spine and scapular region is important because pain from these regions can be referred to the shoulder.

INSPECTION

Inspection of the shoulder region is the initial component of the examination. Observation for muscle atrophy, shoulder asymmetry, soft tissue swelling, ecchymosis, erythema, and overall posture are helpful. Evidence of atrophy of the supraspinatus and the infraspinatus, for example, would suggest the possibility of suprascapular nerve entrapment. A prominent acromioclavicular joint may suggest degenerative changes and spurring with a nontraumatic history or an acute dislocation associated with trauma. Capsular hypertrophy or bone spurs involving the distal clavicle or acromion often cause impingement. Deformities of the contour of the biceps musculature can be easily visualized, such as the "Popeye" appearance in which the lateral head of the biceps retracts distally when the long head of the biceps is ruptured.

PALPATION

Palpation of the shoulder should include all the bony and soft tissue structures, as sites of tenderness may indicate the site of injury. Bony palpation includes the sternoclavicular joint, clavicle, acromioclavicular joint, acromion, greater tuberosity, coracoid process, and the spine of the scapula. Soft tissue structures to palpate are the short and long heads of the biceps, the subacromial bursa, the musculature of the shoulder, the anterior capsule, the posterior capsule, and the periscapular musculature.

RANGE OF MOTION

The examiner needs to evaluate the passive and active range of motion of the shoulder (Fig. 1-3, pp. 10–11). The opposite shoulder should be examined first for the purpose of establishing what is normal for that particular patient. Most patients are fairly symmetric except for the dominant shoulder in "overhead athletes" such as throwers, tennis players, or volleyball athletes, whose dominant shoulder will usually appear different than the nondominant shoulder. For example, the dominant shoulder will usually demonstrate 5 to 10° of increased external rotation with the shoulder in an abducted position and a similar 5 to 10° loss of internal rotation.

Scapulothoracic motion should also be assessed. The normal biomechanics of shoulder abduction require normal scapulothoracic motion. Normal scapulothoracic motion should be 1° of scapular rotation for every 3° of shoulder abduction. Scapulothoracic dysfunction or dyskinesia can be easily seen when shoulder abduction is viewed from behind. This can lead to excessive force transfer to the rotator cuff and subsequent pain.

ROTATOR CUFF STRENGTH

The goal of strength testing of the rotator cuff is to examine the strength of muscle in the cuff and to determine whether pain is produced upon testing (see Fig. 1-3). Testing the strength of the rotator cuff musculature involves isolating each particular muscle.

Subscapularis is best tested using the lift-off test.[2] The lift-off test is performed by having patients internally rotate their shoulders and place the dorsum of their hand against their back. They are then asked to "lift-off" the hand from the back against resistance. The test may need to be modified in a patient with restricted internal rotation by having the patient's hand positioned against the abdomen and resisting internal rotation.

Resisted external rotation tests the infraspinatus and the teres minor muscles. This should be done with the arm at the side with the elbow flexed to 90° as well as with the shoulder abducted to 90°. Careful comparison to the opposite shoulder is needed to discover subtle weakness.

The supraspinatus has classically been evaluated with the shoulder abducted to 90° and in 30° of forward flexion.[3] The shoulder is then internally rotated by pointing the thumb down and the examiner resists abduction. Weakness, especially if it is out of proportion to the pain, is suggestive of a rotator cuff tear. Recent electromyographic studies demonstrate the supraspinatus may be best selected by keeping the thumb up and having the shoulder more forward flexed to 45° (see Fig. 1-3).[4]

The deltoid muscle group is checked with several maneuvers. The anterior aspect is examined by resisting forward flexion. The midportion is checked resisting abduction in a neutral position. The scapula stabilizers also need to be assessed in terms of strength. Having the patient elevate the scapula and "pinch" the scapula checks the rhomboids and the trapezius. "Winging" of the scapula is examined best by having the patient perform a standing wall push-up. Weakness of the serratus anterior muscle seen in injuries to the long thoracic nerve will cause this "winging."

IMPINGEMENT SIGN

The impingement sign has been described in various ways. The intent of the impingement sign is to compress the subacromial space in an attempt to cause pain. The scapula needs to be stabilized and the shoulder is then abducted and/or internally rotated to see if pain occurs. Neer describes abduction with the glenohumeral joint in the plane of the scapula (20° of forward flexion) to determine if pain is elicited.[5] Hawkins and Kennedy perform the test with the shoulder in 90° of forward flexion and then forcibly internally rotating the shoulder (see Fig. 1-3).[6] In addition to causing pain, the classic impingement test described by Neer also involves elimination of the pain by instilling 10 cc of 1 percent lidocaine into the subacromial space.[5]

JOINT STABILITY

The evaluation of the stability of the shoulder is critical, especially in younger athletes because it may be the cause of impingement and rotator cuff pain. The instability can be unidirectional or multidirectional in an anterior, posterior, or inferior plane or planes. The laxity can be physiologic and bilateral or it can be posttraumatic.

The load and shift test of the shoulder is perhaps the most helpful for assessing anterior/posterior stability. This test is performed with the patient supine and the examiner controlling the arm and loading the joint. The other hand then applies anterior and posterior force to the humeral head. Various positions of abduction, adduction, forward flexion, internal rotation, and external rotation allow the translation of the humeral head to be assessed (see Fig. 1-3). Although a definitive classification for the laxity has not been established, a sense as to the degree of instability can be appreciated. The "sulcus sign" assesses inferior laxity (see Fig. 1-3). The patient is seated and downward traction is applied to the shoulder by pulling on the arm and looking for a sulcus just below the acromion. A positive test is 2 cm or more of inferior displacement.

Another test for assessing stability is the "apprehension test." The classic "apprehension test" places the shoulder in abduction and external rotation with a posterior force directing the humeral head anteriorly. This maneuver can cause anterior subluxation of the glenohumeral joint (see Fig. 1-3). In the patient with instability, this will create a sensation that the shoulder is going to dislocate (i.e., a positive test). Pain with this motion and no apprehension is more likely related to impingement.

The relocation test also evaluates the anterior stability of the shoulder.[7] The patient is supine, with the shoulder in abduction and external rotation; an anterior force is applied by having the patient "throw" against the examiner's hand. A positive test suggestive of anterior laxity is when pain and apprehension are created with

Figure 1-3

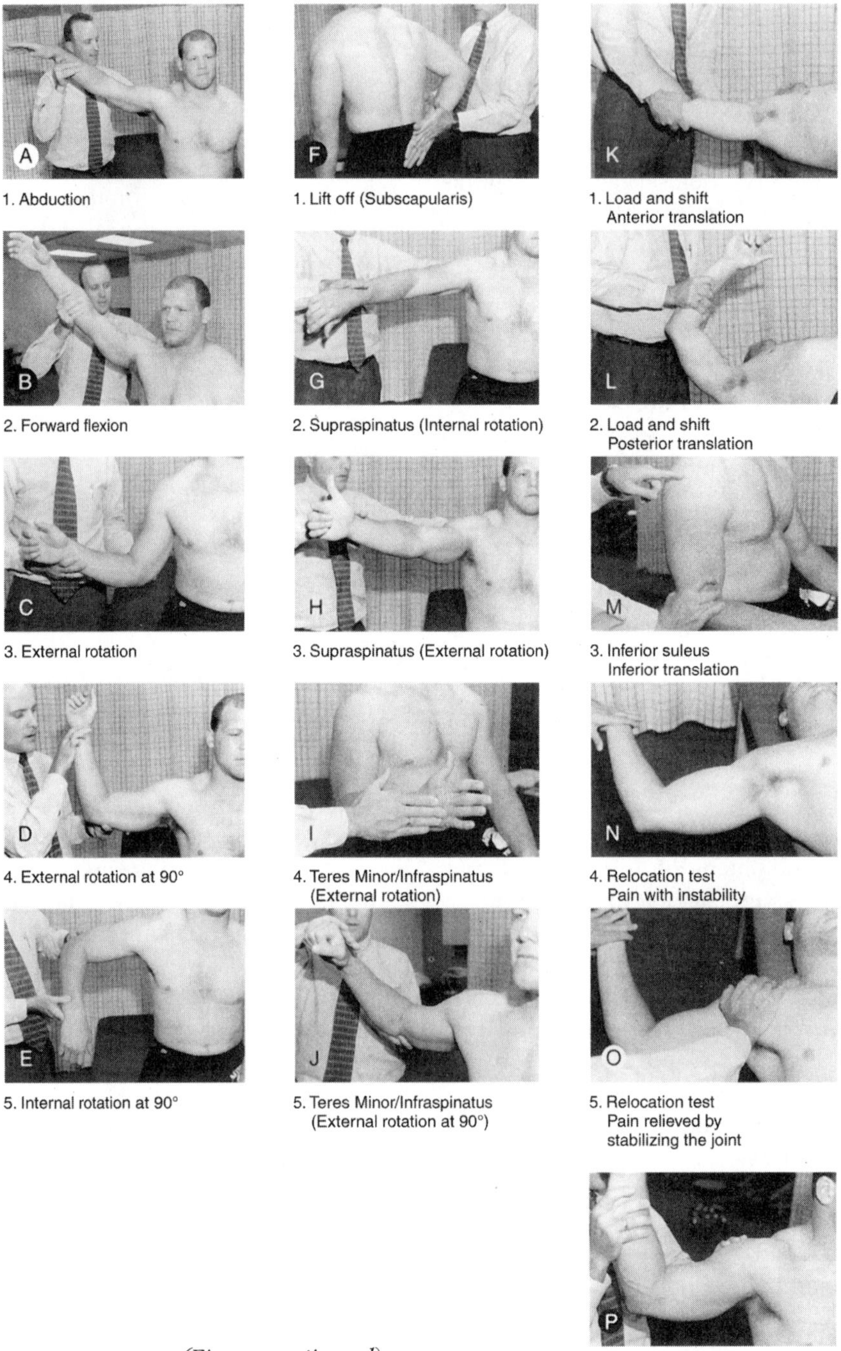

Range of motion

A
1. Abduction

B
2. Forward flexion

C
3. External rotation

D
4. External rotation at 90°

E
5. Internal rotation at 90°

Strength

F
1. Lift off (Subscapularis)

G
2. Supraspinatus (Internal rotation)

H
3. Supraspinatus (External rotation)

I
4. Teres Minor/Infraspinatus
(External rotation)

J
5. Teres Minor/Infraspinatus
(External rotation at 90°)

Stability

K
1. Load and shift
Anterior translation

L
2. Load and shift
Posterior translation

M
3. Inferior suleus
Inferior translation

N
4. Relocation test
Pain with instability

O
5. Relocation test
Pain relieved by
stabilizing the joint

P
6. Apprehension test

(Figure continued)

Figure 1-3 (Continued)

Impingement Signs

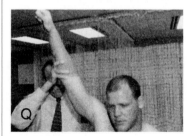

1. Abduction

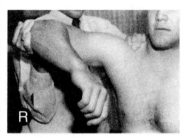

2. Forward flexion and
   Internal rotation

Special Tests

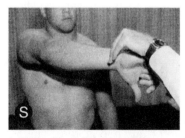

1. Adduction/internal rotation provoking
   pain with a superior labral tear

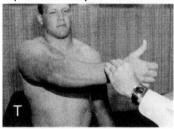

2. Adduction/external rotation
   provoking pain

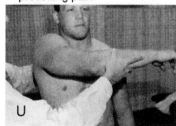

3. Crossover test
   Loads AC joint

A, Abduction. **B,** Forward Flexion. **C,** External rotation. **D,** External rotation of 90°. **E,** Internal rotation at 90°. **F,** Lift off (subscapularis). **G,** Supraspinatus (Internal rotation). **H,** Supraspinatus (External rotation). **I,** Teres minor/infraspinatus (external rotation). **J,** Teres minor/infraspinatus (external rotation at 90°). **K,** Load and shift, anterior translation. **L,** Load and shift, posterior translation. **M,** Inferior suleus, inferior translation. **N,** Relocation test, pain with instability. **O,** Relocation test, pain relieved by stabilizing the joint. **P,** Apprehension test. **Q,** Abduction. **R,** Forward flexion and internal rotation. **S,** Abduction/internal rotation provoking pain with a superior labral tear. **T,** Abduction/internal rotation that does not provoke pain. **U,** Crossover test, loads AC joint.

this maneuver and eliminated when the examiner stabilizes the humeral head with a hand (see Fig. 1-3).

The labrum is difficult to assess with the clinical examination. Several tests are described to evaluate the labrum, but the specificity and sensitivity of these tests are still being determined. The "clunk" test assesses the anterior labrum. The arm is rotated and loaded from a position of extension to forward flexion similar to the McMurray's maneuver of the knee, in an attempt to catch a labral flap or unstable labrum. This is felt as a clunk as the test is done. The superior labrum is evaluated by adducting the shoulder across the body in externally and internally rotated positions.[8] Pain in a position of internal rotation, which is decreased in external rotation, is suggestive of a superior labral tear (see Fig. 1-3). Pain at the acromioclavicular (AC) joint also may be elicited with "crossing" the arm across the body, so it is important to ask the patient to localize the pain to differentiate labral from AC joint pathology.

BICEPS TENDON

The Yergason's test checks the long head of the biceps.[9] In this test, the elbow is flexed to 90° with the forearm pronated. Resisted supination produces pain in the bicipital groove in biceps tendinitis, and a painful "pop" if the long head of the biceps tendon is unstable. Speed's test looks for pain in the area of the bicipital groove during resisted forward flexion of the shoulder with the elbow extended and the forearm supinated. A painful test is indicative of biceps tendinitis.

Neurologic Examination

A complete neurologic examination of the upper extremities is required. Motor strength, sensation to light touch, deep tendon reflexes, and coordination should be evaluated in most cases of shoulder pain.

CERVICAL SPINE

Disorders of the cervical spine may present with shoulder pain, so the cervical spine should also be evaluated. Range of motion can be quickly assessed. The area should also be palpated for any tenderness. Spurling's test is very useful in the evaluation of the cervical spine. In Spurling's test, the neck is extended and laterally flexed to the ipsilateral side, and the head is axially loaded. Shoulder pain produced with this maneuver is highly suggestive of a cervical nerve root process, such as a herniated cervical disc.

Diagnostic Imaging

Imaging techniques are frequently used when evaluating the shoulder.[10] Plain radiographs should be obtained in all cases in which there was a traumatic event, symptoms have been present for more than 8 weeks, the patient is older than age 35 years, or the patient has not responded to treatment. Radiographs may not be necessary in patients under age 35 with no history of trauma.

STANDARD X-RAYS

Standard radiographic views include anterior-posterior (AP) views of the glenohumeral joint with the shoulder both internally and externally rotated. Degenerative changes of the glenohumeral joint and the acromioclavicular joint as well as soft tissue calcifications are seen on these views as are lesions of the humeral head or fractures of the greater tuberosity.

An outlet (arch) view, an axillary view, a modified West Point view, or a Stryker-notch view is indicated depending on the presenting complaint. The outlet view evaluates the acromion and the subacromial space. "Spurs" off the distal clavicle or acromion can be seen. This is a very useful view in patients over 35 years old. Axillary views are useful if the patient presents with a clinical picture of instability, as axillary views will evaluate the glenoid and may demonstrate a defect in the posterior humeral head (Hill-Sachs lesion). An os acromiale is best seen on an axillary view. The Stryker-notch view is useful to better evaluate a Hill-Sachs lesion. The modified West Point view is useful to evaluate degenerative joint disease.

ARTHROGRAPHY

An arthrogram of the shoulder may be of value in assessing the rotator cuff. A radiopaque contrast agent is injected into the glenohumeral joint while imaging the shoulder with fluoroscopy. Leakage of the dye out of the shoulder capsule confirms a rotator cuff tear. Thus, the arthrogram is of use if the clinical question is whether or not the rotator cuff is torn. Although highly sensitive and relatively inexpensive, the shortcoming of this study is that it only evaluates the integrity of the rotator cuff and nothing else. The procedure is also invasive and can be somewhat painful. It is increasingly being replaced by magnetic resonance (MR) arthrography.

MAGNETIC RESONANCE IMAGING AND COMPUTED TOMOGRAPHY

Magnetic resonance imaging is of value in evaluating the subacromial space and the rotator cuff.[11] The MRI can identify full thickness tears, partial thickness tears, and tendinosis of the cuff muscles. The study also details the osseous structures well and small "spurs" can be seen that were not evident on plain radiographs. Additionally, things such as capsular hypertrophy of the acromioclavicular joint causing impingement of the supraspinatus can be seen on MRI. The labrum and glenohumeral ligament/capsule complex is best visualized with MRI or CT arthrography. Contrast in the joint is often necessary for accurate evaluation of the labrum and should be utilized if labral pathology is a concern. The patient in whom the diagnosis is unclear or who is not responding to treatment may warrant a MRI.

Principal Diagnoses

This section discusses each of the common conditions that cause shoulder pain. It is important to keep in mind that the symptoms caused by the same problem frequently vary from person to person.

Impingement Syndrome

PATHOPHYSIOLOGY

Impingement syndrome is one of the most frequent causes of shoulder pain in athletes.[6] In the impingement syndrome, the supraspinatus tendon, the long head of the biceps tendon, and/or the subacromial bursa become "impinged." The structures creating the impingement are the anterolateral acromion, coracoacromial ligament, and/or the acromioclavicular joint. If the biceps is irritated, the pain typically involves the anterior portion of the shoulder. If the subacromial bursa and/or supraspinatus tendon are involved, the pain is seen in the lateral shoulder. Additionally, pain is commonly referred to the upper, outer arm in the area of the deltoid insertion.

The pain of impingement syndrome is associated with overhead activities. This is commonly seen in throwers, swimmers, tennis players (when serving), or hitting in volleyball. Usually, the onset of the pain is insidious and the pain gradually worsens. Rest will typically improve the pain but the pain will recur with a return to activities. Impingement may be primary or secondary in nature.

SECONDARY IMPINGEMENT

It is important to evaluate the glenohumeral stability of an individual presenting with symptoms suggestive of impingement syndrome. The shoulder commonly may have physiological laxity or the laxity may be the result of a traumatic injury. Individuals with laxity require a strong rotator cuff to provide dynamic stability to the glenohumeral joint. Weakness of the rotator cuff allows for migration of the humeral head, especially with the arm in overhead positions, creating "impingement" on the long head of the biceps tendon, the supraspinatus tendon, and the subacromial bursa. This is called secondary impingement, as the impingement results from glenohumeral instability. It is typically seen in younger athletes.

PRIMARY IMPINGEMENT

Primary impingement syndrome is typically seen in athletes over age 35. The pathology is different in primary versus secondary impingement. In contrast to secondary impingement, in primary impingement the subacromial space is compromised by degenerative spurs from the acromion or clavicle. Additionally, the shape of the acromion, as described by Bigliani, may play a role.[12] Bigliani described three acromial types based on morphologic differences. The type-three acromion is hooked anterolaterally, and impinges on the subacromial space.

The athlete with primary impingement will have the same presenting complaints as the athlete with secondary impingement—anterior or lateral shoulder pain that is made worse with overhead activities. Night pain is a common complaint.

PHYSICAL EXAMINATION

In impingement syndrome, the physical examination findings are strikingly similar regardless of whether the impingement is primary or secondary. Tenderness is noted over the involved structures, usually the long head of the biceps or the insertion of the supraspinatus at the greater tuberosity of the humerus. A positive impingement test (described earlier) is present. Weakness and pain with resistance testing to the

supraspinatus, as well as the external rotators (teres minor and infraspinatus), is frequently noted, but the subscapularis is rarely involved. Range of motion is preserved unless there is associated adhesive capsulitis developing. The major difference between primary and secondary impingement on physical examination is that subtle signs of glenohumeral instability will be present in secondary instability.

RADIOGRAPHY

Radiographs of the shoulder will often demonstrate spurs in primary impingement and may show bony changes related to glenohumeral instability in secondary impingement, such as a Hill-Sach's lesion of the humeral head. However, in secondary impingement, the radiographs are usually unremarkable.

TREATMENT

Treatment of impingement syndrome is initially the same whether it is secondary or primary. Anti-inflammatories and icing to control pain are useful. Corticosteroid injections into the subacromial bursa can be effective to decrease pain and inflammation (Fig. 1-4).[13] Three instances in which corticosteroid injections are indicated are (1) uncontrollable pain that keeps the patient awake at night, (2) pain that is preventing the progression of rehabilitation, and (3) failure to improve with the initial treatment. More than two injections should be avoided. Physical therapy should center on strengthening of the rotator cuff and the scapula stabilizers, particularly in secondary impingement.

If conservative treatment is not effective, surgery should be considered. The surgical options are very different for primary and secondary impingement. Subacromial decompression, usually done arthroscopically, is highly effective for the individual with primary impingement. Surgery to decompress the subacromial space is not helpful in secondary impingement. Rather, procedures to stabilize the

Figure 1-4

Subacromial Corticosteroid Injection

1. Complete thorough sterile preparation of the skin. Use sterile gloves.
2. Patient is seated with hands in lap and elbow "hanging" at the end of the table.
3. Prepare a mixture of a local anesthetic and an intermediate-acting steroid: 2 to 4 mL of 1% lidocaine with 2 mL of triamcinolone (10 mg/mL) or 2 mL betamethasone (6 mg/mL) on a 1.5-inch 22-gauge needle.
4. For a posterolateral approach, approximately 1 to 2 cm inferior to the posterolateral acromion, slide the needle into the subacromial space with the needle slightly cephalad.
5. Inject the solution. The solution should inject easily. If resistance is encountered, adjust the needle, as the needle is likely in the tendon.
6. Re-examine the patient to assess if there are decreased pain and improved strength.
7. Prescribe limited activity for 24 to 48 hours and recommend icing. Advise patient that there may be more pain for 24 to 48 hours.

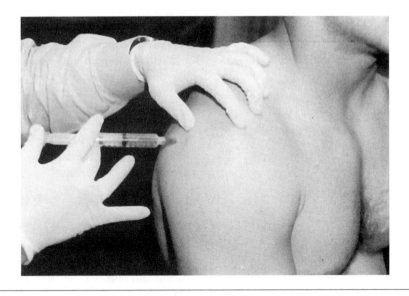

Shoulder injection (posterior–lateral approach).

humeral head are needed. Most patients should be treated nonoperatively for 4 to 6 months before considering a surgical approach.

Rotator Cuff

Injuries to the rotator cuff in sports are frequent. They are often associated with impingement syndrome. The rotator cuff in the impingement syndrome is injured by repetitive microtrauma. Neer classically described impingement as consisting of three stages. Stage I involves edema and hemorrhage of the supraspinatus tendon and subacromial bursa. Stage II disease involves fibrosis and tendinitis. Stage III is the progression to rotator cuff tearing.[5]

Acute, traumatic events may also injure the rotator cuff. Rotator cuff tears result when a sudden eccentric force is applied to the rotator cuff resulting in failure of the tendon. A rotator cuff that has stage II Neer changes is particularly susceptible to acute injury with tear.

Tears of the rotator cuff are uncommon under the age of 40 but strains do occur. In the population over 40 years of age, supraspinatus tears and, less commonly, infraspinatus tears are seen. Tears of the subscapularis tendon are uncommon and are often the result of a shoulder dislocation, but they can occur with a sudden eccentric load to the tendon. The mechanism of injury is similar with strains or disruption of the rotator cuff. Sudden resistance to the arm while catching the body falling or during a forceful overhead motion with the shoulder is frequent.

HISTORY AND PHYSICAL EXAMINATION

The location of pain in injuries to the rotator cuff may be variable, but usually is in the lateral shoulder. Radiation of the pain to the upper, lateral arm is commonly seen. Night pain is frequent.

The physical examination reveals pain and weakness of the involved rotator cuff muscles. Detection of the torn muscle is dependent on the examiner's ability to isolate the muscles during manual testing (see Fig. 1-3).

In tears of the rotator cuff the weakness is profound. But it can be difficult to determine weakness secondary to a disruption of the tendon as opposed to weakness related to severe pain. Injecting the subacromial space with an anesthetic, such as lidocaine, will reduce the pain and if the weakness remains, it is suggestive of a tear.

RADIOGRAPHY

Radiographs are frequently normal. However, fractures may occur in a traumatic injury and need to be excluded. Also, in the athlete over 40 years of age, degenerative or morphologic changes can be noted in the primary impingement syndrome.

Shoulder arthrograms are very accurate in determining rotator cuff tears. However, magnetic resonance imaging is being used more frequently because this study provides more information than the arthrogram, which only evaluates the integrity of the rotator cuff.

TREATMENT

Treatment of rotator cuff injuries depends on the magnitude of the trauma. Most rotator cuff tears in an athletic population will need surgical repair. Less active individuals may do well without surgery, but athletes will not tolerate the loss in strength.

Strains of the rotator cuff can be treated conservatively. Initial conservative care is directed at control of the pain and swelling. Preservation of the range of motion is critical. Rehabilitation to restore rotator cuff strength is equally important. Tendinitis is frequent following a rotator cuff strain due to the loss of muscle strength. The use of corticosteroid injections follows the same guidelines as discussed in the treatment of impingement syndrome.

Other Muscle Injuries

Injuries to the other muscles of the shoulder are less frequent, but strains of the deltoid, pectoralis major, latissimus dorsi, biceps brachii, serratus anterior, levator scapulae, trapezius, and rhomboids occur. Tears in these same muscles are uncommon, with the most frequently torn muscle being the pectoralis major.[14] Pectoralis major tears typically occur when lowering the bar during bench pressing.

Myofascial pain of the trapezius and the rhomboids occurs in patients with poor posture, poor strength, or with disorders of the glenohumeral joint causing scapular substitution patterns for shoulder movement.

The biceps brachii has two heads that act on both the shoulder and the elbow, respectively. Acute strains are uncommon, but biceps tendinitis can occur in association with impingement syndrome. Ruptures of the long head of the biceps can also occur and are, again, usually associated with chronic impingement. The retraction of the muscle distally causes a characteristic "Popeye" bulge of the muscle belly. There is often an associated supraspinatus tear.

Instability of the long head of the biceps can also occur. The tendon becomes unstable in the bicipital groove of the proximal humerus. This can create a "snapping" sensation and pain in the anterior aspect of the shoulder. The Yergason's test and the Speed's test, as described earlier, are helpful to assess the biceps.

Treatment of these various muscle injuries is a combination of resolving the pain and restoring function. Initial treatment is symptomatic, with subsequent progression to a functional rehabilitation program. Strengthening of the scapular stabilizers is helpful to treat the myofascial periscapular pain. Avulsion of a tendon from bony attachment usually requires surgical repair, especially with pectoralis major injuries.[14] Isolated tears of the long head of the biceps tendon results in very little loss of shoulder function and is managed conservatively. Instability or chronic pain involving the long head of the biceps tendon may require a surgical tenodesis.

Glenohumeral Joint

Function of the glenohumeral joint involves a delicate balance of a wide range of motion plus joint stability. Problems with the glenohumeral joint involve instability, which is not covered in this chapter. However, a variety of pain syndromes can be caused by glenohumeral joint dysfunction.

Shoulder pain can be related to degenerative joint disease of the glenohumeral joint. This is seen most often in older athletes. In the younger athlete, degenerative changes are usually related to a history of instability and recurrent dislocations.

Pain associated with arthritis of the glenohumeral joint is a poorly localized, dull ache made worse with activity. Pain at night is uncommon. Stiffness with limitation of abduction and external rotation is characteristic.

PHYSICAL EXAMINATION

Physical examination is most notable for loss of motion and pain with passive motion. Inspection often reveals posterior positioning of the humeral head and atrophy of the supraspinatus and infraspinatus muscles.

RADIOGRAPHY

Radiographs are essential in the diagnosis. A true AP view and the modified West Point view are best to evaluate for arthritic changes.[10] Marginal spurs are visualized involving the glenoid and the humeral head. Joint space narrowing is evident on the modified West Point view.

TREATMENT

Treatment of glenohumeral degenerative joint disease is initially conservative. Nonsteroidal anti-inflammatory agents are used. Maintaining strength and range of motion is important but care must be taken not to irritate the joint. Isometric strengthening of the rotator cuff is the most appropriate.

Shoulder replacement may be indicated if the shoulder pain is uncontrollable. This is rare in young athletes but may be seen in the older athlete. The goal after shoulder replacement surgery is to return the athlete to a recreational level of noncontact activities to include golf, tennis, running, and swimming.

Adhesive Capsulitis

Adhesive capsulitis is caused by prolonged immobility of the glenohumeral joint. Painful conditions that cause the patient to limit motion result in an anatomic restriction of motion. Fractures, tendinitis, or illness may result in this clinical picture. The symptoms include a gradually worsening stiffness of the shoulder. Pain is noted at the limits of the shoulder's mobility. The loss of mobility of the shoulder impairs shoulder function.

PHYSICAL EXAMINATION

The hallmark of the examination of the shoulder in adhesive capsulitis is restricted motion, usually in all planes to some degree. This can variably restrict certain movements more than others and differ from one patient to the next. Additionally, there may be some component of tendinitis of the rotator cuff present.

RADIOGRAPHY

Radiographs are often helpful to determine if there is a bony cause for the limited motion (e.g., degenerative joint disease).

TREATMENT

The treatment consists of pain control and establishing normal shoulder motion. Anti-inflammatory agents can be helpful. Intra-articular corticosteroid injections can also provide pain relief but repeated injections should be avoided.

Physical therapy is required and typically a therapist is needed, as a home program alone will not usually restore function. It is also important for the patient to understand the physical therapy program may be 8 to 12 weeks long before motion is restored and pain relieved. If physical therapy is not of benefit, manipulation of the shoulder under general anesthesia may be needed.

Glenoid Labrum

Tears of labrum can be a diagnostic challenge. A majority of the labral tears are associated with glenohumeral instability. Tears associated with instability are usually located along the inferior aspect of the glenoid from the 4 to 7 o'clock positions. However, isolated labral tears may also occur superiorly or anteriorly. Superior labrum anterior posterior tears of the glenoid labrum were described by Snyder et al in 1990 as SLAP lesions.[15] Four types of SLAP lesions were originally described. The type I lesion is a frayed labrum, with the type II lesion being a tear of the labrum off the glenoid. The type III and type IV injuries are bucket-handle tears of the labrum, with the type IV having an extension of the tear into the biceps tendon. These lesions may be related to traction injuries of the long head of the biceps tendon as it inserts into the superior glenoid labrum during the throwing motion seen in several sports.[16] Also, forceful hyperabduction of the shoulder, seen when landing on the ground after falling with the arm outstretched, has been proposed to create a labral tear.[15]

PHYSICAL EXAMINATION

The pain associated with labral tears is nonspecific. Painful catching of the shoulder may be present, but this can occur in several shoulder disorders. The physical examination is often very similar to the positive findings seen in impingement syndrome. The impingement test is often positive and there is pain elicited with resistance testing of the rotator cuff musculature.

RADIOGRAPHY

Radiographs are nondiagnostic. CT or MRI arthrography is the best choice to evaluate the labrum, as CT is not helpful and conventional MRI has not been reliable. Unfortunately, there are a number of variants of normal anatomy of the labrum, and these may not be distinguishable from a tear on MRI or CT. Therefore, arthroscopy may be the only way to make an accurate diagnosis in many patients.

TREATMENT

Treatment of most symptomatic labral tears requires surgery. Most athletes with labral tears have had extensive conservative treatment at the time of diagnosis. Arthroscopic procedures with bioabsorbable devices or suture anchors provide excellent stabilization of the labral tear, with subsequent healing. Depending on the configuration of the tear, arthroscopic debridement may be warranted, such as with the type I SLAP lesions.

Acromioclavicular Joint Injury

Acromioclavicular joint injury (so-called shoulder separation) is common. Shoulder pain related to the acromioclavicular joint is usually traumatic, but some patients experience insidious onset of the pain. The mechanism of injury in AC dislocation is most commonly associated with a fall landing on the "point" of the shoulder (the lateral acromion) or a direct blow to this same area.

Six grades of injuries have been described by Rockwood, with the majority being grades I, II, or III.[17] In grade I injuries, the acromioclavicular ligament is disrupted either partially or completely, and the coracoclavicular ligament is spared. The grade II acromioclavicular sprain involves partial tearing of the coracoclavicular ligament; with the grade III sprain, the ligament is completely disrupted. Grades IV, V, and VI injuries also involve complete tears of the acromioclavicular and coracoclavicular ligaments with the clavicle displaced from the acromion. Grade IV is a posterior dislocation of the clavicle, whereas in grade V, the clavicle is detached from the trapezius and deltoid resulting in a severe deformity, and the clavicle is dislocated inferiorly below the coracoid in grade VI injuries.

PHYSICAL EXAMINATION

Trauma to the acromioclavicular joint causes pain that is well localized to the joint itself. There is often pain along the trapezius. The range of motion is limited and this limitation is more marked with higher grades of injury.

The physical examination demonstrates a deformity of the superior aspect of the shoulder, which is variable with the grade of injury. The distal clavicle will be more prominent in grade III injuries. Tenderness is well localized to the acromioclavicular joint. Active and passive motions are painful and the crossover test causes pain at the acromioclavicular joint. A thorough neurovascular examination is critical. The type V injury is characterized by significant deformity with the distal clavicle "tenting" the skin.

RADIOGRAPHY

Radiographs are necessary to exclude associated fractures. Views of the acromioclavicular joint will assess the relationship of distal clavicle and acromion. Comparison views of the opposite acromioclavicular joint can be helpful.

TREATMENT

Treatment of most acromioclavicular joint sprains is conservative. Symptomatic treatment with anti-inflammatory agents and ice is indicated for the grades I and II injuries. Restoration of motion and strength is initiated as soon as the pain is controlled. Patients with grade I sprains are able to return to play, depending on the sport, in 2 to 10 days. Grade II sprains return in 2 to 3 weeks for noncontact sports and 3 to 6 weeks for contact/collision sports. The treatment of the grade III acromioclavicular dislocation is more varied. Some practitioners advocate surgical repair acutely, but recently most experts advocate treating grade III nonoperatively, similar to the grade II injuries with a similar return to activity.[18] If an athlete treated conservatively has continued pain and dysfunction of the acromioclavicular joint, excellent results are obtained with a later reconstruction. The grade IV, V, and VI injuries need open reduction and internal fixation acutely.

Acromioclavicular Joint Arthritis

Degenerative joint disease of the acromioclavicular joint is also a cause of shoulder pain. Most patients are older but some younger individuals develop arthritis related to past trauma. Osteolysis of the distal clavicle can also be present in a young athlete. Osteolysis is an avascular necrosis of the distal clavicle related to repetitive stress that is seen in weight lifters or in those with a past history of trauma.[19] As previously discussed, degenerative changes of the acromioclavicular joint may be a cause of impingement syndrome.

HISTORY

The pain will be well localized to the acromioclavicular joint. Overhead activities and activities requiring adduction of the shoulder will create pain. Bench pressing is notorious for causing pain in patients with AC joint problems.

PHYSICAL EXAMINATION

The physical examination is most notable for localized tenderness and a painful crossover test.

RADIOGRAPHY

Radiographs demonstrate degenerative changes with spurring of the distal clavicle or acromion and a narrowed joint space. Osteolysis of the distal clavicle is evident on radiographs of the shoulder, with cystic changes and irregularity of the distal clavicle.

TREATMENT

Treatment is based on the severity of the symptoms. Anti-inflammatory agents, ice, and modification of activities are the initial treatment. Weight lifters can adjust their techniques, such as not lowering the bar to the chest when performing the bench press, thereby reducing the load on the acromioclavicular joint. However, many athletes are not interested in these modifications. Corticosteroid injections into the acromioclavicular joint can be helpful but also may not give lasting improvement, although results of the injection are variable and can provide lasting results for some patients. Surgical resection of the distal clavicle is necessary for athletes with persisting pain and disability. This surgery is extremely successful, with the majority of patients returning to their baseline pre-injury level of activity.

Sternoclavicular Joint

Injuries to the sternoclavicular joint are uncommon. When they occur, these are acute injuries that sprain the sternoclavicular ligament.

The mechanism of injury is usually a force that "squeezes" the shoulders together. In football, this can be the result of having another player fall onto the athlete while he or she is lying on his or her side on the ground.

PHYSICAL EXAMINATION

Pain is localized to the sternoclavicular joint and is elicited by active and passive shoulder motion. The patient may also notice some instability of the proximal clavicle.

Examination reveals point tenderness of the joint and swelling. Increased mobility of the proximal clavicle can be appreciated. Posterior dislocations of the sternoclavicular joint can compromise the airway and adjacent neurovascular structures.

RADIOGRAPHY

Radiographs are indicated to evaluate for a possible fracture but usually do not reveal an altered relationship of the sternoclavicular joint. Computed tomography is useful to image the sternoclavicular joint when a fracture is suspected but not seen on a plain radiograph.

TREATMENT

Treatment of sternoclavicular joint sprains is symptomatic. Even with unstable sternoclavicular joint sprains, most patients do well with conservative treatment. Surgical procedures to stabilize the sternoclavicular joint have frequent complications, and should be avoided. Return to play is variable relating to the severity of the injury and the sport. The athlete may return to noncontact sports when shoulder function is full, but the return to contact/collision sports should be delayed until the joint is nontender.

Fractures

CLAVICLE

Shoulder trauma can result in a fracture. Fractures of the clavicle are very common. Falls on the shoulder or direct blows are common mechanisms, as are falls on an outstretched hand.

Local pain and swelling is obvious. Examination demonstrates local tenderness and often a deformity. A standard AP of the clavicle is adequate to reveal most fractures, but a 45° cephalic tilt view may also be used.

Initial treatment is nonoperative for all clavicle fractures unless the integrity of the skin is compromised or a neurovascular injury is present. Conservative care is directed at pain control and a figure-eight brace or a sling is helpful. Return to collision sports is in 6 to 8 weeks and that decision is based on healing. The most displaced clavicle fractures heal well but a nonunion can occur. Nonunion of clavicle fractures is not predictable and not related to treatment.

PROXIMAL HUMERUS

Avulsion fractures of the greater tuberosity of the humerus are the result of a sudden load being placed on the supraspinatus muscle. This mechanism of injury usually occurs as the athlete is "breaking" a fall. This fracture is much more common in the younger athlete, as an older individual will usually tear the supraspinatus tendon instead. Most avulsions of the greater tuberosity are not displaced, or only minimally displaced, and extent of injury can be seen on an AP radiograph with the shoulder in external rotation.

Treatment is conservative unless there is displacement of more than 1 cm. Treatment consists of a shoulder immobilizer and controlled range-of-motion exercises are started in 10 to 14 days, with controlled strengthening exercises beginning in 3 to 4 weeks.

Other fractures of the proximal humerus are frequently comminuted. Neurovascular examination is essential. Displaced fractures require open reduction and internal fixation.

SCAPULA

Fractures of the scapula, including the acromion and coracoid process, involve significant force. Nonetheless, these fractures are rarely displaced. Treatment involves a sling to immobilize the shoulder until healing is adequate to allow motion in 3 weeks.

Fractures of the scapula can also involve the neck or the body. The athlete is typically very uncomfortable and often has pain with deep inspiration. Radiographs to evaluate the scapula include an AP view, an axillary view, and a tangential oblique view of the scapula. Surgery is rarely needed because displacement almost never occurs. In high-velocity trauma, however, displaced fracture is more likely to be found.

Fractures of the scapula may involve the glenoid. Glenoid fractures are most commonly the result of a shoulder dislocation. Treatment of glenoid fractures is dependent on the extent of injury.

Neurovascular Injury

CERVICAL SPINE

Several neurovascular injuries may present with shoulder pain.[20] For example, cervical spine conditions, such as herniated intervertebral discs, can cause radicular pain in the shoulder. Range of motion of the cervical spine in such patients is usually restricted. A positive Spurling's test, as previously described, will create shoulder and arm pain suggestive of cervical nerve root irritation, which is suggestive of a herniated cervical disc.

PERIPHERAL NERVES

Various peripheral nerves innervate the musculature of the shoulder. Injuries or conditions affecting the suprascapular nerve, axillary nerve, and long thoracic nerve are the most common. Any of these nerves can be injured, depending on the location of a fracture or impingement syndrome.

SUPRASCAPULAR NERVE The suprascapular nerve may be injured at the suprascapular notch or the spinoglenoid notch. At the suprascapular notch, the nerve is susceptible to direct trauma, usually related to a fall. With injury in this location, motor function to the supraspinatus and the infraspinatus muscles is impaired. Injuries to the nerve at the spinoglenoid notch create weakness of the infraspinatus muscle but not the supraspinatus muscle as the supraspinatus is innervated prior to the spinoglenoid notch. Suprascapular nerve injury is seen commonly in volleyball players and has been theorized to result from repetitive stretching of the nerve. Ganglion cysts that arise from the posterior aspect of the glenohumeral joint can encroach on the nerve at the spinoglenoid notch.

When nerve injury is present, physical examination demonstrates atrophy of the muscles innervated by the injured nerve. Weakness of the affected muscles should also be evident. A positive impingement test is typical. Differentiating suprascapular nerve injuries from a rotator cuff tear can be difficult, but with the tears, pain on strength testing is more notable than with suprascapular nerve injury. MRI is helpful to exclude a rotator cuff tear and visualizes a ganglion cyst as well. Electromyography and nerve conduction velocities are diagnostic and can localize the nerve injury.[21]

Initial treatment consists of maintaining shoulder motion and avoiding activities that will create impingement (overhead motions). Modalities and medications to control pain are appropriate. Observation for recovery of nerve function is usually several weeks. Surgical exploration of the nerve may be required if improvement is not evident; serial EMG nerve conduction studies are often useful as an objective measure of recovery. Ganglion cysts can be aspirated and injected with cortisone by the radiologist.

AXILLARY NERVE Axillary nerve injuries are most commonly associated with anterior shoulder dislocations, although blunt trauma has been reported as a mechanism. Chronic entrapment of the nerve can occur, along with entrapment of the posterior circumflex humeral artery in the quadrilateral space located in the posterior aspect of the shoulder. This mechanism of injury occurs in athletes performing repeated overhead movements and is termed "quadrilateral space syndrome."[22]

Acute axillary nerve injuries result in weakness of the deltoid muscle. Sensation is decreased over the lateral upper arm. Pain in athletes with quadrilateral space syndrome is somewhat vague but is aggravated with activities. The examination may reveal tenderness over the posterior aspect of the shoulder and may be otherwise unremarkable. The EMG is of benefit in evaluating the acute injuries but not until after 3 to 6 weeks from the trauma. In quadrilateral space syndrome, however, the EMG is normal. Because this injury involves simultaneous injury to the posterior circumflex humeral artery, the diagnosis is based on an arteriogram of both arms in the adducted as well as the abducted and externally rotated postitions. Surgical decompression is indicated for athletes with persisting complaints.

LONG THORACIC NERVE Weakness of the serratus anterior muscle is the result of traumatic injury to the long thoracic nerve. This has been reported to occur in several different sports, but it also has been reported with the use of backpacks.

Scapular "winging" is the diagnostic finding on the physical examination and an EMG is confirmatory if needed. Conservative treatment consisting of avoidance of the causative activities and physical therapy to preserve motion is indicated. As the nerve recovers, restrengthening of the serratus anterior is necessary.

THORACIC OUTLET SYNDROME

The brachial plexus and subclavian artery and vein exit through the costoclavicular space. The costoclavicular space is bordered on the superior aspect by the clavicle and inferiorly by the first rib. The subclavius and scalene muscles make the borders. Congenital bands may compromise the space but overuse of the musculature may produce tightness and in turn "pinching" of the brachial plexus or vascular structures as they exit. This is known as the thoracic outlet syndrome.

Thoracic outlet syndrome is uncommon in athletes. The syndrome can produce ill-defined shoulder and arm pain. The pain is vague and frequently radiates to the arm. Paresthesias may be present. The pain and paresthesia will not be in a dermatomal distribution and may vary in location on different days.

On physical examination, reproduction of the symptoms by either the Adson's maneuver or the Wright's maneuver is diagnostic. In the Adson's test, the neck is extended and the chin is turned to the affected shoulder that is abducted to 90°.[23] The Wright's test is similar, with the chin is turned to the opposite shoulder.[24] Treatment consists of stretching the muscles of the anterior chest wall and the neck musculature. Strengthening of the scapular stabilizers is of benefit. Surgical intervention is rare.

THROMBOSIS OF THE SUBCLAVIAN VEIN—EFFORT THROMBOSIS

Effort thrombosis is caused when the subclavian vein is repetitively traumatized in the costoclavicular space. This occurs in athletes performing frequent overhead motions. The repeated trauma creates fibrosis around the vein, compromising venous return.

The shoulder and arm pain will be diffuse and achy in nature. Heaviness of the arm is also a common complaint that is precipitated by activity and improves quickly with rest. On examination, the veins are prominent after repeated use of the arm and the arm is swollen diffusely. A venogram is diagnostic. Pulmonary embolism may occur as an uncommon complication.

Treatment of effort thrombosis is initially directed at thrombolysis if the episode is acute. Subsequent coumadinization for 3 to 6 months is necessary. Return to activity after conservative treatment frequently fails because of the extrinsic compression on the subclavian vein by offending anatomic structures. Surgical decompression, which in athletes is typically a transaxillary first rib resection, may be required.

Rehabilitation

In addition to the specific rehabilitation activities discussed earlier for specific shoulder problems, general rehabilitation principles in treating shoulder pain should be followed.[25,26]

Rehabilitation can be divided into three phases. Phase I involves pain control. Pain needs to be controlled with nonsteroidal anti-inflammatory agents, assuming there are no contraindications to using these agents. Local modalities, such as cryotherapy, are also used. Protection of the injured tissue may be needed, such as with a sling or shoulder immobilizer, but

Figure 1-5

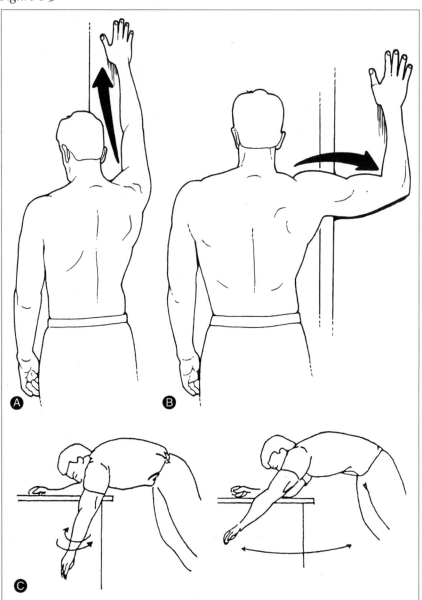

A, Terminal stretching for elevation. **B,** External rotation with a wall. *(Reproduced with permission from Donatelli RA (ed): Physical Therapy of the Shoulder. New York: Churchill Livingstone; 1997:468.)* **C,** Pendulum exercises for range of motion. *(Reproduced with permission from Andrews JR, Wilk KE (eds): The Athlete's Shoulder. New York: Churchill Livingstone; 1994:691.)*

Figure 1-6

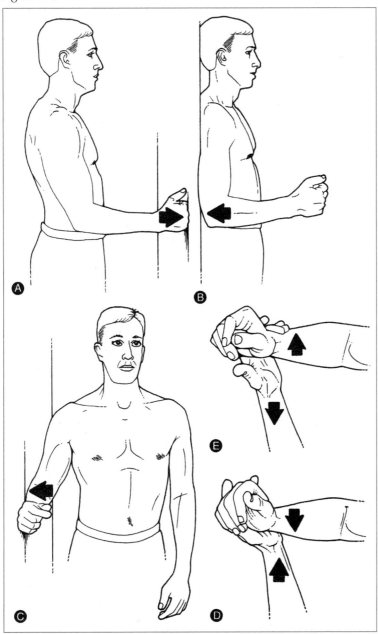

Five-way isometrics for the glenohumeral joint with the elbow flexed at 90°.
A, Flexion. **B,** Extension. **C,** Abduction. **D,** Internal rotation. **E,** External rotation.
(Reproduced with permission from Donatelli RA: Physical Therapy of the Shoulder.
New York: Churchill Livingstone; 1997:465.)

motion should be maintained if possible. However, it is not appropriate to eliminate all shoulder motion for most problems; exercises such as the "pendulum" can be performed (Fig. 1-5). Isometric strengthening can also be done acutely most of the time (Fig. 1-6). This is important for preservation of strength, which will speed recovery time.

Phase II begins 5 to 7 days after the injury, or in an overuse problem, when the pain is diminished sufficiently to allow an increase in activity.

Range of motion is fully restored during this phase. Progressive resistive exercises are initiated to establish normal strength. Rotator cuff strengthening and strengthening of the scapular stabilizers are two examples of exercises done for many causes of shoulder pain (Fig. 1-7). Restoration of the strength and mobility of the shoulder is vital to allow for a successful return to sports.

Phase III rehabilitation involves sports-specific training. To return an athlete to a level

Figure 1-7

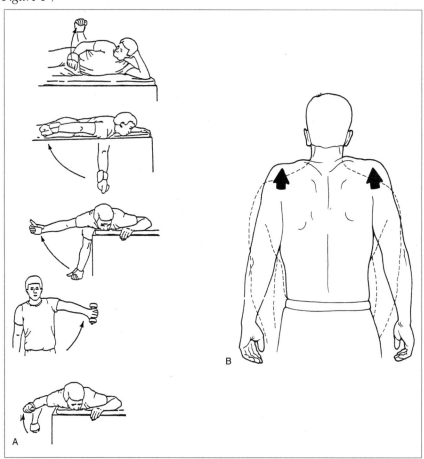

A, Rotator cuff strengthening exercises. Perform two to three sets of 10–15 repetitions with a weight of 1 to 5 lb. **B,** Scapular stabilizing exercises of retraction and elevation. *(Reproduced with permission from Donatelli RA: Physical Therapy of the Shoulder. New York: Churchill Livingstone; 1997:289, 464.)*

Figure 1-7 (Continued)

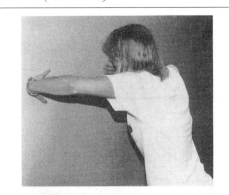

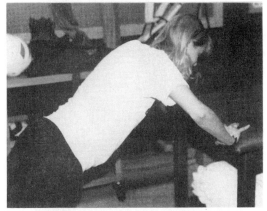

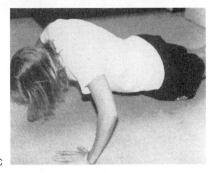

C, Progressive push-up from the wall, a table, the floor. These exercises enhance strength of scapular stabilizers. *(Reproduced with permission from Andrews JR, Wilk KE: The Athlete's Shoulder. New York: Churchill Livingstone; 1994:441.)*

of full recovery and maximal performance, the exercises need to be tailored specifically for the sport. For example, an interval-throwing program is used for the throwing athlete.

References

1. Clark JM, Harryman DT: Tendons, ligaments, and capsule of the rotator cuff. *J Bone Joint Surg (Am)* 74A:713, 1992.
2. Gerber C, Krushell RJ: Isolated rupture of the subscapularis muscle: Clinical features in 16 cases. *J Bone Joint Surg (Br)* 73B:389, 1991.
3. Jobe FW, Jobe CM: Painful athletic injuries of the shoulder. *Clin Orthop* 173:117, 1983.
4. Kelly BT, Kadramas WR, Speer KP: The manual muscle examination for rotator cuff strength. *Am J Sports Med* 24:581, 1996.
5. Neer CS II: Impingement lesions. *Clin Orthop* 173:70, 1983.
6. Hawkins RJ, Kennedy JC: Impingement syndrome in athletes. *Am J Sports Med* 8:151, 1980.
7. Kvitne RS, Jobe FW: The diagnosis and treatment of anterior instability in the throwing athlete. *Clin Orthop* 291:102, 1993.
8. O'Brien SJ, Pagnani MJ, Fealy S, et al: The active compression test: A new and effective test for diagnosing labral tears and acromioclavicular joint abnormality. *Am J Sports Med* 26:610, 1998.
9. Yergason RM: Supination sign. *J Bone Joint Surg (Am)* 13:160, 1931.
10. Rafii M, Minkoff J, DeStefano V: Diagnostic imaging of the shoulder. In: Nicholas JA, Hershman EB (eds): *The Upper Extremity in Sports Medicine.* St. Louis: C.V. Mosby: 1990;91.
11. Iannotti JP, Zlatkin MB, Esterhai JL, et al: Magnetic resonance imaging of the shoulder. Sensitivity, specificity, and predictive value. *J Bone Joint Surg (Am)* 73:17, 1991.
12. Bigliani LU, Morrison DS, April EW: The morphology of the acromion and its relationship to rotator cuff tears. *Orthop Trans* 10:228, 1986.
13. Hollingworth GR, Ellis RM, Hattersley TS: Comparison of injection techniques for shoulder pain: Results of a double blind, randomized study. *Br Med J* 287:1339, 1983.
14. Berson B: Surgical repair of pectoralis major rupture in an athlete. *Am J Sports Med* 7:348, 1979.

15. Snyder SJ, Karzel RP, Del Pizzo W, et al: SLAP lesions of the shoulder. *Arthroscopy* 6:274, 1990.

16. Andrews JR, Carson WG Jr., McLeod WD: Glenoid labral tears related to the long head of the biceps. *Am J Sports Med* 13:337, 1985.

17. Rockwood CA Jr.: Subluxation and dislocations about the shoulder. In: Rockwood CA Jr., Green DP (eds): *Fractures in Adults, Vol. 2,* 4th ed. Philadelphia: J.B. Lippincott; 1996;1353.

18. Tibone J, Sellers R, Tonino P: Strength testing after third-degree acromioclavicular dislocations. *Am J Sports Med* 20:328, 1992.

19. Scavenius M, Iverson BF: Nontraumatic clavicular osteolysis in weight lifters. *Am J Sports Med* 20:463, 1992.

20. Mendoza FX, Main K: Peripheral nerve injuries of the shoulder in the athlete. In: Hershman EB (ed): *Clinics in Sports Medicine: Neurovascular Injuries.* Philadelphia: Saunders: 1990;331.

21. Wilbourn AJ: Electrodiagnostic testing of neurologic injuries in athletes. In: Hershman EB (ed): *Clinics in Sports Medicine: Neurovascular Injuries.* Philadelphia: Saunders: 1990;229.

22. Cahill BR, Palmer RE: Quadrilateral space syndrome. *J Hand Surg* 8:65, 1983.

23. Adson AW, Coffey JR: Cervical rib: Method of anterior approach for relief of symptoms by division of scalenus anticus. *Ann Surg* 85:A39l, 1927.

24. Wright IS: The neurovascular syndromes produced by hyperabduction of the arm. *Am Heart J* 29:1, 1945.

25. Ellenbecker TS, Dersheid GL: Rehabilitation of overuse injuries of the shoulder. *Clin Sports Med* 8:583, 1989.

26. Kibler BW: Shoulder rehabilitation: Principles and practice. *Med Sci Sports Exerc* 30(Suppl):540, 1998.

James Dunlap

Shoulder Dislocations

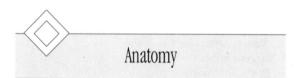

Introduction

Shoulder dislocations account for more than half of all major joint dislocations that require medical care. Although the diagnosis is not difficult, knowing how to manage the injury and to understand the potentially serious consequences that may occur is essential. Once the dislocation is reduced, the examiner must also know when referral to an orthopedic specialist is needed. The purpose of this chapter is to help the clinician become familiar with the steps that must be taken once a shoulder dislocation is identified.

Anatomy

The shoulder joint includes the glenohumeral, acromioclavicular, sternoclavicular, and scapulothoracic articulations. A description of the functional anatomy in shoulder dislocations can be limited to the glenohumeral joint. The humeral head is retroverted 30° (tilted 30° posterior from an imaginary plane drawn up from the more distal epicondyles) and angulated 45° relative to the shaft, which aligns the glenoid fossa with the articular humeral surface and places the arm in a more forward and lateral position.[1] The glenoid fossa has a pear-shaped contour that represents 33 percent of the surface area of the humeral head. The fossa is retroverted 7° and tilted downward 5° relative to the plane of the scapula.[2] **The most important concept to understand is that this anatomic arrangement provides little anterior or inferior bony support.** Additional static and dynamic structures are needed to enhance glenohumeral stability.

Static Stabilizers

GLENOID LABRUM

The fibrous glenoid labrum expands the depth and area of the glenoid by increasing humeral contact surface area by 75 percent in the horizontal direction and 56 percent in the transverse direction.[3] This architecture, when combined with a thin layer of synovial fluid that keeps the surfaces together with intermolecular and viscous forces, creates a relative vacuum with negative air pressure (suction) that maintains the humeral head within the socket.[4]

JOINT CAPSULE

The joint capsule is thin, redundant, and has two times the surface area of the humeral head.[5] This allows tremendous range of motion. Thickenings of the capsule known as glenohumeral ligaments provide the most important static stability (see Chap. 1, Fig. 1-1). Of the superior, middle and inferior glenohumeral ligaments, the **inferior glenohumeral ligament** provides the most important support when the arm is in the throwing or overhead position—abducted and externally rotated[6]. Loss of structural integrity of this ligament is a major reason for anterior instability and recurrent dislocation.

Dynamic Stabilizers

The dynamic glenohumeral stabilizers of the shoulder consist of two layers. The superficial layer includes the biceps, coracobrachialis, and deltoid. The latissimus dorsi insertion forms the floor of the intertubercular groove and may influence glenohumeral stability. The serratus anterior, rhomboids, and trapezius also protect the shoulder but are more important at the scapulothoracic level. The deep layer is the rotator cuff. The supraspinatus, infraspinatus and teres minor insert on the greater tuberosity and the subscapularis inserts on the lesser tuberosity.

Figure 2-1

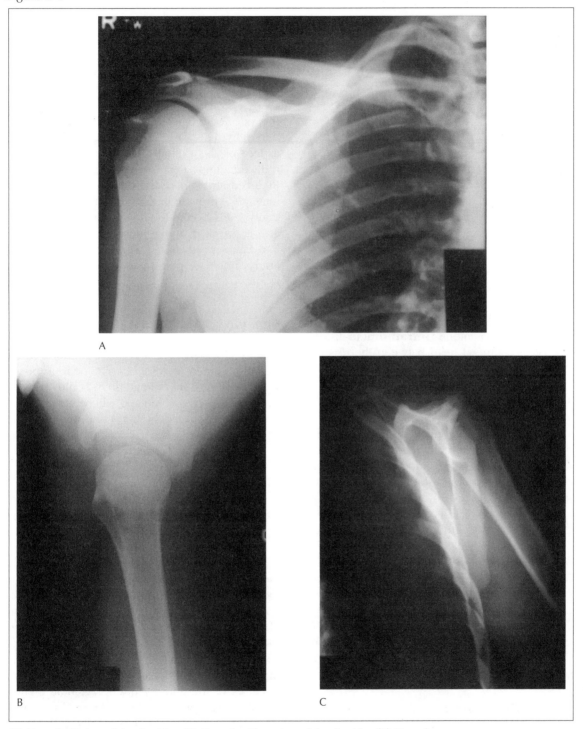

(A) Normal AP view of the shoulder. (B) Normal axillary view of the shoulder. (C) Normal scapular Y view of the shoulder.

Anterior Glenohumeral Dislocation

Classification by Humeral Head Position

More than 95 percent of glenohumeral dislocations are anterior, meaning that the humeral head moves anteriorly in relation to the glenoid fossa. As many as 90 percent of these dislocations are **subcoracoid**, in which humeral head displacement is anterior to the glenoid and inferior to the coracoid.[7] **Subglenoid** dislocation is next most common. In this case, the humeral head lies anterior and below the glenoid. With **subclavicular** dislocation, the humeral head lies medial to the coracoid process and beneath the clavicle. Least common is **intrathoracic** dislocation of the humeral head between the ribs and thoracic cavity.

Mechanism of Injury and Presentation

The mechanism of the injury, for example, a fall when the arm is externally rotated, abducted, or extended, provides one important clue to the direction and type of dislocation. When atraumatic dislocations occur, the clinician should look for signs of joint laxity (Marfan's syndrome, Ehlers-Danlos, nonpathological joint laxity, etc.).

The manner in which the patient presents also helps. After anterior dislocation, the arm may be held in abduction and slight external rotation. Adduction and internal rotation are difficult to perform. The normal round contour of the shoulder is lost and the distal acromion becomes more prominent. The anterior area of the shoulder will appear full, with loss of coracoid process distinction.

Physical Examination

Although injury history and observation usually provide immediate diagnosis, several areas must still be carefully assessed. Manual testing of muscle strength can be difficult because the patient splints the injury and has weakness secondary to pain.

The axillary nerve is the most frequently injured neurologic structure. Test the axillary nerve by checking sensation over the lateral aspect of the deltoid. After the dislocation is reduced, this area should be tested again. Reduced strength of the deltoid after reduction may also provide indication of axillary nerve injury. Sensation to the dorsal aspect of the forearm is supplied by the musculocutaneous nerve and can be easily tested. Palpation of the axillary artery should be performed, although injury to it is rare.

Imaging

After the dislocation has been reduced, radiographs should always be obtained. If possible, pre-reduction radiographs should also be obtained. However, the site where the injury is diagnosed (e.g., athletic field) and the expertise of the examiner often dictate the appropriateness of obtaining pre-reduction x-rays. On the field, it is usually easier to try to reduce the shoulder through techniques discussed later and obtain radiographs after the game. If the neurovascular examination is abnormal or in question, however, obtain radiographs as quickly as possible.

Shoulder x-rays for traumatic injury typically include a **true anterior-posterior (AP), an axillary, and outlet or scapula Y view** (Fig. 2-1A, B, C). These radiographs not only confirm glenohumeral integrity but also can be used to look for associated injuries such as Hill-Sachs compression fracture of the humeral head, humeral shaft fractures, and Bankart avulsion fractures of the anterior inferior glenoid. When the films are examined, the outlet or Y view will show the scapula as the body of the Y, the coracoid process as the anterior arm, and the spine and acromion as the posterior arm. The humeral

Figure 2-2

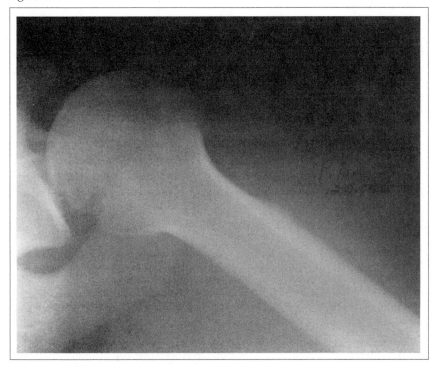

Hill-Sachs lesion seen on the axillary view of shoulder.

head is anterior to the Y in an anterior dislocation and posterior to the Y with posterior dislocation. The axillary view demonstrates compression fractures of the humeral head (Hill-Sachs lesions) and fractures of the glenoid as well as the position of the humeral head in relation to the glenoid. As many as 38 to 55 percent of anterior dislocations will have Hill-Sachs fractures (Fig. 2-2). Another 15 percent may have greater tuberosity fractures.[7,8]

Reduction of Shoulder Dislocations

There are a variety of methods for reducing a dislocated shoulder. The best techniques require no countertraction, the use of a bed sheet, or another assistant. These include the Milch and Hennipen techniques, and the Stimson and scapula manipulation methods.

The scapula manipulation and modified Stimson techniques in the prone position are probably the easiest to master and least painful. In the modified Stimson technique, rather than using weights, the examiner places the patient in a prone position and uses gravity and longitudinal traction from a free hand before gently externally or internally rotating the humerus (Fig. 2-3). The scapula manipulation technique only differs from the modified Stimson maneuver in the use of the heel of the other free hand to put medial pressure on the inferior border of the scapula to reposition the glenoid fossa downward while longitudinal traction is maintained (Fig. 2-4). This technique can also be performed with the patient seated and the arm forward flexed at 90°.

In the Milch maneuver, the seated or supine athlete is asked to reach up to "pick an apple off the tree." Once the arm is fully abducted and for-

Figure 2-3

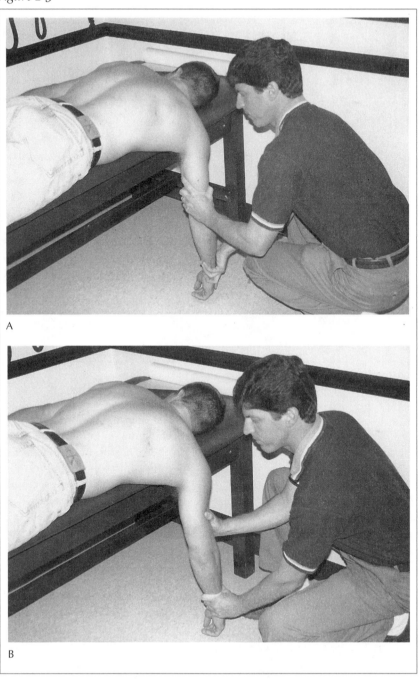

Modified Stimson maneuver. Gravity, longitudinal traction, and gentle external or internal rotation are used to reduce the shoulder.

Figure 2-4

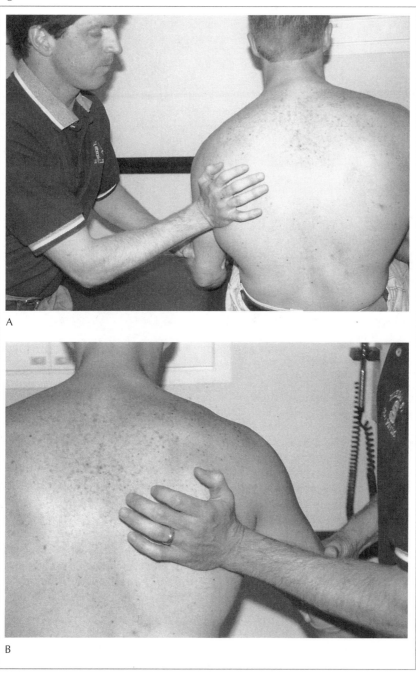

A

B

Scapula manipulation maneuver. Notice the position of the heel of the hand as it pushes the scapula border medially. The arm should be in forward flexion with longitudinal traction applied.

Figure 2-5

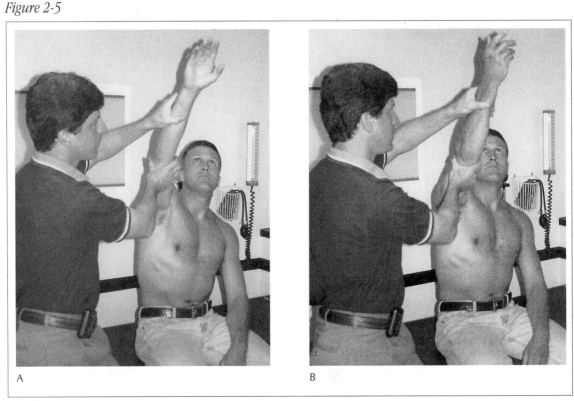

A   B

Milch maneuver. The arm "grasps for an apple" **(A)** and then is externally rotated while traction is maintained **(B)**.

ward flexed, gentle external rotation and longitudinal traction are applied (Fig.2-5).

The Hennepin technique requires no traction.
From the supine position, the elbow is flexed to
90° and held tight to the body—adducted, while
the examiner slowly externally rotates the arm
(Fig. 2-6). This technique is useful for the athlete
lying on the ground, or in a similar setting, with
no chairs or benches. A dislocation may also be
easily reduced on the field if the shoulder is
placed in slight abduction, forward flexion, and
internal rotation.

It should be obvious from the descriptions of
these techniques that many maneuvers will work.
Remembering two techniques is sufficient. Finally,
several authorities have reported anecdotal success using a patient-driven technique developed
for those occasions. when nobody is around or

knows how to reduce a shoulder dislocation. The
seated patient grabs the wrist of the arm of the
injured shoulder (or clasps the fingers together),
extending the injured arm so that the hands can
clasp around the ipsilateral knee. When the
patient leans back, the knee then serves as a fulcrum on the uninjured wrist (or clasped hands),
introducing traction on the injured shoulder,
which causes reduction (Fig. 2-7).

In most dislocations, anesthesia is not
required. In difficult reductions, 5 to 10 mL of
1 percent lidocaine without epinephrine can be
injected into the joint, and is efficacious as intravenous narcotics or benzodiazapines such as
diazepam, midazolam, or lorazepam.[9] To perform the shoulder injection, find the posterior-
lateral tip of the acromion and the coracoid
process, aiming the needle (22 to 25 gauge)

Figure 2-6

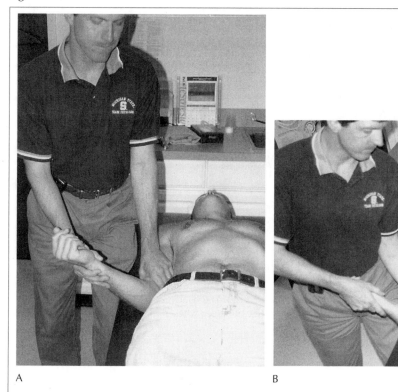

A   B

Hennipen technique. The arm is held close to the body while the examiner slowly externally rotates the shoulder.

toward the coracoid. Wait at least 10 min before attempting the reduction maneuver.

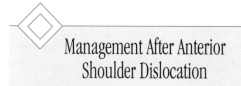

Management After Anterior Shoulder Dislocation

Natural History

Not long ago, researchers discovered that the future behavior of primary traumatic shoulder dislocations depends on the age at the time of injury. Most studies report a recurrence rate of 90 to 95 percent in athletes younger than 20 years.[10,11] A more recent study, however, suggests that this number may be closer to 66 percent.[8] Immobilization has not been shown to reduce the number who have recurrent dislocations, and symptoms of instability persist for as many as 50 to 60 percent. In those patients that eventually do require surgery, 80 percent will have a complete tear of the capsulolabral complex.[8,10] Approximately half of anterior dislocations in this age group will have Hill-Sachs lesions.[8] These are associated with a higher frequency of recurrent dislocations, instability, and eventually, surgery. The need for shoulder dislocation reduction has also been associated with a higher likelihood of instability and surgical repair.[12] Contrary to expec-

Figure 2-7

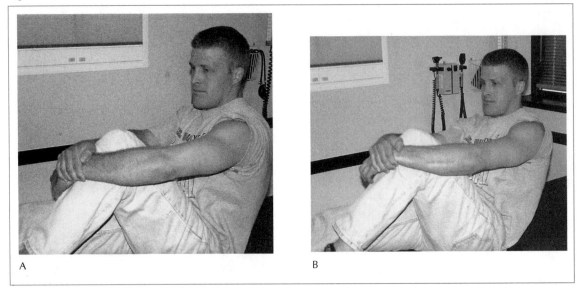

A
B

Self-reduction technique. The uninjured arm clasps the other wrist or hand. The hands are placed around the knee, allowing it to act as a fulcrum, reducing the shoulder when the patient leans back.

tation, shoulder dominance does not appear to play a significant role in either the rate of recurrence or the need to repair a dislocation. Very few in this age group have rotator cuff tears.

In shoulder dislocations in patients over 30 years old, the natural course is much more favorable. Studies have reported a recurrence rate of 20 to 25 percent.[9,11] Most do quite well with a brief 2-week course of immobilization to diminish pain and limit extreme external rotation and abduction, followed by aggressive physical therapy. Because concomitant rotator cuff tears after dislocations are more prevalent in this population, any dysfunction after 3 weeks should lead to further clinical and radiographic investigation.

Controversy in Anterior Dislocation Management

The importance of understanding the natural history of shoulder dislocations in various age groups lies in the decision of whether or not referral to an orthopedic surgeon is necessary. Even into the early 1990s, surgical intervention was favored in athletes younger than 20 who sustained a first traumatic dislocation because the recurrence rate was tremendously high. Many orthopedists have now made a fundamental shift from that aggressive surgical approach to one that encourages patient selection based on clinical evidence of instability with serial examinations.

A summary of two studies can help to demonstrate why this philosophical change has occurred and shed light onto the current controversy in this area. In 1977, Hovelius began a landmark, long-term, prospective trial evaluating the initial treatment of primary shoulder dislocations in Sweden. He evaluated 245 dislocators over 10 years, with only 10 lost to follow-up (9 died). Of the 235 patients, 211 were examined again after 10 years. The remaining 24 patients received a questionnaire or answered a telephone interview. In the group with initial dislocation between the ages of 12 to 22 years, 34 of 99 eventually required operative stabilization for recurrent dislocation. Operative stabilization decreased to 28 percent in patients 23 to 29 years old and to 9 percent in patients 30 to 40 years old. Of most interest, however, was the finding in the 12 to 22-year group that 34 of 99 had no recurrence and another 13 of 99 were completely healed. Although it is unclear as to the reason, 24 of 107 of all the dislocators who had at least one recurrence stabilized over time and required no surgical intervention. In summary, Hovelius reported a 66 percent recurrence rate in the 12 to 22 age group, much lower than in many studies, and he concluded that some young shoulders stabilize over time.[8,13]

In the other study, Arciero et al. came to the opposite conclusion after looking at a completely different population at the United States Military Academy—a group that cannot modify its physical activity. The original study design was a 4-week, nonrandomized comparison of arthroscopic repair versus 4 weeks of immobilization in 36 patients.[14] Fifteen patients opted for nonoperative treatment and 21 selected surgery. Follow-up in the nonoperative group averaged 23 months (range 15 to 39) and 32 months (range 15 to 45) in the operative group. The recurrence rate was 80 percent (12 of 15) in the nonoperative group, and 7 of those 12 went on to open surgical treatment. In the operative group, 18 of 21 had no recurrent instability. Although the recurrence rate with early arthroscopic surgical repair was lower than in the conservatively treated group, there were 3 treatment failures. When the 3 failures in the surgical group are added to the 3 out of 15 in the nonoperative group who did well, 6 of 36 did not benefit from early operative treatment. A publication 2 years later, comparing 53 who chose conservative treatment with 63 who chose surgery, reported essentially the same findings,[15] except the number who had recurrent instability in the conservative group increased to 48 of 53

(90 percent). The controversy that is raised in these two studies stems from the push to repair young dislocators early with the arthroscopic technique. The controversy would end if the success rate of this technique was as high as the open repair—95 percent.

At this time, the best candidates for early surgical treatment would be those in a high-demand sport (throwers, volleyball, basketball, etc.) and those that do not want to face the significant possibility that a recurrence will lead to more time missed. Table 2-1 summarizes those who should probably see an orthopedic surgeon.

Surgical Repair of Anterior Shoulder Dislocations

Bankart is the name most commonly associated with this repair because of his work between 1925 and 1954.[16] The basic idea behind this surgical technique is the reattachment of the glenoid labrum and capsule to the anterior glenoid neck. Today, whether the procedure is performed through a scope or openly, absorbable suture anchors are used to reattach the labrum to the glenoid and more sutures are used to reattach the capsule to the labrum. The primary static

Table 2-1

Shoulder Dislocations

INDICATIONS FOR REFERRAL TO AN ORTHOPEDIC SURGEON
Bankart avulsion fracture of the glenoid.
Hill–Sachs compression fracture of the humeral head.
Humeral fractures.
Significant difficulty reducing the dislocation.
Neurological or vascular compromise.
Recurrent dislocation.
Posterior dislocations that cannot be reduced.
Young patient age, high-demand sport, reluctance to modify activity.
Clinical instability after conservative treatment.

stabilizer, the inferior glenohumeral ligament, is also frequently reconstructed in this process. In some cases, if there is excessive capsule redundancy, the capsule incision is converted into a T (T-plasty), in which the inferior flap is brought superiorly, and the superior flap is transposed downward to reduce the laxity. Once the stabilization is completed, the patient is maintained in internal rotation for 4 weeks, but elbow motion is allowed. At 4 weeks, shoulder active-assisted and passive range-of-motion movement are initiated. Once full range of motion is established, resistance exercises are started. At 4 to 6 months, throwing and contact sports can be resumed.

Conservative Treatment of Primary Anterior Dislocations

After a period of immobilization to decrease pain and allow some healing (2 to 4 weeks), aggressive rehabilitation of the rotator cuff and scapular rotator muscles is undertaken. Positions of extreme external rotation and abduction are limited for about 3 months after sling removal. Serial examination is essential, especially in the athletes whose activity requires overhead motion or throwing. If, after serial examinations, no clinical instability is noted, the decision to repair the shoulder can be deferred. The physical examination should assess for anterior-posterior and inferior instability (the sulcus sign when longitudinal traction is placed on the arm). If both are present, multidirectional instability is diagnosed and referral to a sports medicine specialist should be made, not for surgery, but for aggressive sports-specific physical therapy and close follow-up.

Not infrequently, the labrum is torn after a dislocation. The presence of a labral tear can be made by a positive O'Brien test, in which the shoulder is horizontally adducted at 90° of forward flexion (be careful not to mistake pronation at the elbow as horizontal glenohumeral adduction and internal rotation) and placed in internal rotation (emptying a can). Pain in this position when resistance against further forward flexion is applied, that decreases when the palm is held up (supinated) is a positive test that approaches 90 percent sensitivity and specificity.[17] Patients with a positive test should be referred to a shoulder specialist.

In the older patient, especially those over age 40, immobilization in a sling is usually only continued for 7 to 10 days, until pain subsides. Rehabilitation is begun earlier, to protect the patient from adhesive capsulitis (joint stiffens) and because the risk of recurrence is minimal. The therapy program does not differ from the prescription in a young dislocator.

Posterior Glenohumeral Dislocation

Posterior shoulder dislocations are exceptionally rare compared with anterior dislocations, with percentages ranging from 2 to 4 percent of all shoulder dislocations. Of these posterior shoulder dislocations, 95 percent are subacromial, in which the humeral head lies beneath the acromion and behind the glenoid.[18] Another 5 percent are either subglenoid—posterior and inferior to the glenoid, or subspinous—adjacent to the scapula.

The typical mechanism for posterior dislocation is an axial loading force to an adducted and internally rotated arm. Tonic-clonic seizures and electric shocks or lightning strikes are common mechanisms for this injury. Traumatic dislocations are less common but would occur as a result of posterior directed force on the outstretched arm.

The typical presentation of a posterior dislocation is the sling position—the patient holds the arm adducted and internally rotated. The glenoid fossa is empty and the coracoid process is prominent. On physical examination, external rotation will be painful and difficult. Supination from a forward flexed position will be impaired. Be careful to avoid a misdiagnosis of "frozen shoulder" because of older age of a patient and limited range of motion or because the signs described previously may not be obvious.

Radiography

Although the scapula Y view will show obvious signs of dislocation, the AP film also provides clues to the diagnosis. The glenoid may be empty and a space of more than 6 mm between the anterior rim of the glenoid and the humeral head is diagnostic of posterior dislocation.[19] A humeral head shaped like a light bulb (symmetrical) from internal rotation versus the normal club shape is another clue. Radiographic complications often seen after posterior dislocation include fractures of the posterior glenoid rim and lesser tuberosity, and reverse Hill-Sachs impaction fractures.

Reduction

The patient is positioned supine, longitudinal traction is applied to the arm, and gentle internal rotation is used to unlock the impaction fracture from the glenoid. **Do not use external rotation force** because of the risk of displacing a fracture. Posterior pressure is then applied to the head while longitudinal traction is maintained on the adducted arm. Having an assistant provide longitudinal traction while the other maneuvers are performed is helpful. Suitable sedation with an intravenous benzodiazepine or narcotic (perhaps even general anesthesia) is usually needed. Pre-reduction radiographs are again recommended.

Management After Reduction

The management is usually the same as in anterior dislocations. Operative treatment indications include failed closed reduction and displaced fractures. Postoperatively, the arm is splinted in neutral rotation, slight abduction, and extension for 6 weeks. The usual rehabilitation to restore range of motion and, eventually, strength is then implemented.

Recurrent Subluxation

Although the diagnosis of recurrent dislocation becomes obvious from the history of the shoulder popping out, the presentation in athletes with chronic subluxation is more subtle. Certain movements may produce clicking or pain or sloppiness that is difficult to describe. The athlete may describe a "dead arm" that began with a sharp pain when the shoulder was externally rotated or a direct blow was sustained. The severe pain subsides quickly, but weakness and soreness persist. Throwers in the cocking and acceleration phases, volleyball spiking and serving, overhead tennis serves and volleys, backstrokers, and water polo players are a few examples of individuals in whom recurrent subluxation occurs.

The physical examination findings are subtle as well. Posterior shoulder tenderness is often present. Mild bicipital and mid-deltoid tenderness may be seen. In throwers, a 10 to 15° loss of internal rotation and equivalent gain in external rotation may be seen, but this is often a physiologic adaptation. Impingement testing is often positive, not necessarily because of true impingement but more likely as the result of eccentric damage to the biceps tendon when it tries to keep the loose shoulder in the socket during deceleration. Apprehension testing may be positive with reduction of the pain with the relocation maneuver. Radiographs may show Hill-Sachs lesions or calcification of the anteroinferior glenoid margin.

The mainstay of treatment is physical therapy. If compromise of the inferior glenohumeral ligament or the glenoid labrum is suspected, the patients will usually do better with surgery first and then physical therapy.

Physical Therapy

The management of recurrent subluxation, multidirectional instability, conservatively treated dislocations, and postoperative shoulder dislocations that have achieved full range of motion begins with aggressive physical therapy. The rotator cuff and scapula stabilizing muscles are strengthened through a combination of proprioceptive exercises, theraband tubing, and weights. Resisted internal and external rotation, resisted forward flexion with the thumb pointing down (the empty can position), reverse butterflies in which the shoulder blades are brought together with the arms at shoulder height and above the head, and inside push-ups (hands together) are a few examples. Athletes must understand that they must perform home versions of this program in an ongoing fashion until such time that they decide to give up the sports that exacerbate the shoulder problem.

Surgical Management of Instability

In cases of instability that fail to respond to physical therapy, a variety of surgical techniques are available. None are perfect, and most involve a shift of the shoulder capsule to decrease laxity and modification of the Bankart repair. The inferior glenohumeral ligament is frequently reconstructed. Knowing how much tension to place on the capsule and ligaments is difficult. Many athletes, especially those with multidirectional instability, are unable to return to the same high competitive level. A new approach that may offer hope in these athletes is thermal capsular shrinkage, in which radiofrequency pulses are used to heat the capsule to about 65°C, causing

the collagen in the capsule to shrink. Many orthopedists have reported 90 to 95 percent success rates at 2 years (unpublished data) and are cautiously optimistic about the long-term success of the procedure.

The athletes who most benefit from this procedure appear to be those with multidirectional instability, overhead throwers who sublux and do not truly dislocate, those who dislocate and have ligamentous laxity but do not want an open procedure, and posterior subluxers. Several questions remain, however. For example, there is significant individual variation in the amount of scarring that occurs after the procedure. Some individuals may scar excessively, with potentially severe loss of range of motion. If a revision is necessary, this scar tissue makes operative success more difficult. Older individuals do not respond to the procedure, probably because of age-related mechanical property changes in the collagen. Unless extreme care is used, the axillary nerve and vessels can be injured by the heat. Finally, the long-term success of the procedure is still unknown.

Return to Play Criteria

The decision to return to play after shoulder dislocations does not depend on whether the athlete has had surgery to repair the shoulder. Instead, return to play should be individualized, based on the skill level of the athlete, the type of competition, and the intensity of the sport. After shoulder dislocation, an athlete can **return to practice** if active range of motion is full and pain-free and strength of all shoulder muscles is intact.

An assessment of endurance should also be made. For example, a pitcher may begin by simulating the throwing motion with theraband tubing. If that effort is pain-free, 20 to 40 soft tosses from varying distances are made. Once that test is passed, the intensity and the number of throws are increased over the course of the next few days to weeks. An athlete can return to **full contact-collision sports** if the demands of the sports-specific activities can be met **and** the athlete has the confidence to compete.

References

1. Inman VT, Saunder M, Abbott LC: Observation of the function of the shoulder joint. *J Bone Joint Surg* 26:1, 1944.
2. Freedman L, Munro RR: Abduction of the arm in the scapular place: Scapular and glenohumeral movements. *J Bone Joint Surg* 48A:1503, 1966.
3. Saha AK: Dynamic stability of the glenohumeral joint. *Acta Orthop Scand* 42:491, 1971.
4. Kumar VP, Balasubramianium P: The role of atmospheric pressure in stabilizing the shoulder: An experimental study *J Bone Joint Surg* 67B:719, 1985.
5. DePalma AF: *Surgery of the Shoulder* (3rd ed.). Philadelphia: J.B. Lippincott; 1983.
6. O'Brien SJ, Neves MC, Arnoczky SP, et al: The anatomy and histology of the inferior glenohumeral ligament complex of the shoulder. *Am J Sports Med* 18:449, 1990.
7. Rowe CR: Prognosis in dislocation of the shoulder. *J Bone Joint Surg* 38A:957, 1956.
8. Hovelius L, Ericksson K, Fredin H, et al: Recurrences after initial dislocation of the shoulder: Results of a prospective study of treatment. *J Bone Joint Surg* 65:343, 1983.
9. Matthews DE, Roberts T: Intrarticular lidocaine versus intravenous analgesia for reduction of acute anterior shoulder dislocations: A prospective study. *Am J Sports Med* 23:54, 1995.
10. Rowe CR: Acute and recurrent anterior dislocations of the shoulder. *Orthop Clin North Am* 11:253, 1980.
11. Lill LH, Verhegden P, Korner J, et al: Conservative treatment after a first traumatic shoulder dislocation. *Chirurg* 69:1230, 1998.
12. Henry JH, Genung JA: Natural history of glenohumeral dislocation—Revisited. *Am J Sports Med* 10:135,1982.
13. Hovelius L, Augustini BG, Fredin H, et al: Primary anterior dislocation of the shoulder in young patients: A ten-year prospective study. *J Bone Joint Surg Am* 78:1677, 1996.
14. Arciero RA, Wheeler JH, Ryan JB, McBride JT: Arthroscopic Bankart repair versus nonoperative treatment for acute, initial anterior shoulder dislocations. *Am J Sports Med* 22:589, 1994.
15. Taylor DC, Arciero RA: Pathological changes associated with shoulder dislocations. Findings in first time, traumatic shoulder dislocations. *Am J Sports Med* 25:306, 1997.
16. Bankart ASB: The pathology and treatment of recurrent dislocation of the shoulder joint. *Br J Surg* 26:23, 1938.
17. O'Brien SJ, Pagnani MJ, Fealy S, et al: The active compression test: A new and effective test for diagnosing labral tears and acromioclavicular joint abnormality. *Am J Sports Med* 26:610, 1998.
18. Malgaigne JF: *Traité des Factures et des Luxations*. Paris: J.B. Bulliere; 1855.
19. Arndt JH, Sears AD: Posterior dislocation of the shoulder. *Am J Roentgenol* 94:639, 1965.

Robert G. Hosey

Elbow Pain

Introduction

Elbow pain is a common complaint among athletes, especially those involved in throwing and racquet sports such as baseball, softball, and tennis. Injuries to the elbow may occur as the result of an acute traumatic event or from overuse. Nerve, muscle, tendon, ligament, bone, or cartilage that constitute and surround the joint can all be affected. Elbow pain in an athlete can be a symptom of a common, relatively benign process like tendinitis or it can signify a potentially devastating career-threatening injury such as osteochondritis dissecans. This spectrum of disease necessitates a thorough understanding of the elbow joint in order to make an accurate diagnosis and institute proper management.

This chapter deals with injuries sustained by the elbow in athletes. A review of elbow anatomy and biomechanics is discussed followed by history and physical examination. Specific injuries are addressed in the sections devoted to throwing-related injuries, tendonopathies and bursitis, entrapment neuropathies, and traumatic injuries of the elbow.

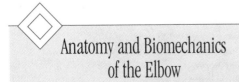

Anatomy and Biomechanics of the Elbow

The elbow is basically a simple "hinge joint," with flexion and extension its primary movement. The ability of the elbow to allow for pronation and supination further increases the variety of motions that can be performed and that are necessary for many athletic activities.

Bony Anatomy

The bony framework consists of the humerus, radius, and ulna and their respective articula-tions. The distal aspect of the humerus flares as it approaches the forearm to form the medial and lateral condyles and the articular surfaces of the capitellum and the trochlea (Fig. 3-1). The spheroidal shaped capitellum articulates with the radial head on the lateral side of the joint. The radius, in turn, articulates with the proximal ulna constituting the proximal radial-ulnar joint. Medially, the ulna forms the olecrenon fossa, which consists of the coronoid process distally and the olecrenon process proximally. The trochlea of the humerus lies within the olecrenon fossa articulating with the olecrenon and coronoid processes. The posterior aspect of the trochlea extends obliquely accounting for the valgus carrying angle of the arm when it is in extension. The normal carrying angle varies from between 10 to 15° of valgus in the general population, with women having a slightly higher average angle.[1]

Soft Tissue Anatomy

The stability of the elbow is enhanced by its ligamentous architecture. The medial aspect of the elbow may be subjected to considerable repetitive tension forces and stability of the joint depends on the well-developed medial collateral ligament(s). The medial or ulnar collateral ligament is composed of three discrete bands, the anterior, transverse, and posterior bands. This "ligament complex" spans the joint originating along the inferior surface of the medial epicondyle and inserting on the proximal ulna (Fig. 3-2). The lateral collateral ligament complex consists of the radial collateral ligament (RCL), lateral ulnar collateral ligament (LUCL), and the annular ligament (Fig. 3-3). The radial collateral ligament and the lateral ulnar collateral ligament originate on the lateral epicondyle of the humerus. The RCL inserts on the annular ligament whereas the LUCL inserts on the lateral aspect of the ulna providing resistance to varus stress. The annular ligament, meanwhile, makes up 80 percent of a fibro-osseous ring that retains the radial head

Figure 3-1

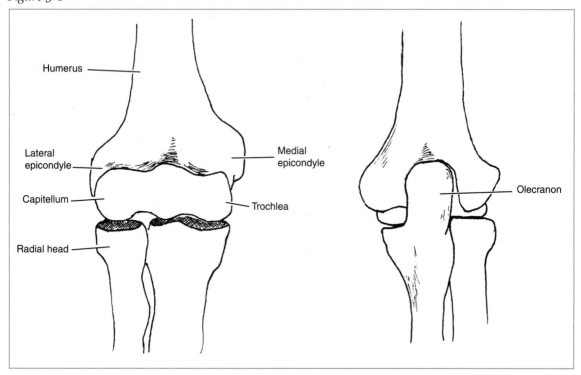

The bony anatomy of the elbow. Anterior (*left*) and posterior (*right*) views.

Figure 3-2

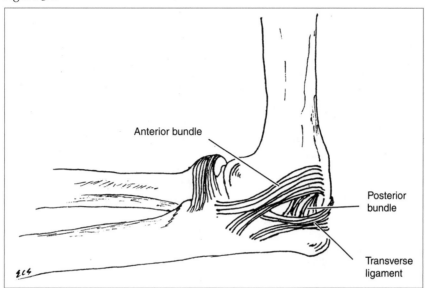

Ligamentous structure of the medial collateral ligament of the elbow. (*Courtesy of Ellsworth C. Seely, M.D.*)

Figure 3-3

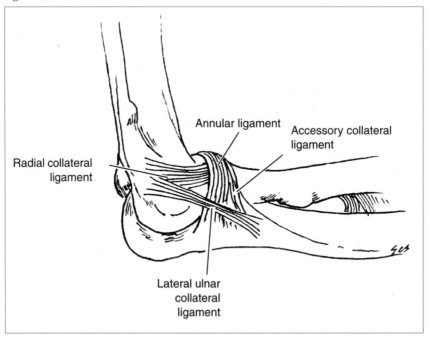

Ligamentous restraints of the lateral elbow. *(Courtesy of Ellsworth C. Seely, M.D.)*

while allowing for pronation and supination to occur.[2]

The elbow is flanked posteriorly by the triceps muscle as it inserts on the olecranon process. Anteriorly, the biceps brachii, brachioradialis, and the brachialis pass the joint on their way to their insertions in the proximal forearm. The extensor muscles of the forearm and wrist share a common origin at the lateral epicondyle of the humerus. Similarly, the flexors arise from the medial epicondyle with the humeral head of the pronator teres lying just superior. The pronator teres (ulnar head) and the supinator muscles originate distal to the joint.

The radial, median, and ulnar nerves all traverse the elbow joint prior to supplying motor and sensory innervation to the forearm and hand. Each nerve and its branches are susceptible to compression or entrapment. The specific anatomy and symptomatology of these entrapment neuropathies are discussed later in the chapter.

Elbow Stability

The stability of any joint depends on both static and dynamic components. Static stabilizers include the articular surface as well as the joint capsule and ligaments, while the muscles provide dynamic stabilization. The elbow relies mainly on its static components for joint stability.

Because of its anatomy, the elbow is most susceptible to injury from varus and valgus forces. These forces are resisted by the static components to varying degrees depending on the position of the elbow. In general, the articular surfaces provide approximately half of all elbow stability, with the collateral ligament complexes providing the other half.

Bony stability is at its maximum when the elbow is in full extension. As the elbow flexes, the collateral ligaments provide a greater percentage of the resistance to varus and valgus stress forces. The primary ligamentous restraint to varus forces is the radial collateral ligament complex (see Fig. 3-3), whereas the anterior band of the ulnar collateral ligament is immensely important in resisting valgus forces (see Fig. 3-2). In fact, in anatomic sectioning studies, the anterior band of the UCL was found to be the dominant stabilizing structure of the medial elbow.[3,4,5] Transection of the anterior band results in significant valgus instability, especially from 30 to 110° of flexion, the elbow's position of function.[5] This finding has tremendous clinical importance in throwing athletes who generate significant valgus forces on the elbow during the throwing motion.

Biomechanics of Throwing

The action of overhand throwing can be divided into at least four phases, which include the wind-up, cocking, acceleration, and follow-through.[6] The wind-up varies among players but acts to prepare the upper extremity and body to launch the object being thrown. In baseball and softball players, this phase ends when the ball leaves the glove. The cocking phase consists of the shoulder progressing through movement of abduction and external rotation and ends when maximal external rotation is achieved. As the shoulder begins to internally rotate, the acceleration phase begins which ends when the ball is released. Finally, follow-through commences with release of the ball and ends when the athlete's motion is terminated.[6]

Throughout the throwing cycle, the elbow has considerable stresses placed on it, which threaten the integrity of the joint. In the late cocking phase, the elbow is flexed somewhere between 90 and 100° and the forearm is supinated, producing a valgus stress on the elbow.[7,8] Maximum valgus stress occurs during late cocking and as the arm begins to accelerate. During this time, the elbow flexes an additional 20 to 30° and the shoulder begins its forceful internal rotation. Varus compression is also occurring during this phase, resulting in contact between the radial head and the capitellum. Posteriorly, tensile

forces are occurring as the triceps contracts and the olecrenon impacts with the olecrenon fossa.

With continued acceleration and ball release, the elbow rapidly extends and the angular velocity peaks near 5,000° per s, a speed that would be equivalent to the elbow making 14 full-circle movements in 1 s.[9] Rapid extension of the elbow coincides with pronation of the forearm, which redirects the valgus force to the lateral aspect of the joint. Also during this motion, the radial head pronates and impacts the inferomedial aspect of the capitellum (Fig. 3-4).[8]

After release of the ball, deceleration of the elbow is coordinated by eccentric contraction of the biceps and brachialis as well as by concentric contraction of the triceps. Posteriorly, the olecrenon may impact with the humerus if deceleration is uncoordinated, resulting in irritation and possible osteophyte formation. Although the biceps, brachialis, and triceps are important in coordinating deceleration, muscles play only a small role in attenuating joint forces at the elbow during throwing. In fact, EMG studies of the elbow in baseball pitchers have shown only low to moderate activity of all surrounding muscles throughout the entire pitching sequence.[10] This indicates that the muscles around the elbow supply little protection against forces occurring during overhand throwing and that the ligaments are required to resist the majority of the force.

History and Physical Examination of the Elbow

The ability to perform an accurate and detailed history and physical examination is essential in the diagnosis and management of elbow disorders. Although a thorough history and physical will often lead to the correct diagnosis without the need for additional tests, they may also reveal that focused ancillary tests are warranted.

Figure 3-4

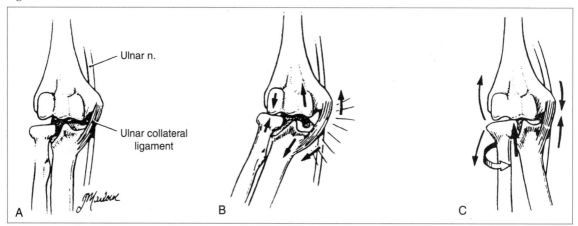

Forces on the elbow during the act of throwing. (**A**) The elbow in neutral position. (**B**) The elbow during late cocking and early acceleration generates valgus forces applied to the structures on the medial aspect of the elbow and varus compression forces across the radiocapitellar articulation. (**C**) Following ball release in the late acceleration and deceleration phases, the valgus force is shifted to the lateral elbow. Also during this time, the radial head pronates and impacts with the inferomedial capitellum. *(Reproduced with permission from Pappas AM, Vitolo J: Elbow anatomy and function. In: Pappas AM (ed):Upper extremity injuries in the athlete. New York: Churchill Livingstone, 1995;317.)*

History

A systematic approach to the history taking in a patient who presents with elbow pain allows for maximal information acquisition. Pain location, nature, and aggravating and alleviating factors should be sought. Determination of associated wrist, neck, or shoulder pain, parasthesias, muscle weakness, clicking, catching, or locking of the joint should also be noted. When did the symptoms start? Did a specific incident occur or was there a gradual onset of symptoms? Was there a repeat injury? In addition, it is essential to inquire about the patients' athletic activity. In what sport do they participate? What position do they play? What is their dominant hand? For throwing athletes, the specific phase of the throwing cycle where discomfort is felt should be determined. Furthermore, it is imperative to ask about any recent changes in training volume (number of pitches thrown) or technique (started throwing side-arm). Finally, a history of

previous treatment and any benefits received may aid in planning future treatment.

Physical Examination

Physical examination of the elbow should involve careful inspection, palpation, and an assessment of the range of motion. In addition, an investigation of elbow stability and a careful neurovascular examination should be performed.

On inspection, the elbow is noted to normally have a valgus carrying angle of approximately 10 to 15°. Differences in limb size may be apparent. This is recognized as a common consequence of exercise hypertrophy in overhand athletes.[11] Joint or bursal swelling, surrounding ecchymosis, and muscle atrophy may also be appreciated on visual inspection. Palpation of the elbow joint requires knowledge of the bony and soft tissue anatomy previously described. Determination of the specific location of tenderness should be attempted. The presence of a joint effusion can be determined by palpating the triangular shaped area formed by the lateral epicondyle, radial head, and the tip of the olecrenon. Fullness in this area signifies the presence of an effusion.

The extent of elbow motion, both passive and active, should be recorded. The elbow normally is able to extend to 0 degrees, flex to 150°, pronate 90°, and supinate 90°. Some individuals with "loose joints" are able to extend beyond 0°. This "laxity" does not represent instability in the majority of cases. It is important to assess the opposite elbow and other joints to determine if the patient has generalized joint laxity. Any pain, clicking, or crepitus during motion testing should be pinpointed as to location.

As previously discussed, elbow stability is extremely important for normal functioning of the joint. Instability that results from an acute elbow dislocation should be immediately obvious because of extreme pain and swelling. On the other hand, medial instability that occurs as the result of a partial or complete tear of the ulnar collateral ligament can be very subtle. To test the integrity of the ulnar collateral ligament a valgus stress is applied to the elbow with the elbow in 20 to 30° of flexion (Fig. 3-5). At this angle, the anterior band of the UCL is the major restraint to a valgus-directed force. The lack of a firm endpoint indicates injury to the ligament. Varus stress testing can also be performed in the same manner to assess the radial collateral ligament complex.

Neurovascular examination should include resisted muscle testing of the upper extremities, a thorough sensory examination, assessment of deep tendon reflexes, and documentation of vascular pulse quality. Examination of the neck, shoulder, wrist, and hand are needed as well.

Figure 3-5

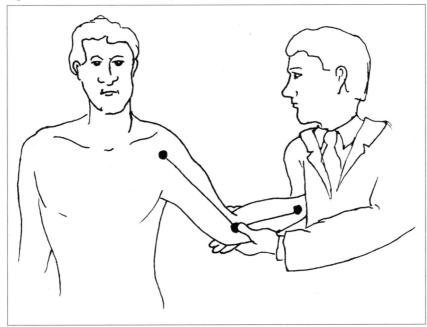

Technique for examining the integrity of the ulnar collateral ligament.

Throwing-Related Injuries

Injuries to the elbow are common among the throwing athletes. Because of the biomechanics involved in throwing, the structures on both the medial and lateral aspects of the elbow are placed under significant stress. Injuries can occur to these tissues as the result of an acute injury, but more frequently occur as the result of repetitive forces and overuse.

Ulnar Collateral Ligament Injury

HISTORY

Injury to the ulnar collateral ligament typically occurs in baseball pitchers and javelin throwers but may be seen in other throwing athletes. In the throwing athlete, excessive valgus forces on the medial compartment of the elbow are encountered during the late cocking and early acceleration phases of throwing. These forces are primarily focused on the anterior bundle of the ulnar collateral ligament. Repetitive microtrauma from overloading the ligament can lead to inflammation and microscopic tears in the ligament. As a result, the ligament can weaken and rupture at this site.[12] Injuries to this ligament can be devastating to the throwing athlete and require prompt identification and management.

Jobe et al have reported that up to 50 percent of athletes with a rupture of the ulnar collateral ligament recall a sudden event at the time of rupture.[13] Most patients, however, reported pain or loss of function prior to the sudden event. Baseball pitchers, specifically, may report months of pain, tenderness, and loss of control leading up to the eventual rupture of the ligament. These symptoms may only be present during the throwing motion and may resolve with abstinence from throwing.

PHYSICAL EXAMINATION

On physical examination, there is usually tenderness over the ligament complex, particularly on the ulnar aspect because the ligament usually tears off of the medial aspect of the coronoid process. If the tear is acute, an ecchymotic area is usually present along the medial joint. The athlete may also have pain with full extension of the elbow. Ulnar nerve symptoms can be elicited in some of these patients due to injury of the nerve that occurs with an incompetent ulnar collateral ligament. In a study by Conway and Jobe, 40 percent of patients with a ruptured UCL demonstrated impairment of the ulnar nerve.[12]

The hallmark of UCL rupture is the presence of valgus instability. Applying a valgus force with the elbow in approximately 25° of flexion and the humerus in external rotation can best assess integrity of the ligament. This position unlocks the olecrenon from its fossa and locks the shoulder in place. The examiner then uses one hand to apply the valgus force while the other may be used to palpate along the joint line. The opposite elbow is used as control to discern any opening of the affected elbow (see Fig. 3-5).

ANCILLARY TESTS

Routine radiographs of the elbow may show calcification within the ulnar collateral ligament indicative of a more chronic process leading to rupture. In addition, ulnar traction spurs and loose bodies may be seen. The use of valgus-stress radiographs to aid in diagnosis of a ruptured UCL has been advocated and may provide additional information in some cases.[14,15] Care should be taken in the interpretation of these studies because uninjured throwing athletes can demonstrate some degree of medial laxity as well.[16]

Most recently, MRI and CT arthrography have been shown to be useful diagnostic tools (Fig. 3-6).[17,18] In one study, MRI was 100 percent sensitive in picking up complete tears but failed

Figure 3-6

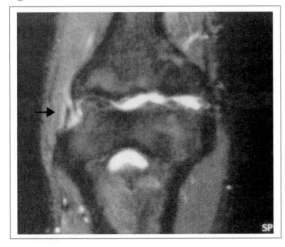

Magnetic resonance image demonstrating complete tear of the ulnar collateral ligament.

to consistently identify partial tears. CT arthrography also had 100 percent sensitivity for complete tears and was better at identifying partial tears.[18] With the addition of contrast media, MRI may improve in its ability to identify partial tears.

TREATMENT

Once a diagnosis has been solidified, treatment decisions need to be addressed. Treatment will vary depending on the patient's level of competition and expectations regarding the athlete's return to participation.

Patients who are not involved in sports requiring repetitive overhead throwing motion rarely require surgical management. Conservative management in these patients consists of rest, ice, and anti-inflammatory medication. A sling may be used for comfort initially if there is significant pain with range of motion. Rehabilitation should concentrate on stretching and strengthening of the forearm extensor and flexor muscles. Strengthening of the flexor/pronator muscles, specifically, may decrease symptoms of instability.[19] Conservative measures can be attempted

in throwing athletes, with a gradual return to throwing activities once the patient has achieved normal strength. Rehabilitation in the overhead athlete may take 3 to 6 months.

Surgical management of the patient with a torn UCL is indicated for athletes who fail conservative management and in the majority of athletes dependent on a stable elbow for continued athletic participation. This latter category most notably includes baseball pitchers and javelin throwers. Operative therapy may consist of primary repair of the injured ligament or reconstruction using a tendon graft (palmaris longus, plantaris, or lateral edge of the Achilles tendon have been used). In a study of professional baseball players comparing these two techniques, reconstruction using a free tendon graft allowed a higher percentage of athletes to return to their previous level of participation.[12] Following surgery, a long rehabilitation process is undertaken, with return to pitching in approximately 12 to 18 months.

Valgus Extension Overload Syndrome

In addition to causing injury to the UCL, repetitive valgus forces can lead to impingement of the olecrenon process onto the medial wall of the olecrenon fossa. Impingement is thought to occur as the result of a combination of valgus stress occurring in a setting of cubitus valgus and hypertrophy of the olecrenon fossa and the humerus.[11] This situation is seen primarily in overhead athletes. Recurrent impingement leads to the formation of posterior and posteriormedial osteophytes and may cause injury to the articular cartilage and loose body formation.[20]

HISTORY

Patients with valgus extension overload syndrome usually present with pain that occurs with forced extension or application of valgus load. Pain is commonly localized posteriorly or pos-

Figure 3-7

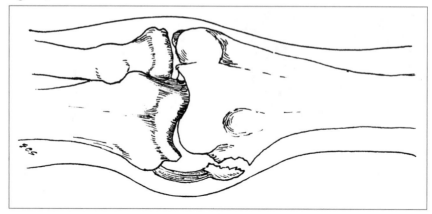

Drawing depicting avulsion of the medial epicondyle.

teromedially. In baseball pitchers, these symptoms are typically produced during the early acceleration phase of throwing.[20] Futher history may reveal that they feel fine throwing for a short period of time but then gradually lose control of their pitches and symptoms increase in severity.

PHYSICAL EXAMINATION

On physical examination, cubitus valgus and a flexion contracture of the affected arm may be present. Pain, which is increased with valgus stressing of the elbow, is usually localized to the posterior aspect of the olecrenon.

ANCILLARY TESTS

Plain radiographs may illustrate a posteromedial osteophyte on the lateral view. Special views are often required to best visualize these lesions.[20] Occasionally, these osteophytes are purely formed of cartilage and will not be visible on plain radiography.

TREATMENT

Conservative therapy should be attempted initially. Treatment should consist of an isotonic strengthening and stretching regimen in conjunction with the use of NSAIDs. In addition, ultrasound and heat application may be beneficial. Patients who are unable to return to prior level of activity should be considered for surgical intervention. Arthroscopic techniques allow for removal of the osteophytes and any associated loose bodies without any incisions into the elbow itself.

The Skeletally Immature Athlete

Skeletal maturity is often not reached until the beginning of the third decade of life in males and the latter part of the second decade in females. Imbalances in strength and flexibility are often present during this growing phase of life. In the elbow, the presence of ossification centers occurs sequentially with presence first at the capetillum around 1 year of age and occurring last at the lateral epicondyle at approximately age 10. This process is delayed an average of 2 years in boys compared to girls, with the exception of the capitellum.[21] The resulting forces across open growth plates can lead to injuries in the immature throwing athlete.

Little League Elbow

Brogdon and Crow originally coined the term "little leaguer's elbow" in 1960.[22] They described avulsion of the medial epicondyle with soft tissue swelling in three little league pitchers. Since that time, "little league elbow" has been used to characterize nearly any pain that occurs in the elbow of young throwing athletes. The actual injury is an apophysitis that occurs at the medial epicondyle as a result overuse. It is seen predominately in baseball players because of the valgus forces applied during the late cocking and early acceleration phases of throwing. As a result of overuse, a medial traction apophysitis produces pain and swelling at the medial epicondyle. With persistent throwing, the pull of the common flexor and pronator muscles can lead to separation and fragmentation of the medial epicondyle (Fig. 3-7). Additionally, a portion of, or the entire medial epicondyle can be avulsed in an acute manner. Avulsion of the entire epicondyle is more common in the younger athlete.[23]

PHYSICAL EXAMINATION

On clinical examination, these patients have tenderness and swelling over the medial epicondyle. Loss of full extension is usually apparent, and range of motion is typically limited secondary to pain. In an acute avulsion, ecchymosis is also likely to be present. Pain and instability are usually noted on valgus stress testing.

ANCILLARY TESTS

Radiographs of the elbow may demonstrate complete avulsion or fragmentation of the medial epicondyle and soft tissue swelling. Comparison views of the unaffected elbow should also be obtained to help diagnose minimal separation.

TREATMENT

Treatment is dependent on the amount of separation observed on x-rays. If only minimal widening of the apophysis is noted, the athlete may be treated with rest for 2 to 3 weeks (or until pain free), followed by gradual return

to throwing activities over the following 4 to 6 weeks. If the medial epicondyle is avulsed a distance of greater than 5 mm, surgery is indicated for open reduction and internal fixation. Surgical intervention in these cases has allowed for return to sports participation.[24] Avulsion with displacement less than 5 mm can be managed with immobilization for 2 weeks.

Post-surgical and conservative treatment options should include rehabilitation consisting of range-of-motion exercises, triceps strengthening, and an evaluation of the patient's throwing mechanics.[25] Patients should be re-examined throughout the rehabilitation process to assess healing and medial stability of the elbow.

Panner's Disease

As previously discussed, the lateral side of the elbow experiences compressive forces during the act of throwing. These repetitive forces can lead to injury of the radiocapitellar articulation. Panner's disease is a disorder that affects ossification centers in the skeletally immature individual. It is characterized by degeneration or necrosis of the capitellum followed by regeneration and recalcification.[26] Panner originally described a localized lesion of subchondral bone of the capitellum and its overlying articular cartilage.[27]

HISTORY AND PHYSICAL EXAMINATION

Children are usually affected between the ages of 7 and 12. They usually present with pain that is localized to the lateral aspect of the joint and is exacerbated by the throwing motion. The elbow may also appear swollen, but full extension is generally achieved.

ANCILLARY TESTS

Radiographically, the capitellar ossification center is fragmented and the epiphysis may be irregular and smaller compared to the unaffected side. The fragmented appearance of the ossification center due to the varying stages of sclerosis and recalcification that occur are characteristic of Panner's disease. The natural history of this disorder is for the capitellar epiphysis to remodel with restoration of normal appearance and architecture as growth progresses. As such, it is a self-limiting disease.[26]

TREATMENT

Because it is a self-limiting disease, the mainstay of treatment involves rest and discontinuation of throwing. Posterior splinting of the elbow may be helpful in the acute setting to alleviate pain. Ice and anti-inflammatory medications can also be useful. Radiographic follow-up is needed to document healing.

Osteochondritis Dissecans

Strictly defined, osteochondritis dissecans (OCD) is an inflammation of both bone and cartilage that may result in the separation of pieces of cartilage into the joint.[26] However, the term osteochondritis can be misleading because signs of inflammation have never been documented in histologic studies.[28] Just as confusing is the underlying etiology of the disease. The most plausible theories seem to indicate that it is associated with trauma or vascular impairment. In the elbow, OCD mainly affects the central and lateral regions of the capitellum.[28,29] Athletes who experience compressive forces across the radiocapitellar joint, such as throwing athletes and gymnasts, appear to be susceptible to develop OCD.[28,30]

HISTORY AND PHYSICAL EXAMINATION

The presenting complaint in these patients is usually insidious onset of pain that may be increased with throwing motion and relieved with rest. Mechanical symptoms, such as clicking or locking of the joint, along with restricted range of motion can also be encountered, especially if there are loose fragments. Patients are typically older than those with Panner's disease, with common presentation between the ages of 13 to 16.

ANCILLARY TESTS

Radiographs commonly show the characteristic radiolucent focal defect in the capitellum along with irregular ossification (Fig. 3-8). Occasionally, loose bodies can be seen within the joint. Magnetic resonance imaging can be helpful in identifying early osteochondral lesions and identifying cartilagenous loose bodies.[31,32]

TREATMENT

Treatment is aimed at preserving the normal configuration of the articular cartilage. In general, the younger the patient, the more favorable the outcome. OCD lesions are typically classified into one of three types. Type I lesions have intact articular cartilage and may be a variant of normal ossification. Type II lesions demonstrate evidence of disruption of the articular cartilage whereas type III lesions involve the formation of loose bodies within the joint.[26] Another classification system based on arthroscopic evaluation has also been reported.[33] Type I lesions are treated conservatively with cessation of throwing and splinting for comfort. Active range of motion may begin when symptoms have resolved. Radiographic healing should also be documented in follow up prior to full return to activity.[26,28,30] Treatment of types II and III lesions typically involve a surgical approach to remove loose bodies and attempt to retain articular architecture. Despite recent advances in arthroscopic techniques, individuals with more advanced disease and those who have reached skeletal maturity at time of diagnosis tend to have a poorer prognosis.[34]

Figure 3-8

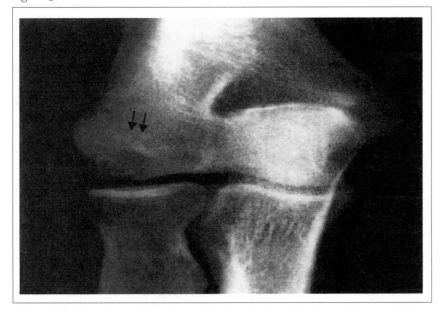

Plain radiograph demonstrates an osteochondritis dissecans lesion of the capitellum. Note the surrounding ring of bony sclerosis.

Tendonopathies and Bursitis

Lateral Epicondylitis

Lateral epicondylitis, commonly known as "tennis elbow," is the leading diagnosis in complaints of pain and disability of the elbow.[35,36] The origin of the extensor carpi radialis brevis has been implicated as the primary source of pathology in tennis elbow.[36] As with other overuse injuries, tennis elbow results from repetitive microtrauma. Repetitive microtrauma refers to a process of repetitive bouts of submaximal loading of a tissue without adequate recovery time. As a consequence, injury to the tissue occurs.

The term epicondylitis suggests the presence of an inflammatory component. Histologic studies, however, have failed to consistently demonstrate inflammatory cells.[37] Instead, Nirschl has noted what he terms "angiofibroblastic tendinosis" in his histologic studies of patients with lateral epicondylitis. Specifically, he found vessel proliferation and fibroblastic changes with a lack of inflammatory cells. These tissue changes are more consistent with a picture of tendinosis than tendinitis. In reality, a spectrum of disease may exist. It is possible that early on in tennis elbow an inflammatory component exists that may be subclinical followed by the more chronic changes of tendinosis noted by Nirschl.

HISTORY

The majority of individuals with lateral epicondylitis present with the acute or gradual onset of lateral elbow pain. History may reveal a pattern of repetitive pronation-supination, or flexion-extension activity. Pain provoking activities can include simple tasks of turning a door handle or shaking hands. Athletes participating in racquet sports often recognize the backhand motion as the most likely to cause pain. Work-related activities should also be explored as a possible etiology for symptom production.

PHYSICAL EXAMINATION

Clinical examination reveals point tenderness at the lateral epicondyle. Elbow range of motion is usually without limitation. Pain is likely to be elicited with testing of grip strength as well as with resisted wrist extension. Provocative tests may be helpful in diagnosis. For instance, having the patient lift an object, such as a chair, with the forearm pronated reproduces pain at the lateral epicondyle.[38]

ANCILLARY TESTS

Radiographs are not generally useful in un-complicated cases, but may be useful in in-stances where the diagnosis is in doubt.

TREATMENT

Treatment of the individual with tennis elbow should begin with the avoidance of painful activities. In the case of everyday tasks, this may be accomplished by modification of lifting technique. Lifting with the forearm in supination as opposed to pronation will decrease the strain on the extensor muscles. Ice and anti-inflammatory medications are employed to help with pain relief.

Consideration should also be given to a course of physical therapy. Modalities such as ultrasound, iontophoresis, phonophoresis, and galvanic stimulation are thought to decrease pain, inflammation, and promote healing. In recalcitrant cases, corticosteroid injection may be beneficial and can be performed safely in the office setting.

After pain has been relieved, an exercise pro-gram focused on strengthening of the wrist extensors should be instituted. In racquet sport athletes, stroke technique may need to be cor-rected to avoid placing the forearm in a fully pronated position while striking the ball. Adjust-ing the racquet grip and string tension can also lessen forces at the lateral epicondyle. Finally, the use of a counterforce brace, which inhibits maximum contraction of the hand and wrist extensors, has also been advocated in the treat-ment of tennis elbow.[37,39] In cases of resistant chronic lateral epicondylitis lasting more than a year, surgical therapy remains a viable alterna-tive.

Medial Epicondylitis

Medial epicondylitis is similar in presentation, pathology, and treatment compared with lateral epicondylitis, with the obvious exception that it involves the medial aspect of the elbow. Also known as medial tennis elbow, or golfers elbow, it occurs less frequently than tennis elbow. The origin of the pronator teres, palmaris longus, and flexor carpi ulnaris at the medial epi-condyle are primarily involved. An overuse syn-drome involving these muscles can result from repetitive valgus stress and pull of the forearm flexors. Sports that are frequently associated with this condition include racquet sports, throwing sports, and golf.

HISTORY AND PHYSICAL EXAMINATION

Clinically, patients are likely to report a dull aching pain in the area of the medial epicondyle. As with lateral epicondylitis, a history of repeti-tive pronation-supination or flexion-extension is usually elicited. In contrast to tennis elbow, it is the forehand stroke and serving in racquet sports that are problematic. Examination is apt to reveal pain with grip and resisted wrist flexion and ten-derness at the medial epicondyle. Care should be taken during the examination to exclude injury to the ulnar collateral ligament and ulnar nerve, radiculopathy, or avulsion of the common flexor origin.

ANCILLARY TESTS

Radiographs are not routinely necessary for diagnosis or management. In chronic cases, however, an ulnar traction spur may be present on plain x-rays.

TREATMENT

Treatment of medial epicondylitis is similar to that of lateral epicondylitis. First and foremost is the need to control pain. Again, ice, anti-inflammatory medications, and the avoidance of painful activity are the initial measures taken. Soft-tissue modalities and corticosteroid injection can also be used.

Rehabilitation focuses on stretching followed by strengthening of the wrist flexors and pronators. Initially, isometric exercises are used, with progression to eccentric and concentric resistance exercises of the common forearm flexors and pronators. Once again, sport technique and biomechanical analysis is important to identify abnormalities that may be involved in injury origination. Refractory cases of medial epicondylitis may be amenable to surgical intervention, which involves the excision of degenerative tissue and re-approximation of the flexor/pronator muscles.

Olecrenon Bursitis

The olecrenon bursa lies posterior and superficial to the olecrenon process. This tenuous position predisposes the bursa to injury as a result of direct trauma. Sports that seem to have a relatively high rate of injury to this area include football and hockey. Olecrenon bursitis has also been referred to as student's elbow and miner's elbow. These occupations have a requirement for large amounts of time spent leaning on the elbows, which may predispose the individual to develop this disorder.

ACUTE

In the acute setting, prolonged pressure over the bursa or repeated episodes of trauma can lead to an acute inflammatory response. As a result, there may be overproduction of bursal fluid with subsequent distension of the bursa. Alternatively, a macrotraumatic event can result in a hemorrhagic fluid accumulation within the bursa. Treatment of acute bursitis is aimed at prevention. The use of elbow pads is essential to help dissipate forces that would otherwise be absorbed by the bursa. If an injury does occur, a compressive wrap and ice should be instituted for the first 24 hr, followed by heat application. If swelling is present and painful, aspiration of the bursa can be performed under sterile conditions to relieve pressure. Because even mild repeat trauma can cause recurrence of symptoms, additional padding should be employed prior to return to activities. Olecrenon bursitis can be classified as acute, chronic, or suppurative.

CHRONIC

Chronic olecrenon bursitis is characterized by thickening of the bursal walls. Repetitive trauma leads to the formation of granulation tissue, which tends to grow into the bursal sac gradually filling the space.[40] Clinically, a firm rubbery mass may be palpated over the olecrenon with or without the presence of fluid. A typical presentation involves an athlete who has had numerous episodes of falling on a partially flexed elbow. Often, an acute injury is superimposed on a more chronic process. In cases where bursitis is a recurrent problem and is associated with decreased performance or symptoms, surgical excision of the bursa is recommended.

SUPPURATIVE

Suppurative olecrenon bursitis results from bacterial invasion of the bursa. Bacteria can be introduced via a puncture wound or superficial abrasion. Once in place, the bursa provides an optimal environment for bacterial growth.

Patients will generally develop an associated cellulitis with erythema, warmth, and bursal distension. Although pain and limited motion are often present, systemic symptoms of malaise, fever, and chills are less common. Diagnosis requires fluid aspiration with analysis for cell count, crystals, and culture. The most commonly cultured organism is *Staphylococcus aureus*, which accounts for approximately 94 percent of cases.[41] Septic bursitis necessitates drainage of bursal contents and administration of systemic antibiotics. Usually, this can be accomplished with needle aspiration and oral antibiotics; however, incision and drainage followed by intravenous antibiotics are occasionally needed.

Entrapment Neuropathies

Several areas of potential entrapment mark the route taken by the nerves supplying the upper extremity. The bony and soft tissue anatomy of the elbow joint serves as a conduit for the nerves as they pass from the proximal arm to the forearm. Within this area, the main nerve or branches of the radial, median, and ulnar nerve can be entrapped or injured producing symptoms locally as well as distally.

Radial Nerve

As a continuation of the posterior cord of the brachial plexus, the radial nerve receives contributions from the C5-C8 spinal roots. In the proximal arm the nerve travels in the spiral groove of the humerus, then courses anteriorly at the elbow where it bifurcates forming the posterior interosseous nerve and the superficial radial nerve. The radial nerve and its branches are responsible for innervating muscles involved in elbow, wrist, and metacarpophalangeal extension, as well as for supination of the forearm. At the elbow, the radial nerve and the posterior interosseous nerve are susceptible to compression or entrapment.

RADIAL TUNNEL SYNDROME

The most common site of radial nerve compression occurs at the radial tunnel.[42] Several sites of potential compression and subsequent clinical symptoms and signs have been identified (Table 3-1).[42–44] Diagnosis is often difficult as symptoms are easily confused with lateral epicondylitis. In radial tunnel syndrome (RTS), however, the pain tends to be of a dull ache compared to the sharp stabbing pain commonly encountered in tennis elbow. In addition, tenderness is located distal to the lateral epicondyle over the extensor muscle mass in RTS. Conservative treatment of RTS includes rest, splinting, and use of anti-inflammatory medications. Patients with symptoms continuing longer than 6 months should be considered candidates for surgical decompression.

POSTERIOR INTEROSSEOUS NERVE SYNDROME

The posterior interosseous nerve branches from the radial nerve at the level of the radiocapitellar joint. As it passes under the supinator muscle, it is susceptible to compression by the fibrous arch of the supinator muscle; the so-called arcade of Frohse (Fig. 3-9). The nerve may also be compromised as a result of repetitive pronation-supination motions leading to overuse of the extensor muscles of the forearm. Compression of the posterior interosseous nerve results in symptoms similar to those encountered in RTS and may even be considered as a spectrum of disease (see Table 3-1). The posterior interosseous nerve, however, is a purely motor

Table 3-1

Entrapment Neuropathies of the Elbow

INVOLVED NERVE	ENTRAPMENT SITE(S)	SIGNS AND SYMPTOMS
RADIAL NERVE		
Radial tunnel syndrome (RTS)	Prominent edge of ECRB Vascular arcade (lease of Henry) Arcade of Frohse	Pain at lateral elbow Pain with resisted supination and resisted extension of middle finger Tenderness over extensor muscle mass 4 cm from elbow
Posterior interosseous nerve	Arcade of Frohse	Same as RTS but without sensory symptoms; (may represent spectrum of disease)
MEDIAN NERVE		
Pronator syndrome	Thickened lacertus fibrosus Hypertrophy of pronator teres Fibrous arch of flexor digitorum superficialis	Parasthesias of radial 3½ digits Tenderness over pronator teres with reproduction of symptoms
Anterior interosseous nerve	Ligament of Struthers Anomolous musculature	Proximal volar forearm pain Weakness of flexor pollicus longus, pronator quadratus, and flexor digitorum profundus to index finger Inability to form "OK sign"
ULNAR NERVE		
Cubital tunnel syndrome	Below arcade of Struthers Ulnar groove of medial epicondyle Between two heads of the flexor carpi ulnaris	Pain at medial aspect of elbow that is increased with elbow flexion Parasthesias of fourth and fifth digits Positive Tinel's sign at cubital tunnel

ECRB, extensor carpi radialis brevis.

nerve. Therefore, unlike in RTS, pain is not typically the most prominent symptom. Furthermore, patients can exhibit weakness of wrist and thumb extension without sensory changes.[42] Treatment is essentially identical as that for RTS.

Median Nerve

The median nerve receives contributions from the spinal roots of C6-T1 by way of the medial and lateral cords of the brachial plexus. Proximal to the elbow, the median nerve runs on the medial aspect of the arm. As it crosses the antecubital fossa the nerve lies medial to the brachial artery and biceps tendon. From there it courses under the lacertus fibrosus and proceeds distally between the heads of the pronator teres (Fig. 3-10). On its path to the wrist, at the distal aspect of the pronator, the anterior interosseous nerve arises as a branch of the median. The median nerve and its branches are responsible for innervation of the majority of flexors in the forearm and the muscles of the thenar eminence in the hand. In addition,

Figure 3-9

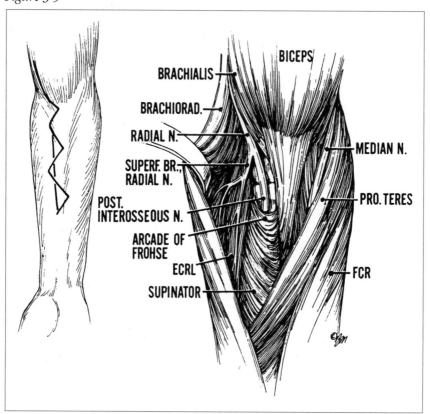

Anatomy of the radial tunnel with possible sites of nerve entrapment. *(Reproduced with permission from Eversman WW: Entrapment and compression neuropathies. In: Green DP (ed): Operative hand surgery, 2nd ed. New York: Churchill Livingstone, 1988;1458.)*

sensation is supplied to the lateral cutaneous region of the palm and the volar aspect of the first three digits and lateral half of the fourth digit.

PRONATOR SYNDROME

Pronator syndrome involves compression of the median nerve prior to the branching of the anterior interosseous nerve. The exact site of compression is often difficult to identify on clinical examination as the nerve may be compromised at different sites (see Table 3-1).

Symptoms exhibited in pronator syndrome include those listed in Table 3-1 as well as a dull, aching pain in the proximal forearm, hand numbness, and premature tiring of the forearm flexors. All of these symptoms can include an exertional component.[45] Pronator syndrome is often encountered most frequently in athletes required to perform repetitive forearm pronation, such as in throwing and racquet sports. Direct trauma to the nerve may also lead to symptoms consistent with pronator syndrome.

Diagnosis is often difficult as symptoms may remain vague and EMG studies are rarely diagnostic.[46] If pronator syndrome is suspected, conservative management should be instituted, which consists of rest, anti-inflammatory medication, and physical therapy. Biomechanical modification of the athlete's activities (such as throwing technique) may also prove beneficial. Failure of conservative management suggests the need for operative decompression.

ANTERIOR INTEROSSEOUS SYNDROME

Anterior interosseous syndrome can result from a single acute trauma or, more commonly, from cumulative trauma. Cumulative trauma to the forearm sufficient to cause this syndrome may occur in gymnasts and weight lifters.[45] Although a pure motor palsy is the general presentation, patients may initially describe volar forearm pain. Clinically, these patients exhibit weakness of the thumb and index finger flexors (see Table 3-1). As a result, they are unable to make the normal "OK" sign with their thumb and index finger (Fig. 3-11).

Electromyography testing is often helpful in diagnosis, showing denervation of the affected muscles approximately 3 weeks after onset of symptoms. Conservative management includes rest and tapering doses of oral steroid medications. Treatment may continue for up to 8 weeks prior to considering surgical intervention.[42]

Figure 3-10

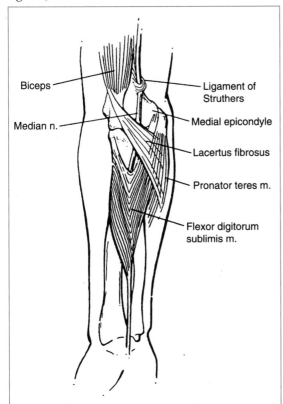

The anatomy of the median nerve in the elbow region. *(Reproduced with permission from Butters KP, Singer KM: Nerve lesions of the arm and elbow. In: DeLee JC, Drez D Jr (eds): Orthopaedic sports medicine: Principles and practice. Philadelphia: WB Saunders Co.; 1994;807.)*

Ulnar Nerve

The ulnar nerve has its origin from the medial cord of the brachial plexus and carries nerve fibers derived from the C8 and T1 spinal roots. It ultimately innervates the majority of the intrinsic muscles of the hand, the flexor carpi ulnaris, the flexor digitorum profundus (fourth and fifth digits), and provides sensation to dorsoulnar aspect of the hand fifth digit, and half of the fourth digit. In the distal part of the arm the nerve passes through the arcade of Struthers before entering the elbow behind the medial epicondyle and into the cubital tunnel. Exiting the elbow, the nerve navigates its way between the two heads of the flexor carpi ulnaris on its way to the wrist (Fig. 3-12).

CUBITAL TUNNEL SYNDROME

The ulnar nerve enters the cubital tunnel after emerging from behind the medial epicondyle. At this site, the ulnar collateral ligament forms the floor, the triangular arcuate ligament the roof, and the humeral and ulnar heads of the flexor carpi ulnaris, the lateral boundaries of the cubital tunnel. Here, the nerve is subject to injury from traction forces, compression, and direct trauma. Common signs and symptoms of cubital tunnel syndrome are noted in Table 3-1. In addition, physical examination may reveal a fullness and

Figure 3-11

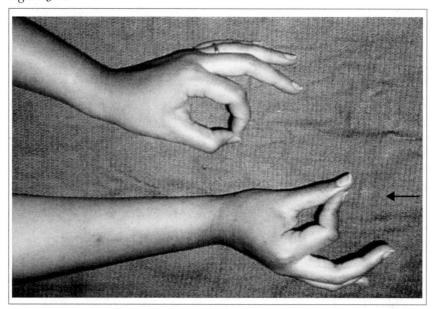

Photograph depicting the inability to make the "OK" sign secondary to anterior interosseous nerve syndrome. *(Reproduced with permission from Vigil, DV.)*

Figure 3-12

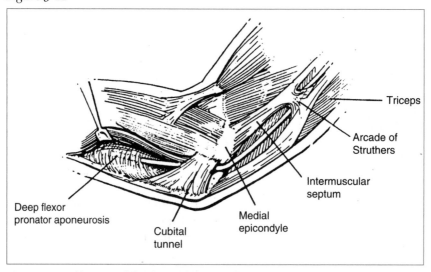

The anatomy and course of the ulnar nerve in the elbow region. *(Reproduced with permission from Butters KP, Singer KM: Nerve lesions of the arm and elbow. In: DeLee JC, Drez D Jr (eds): Orthopaedic sports medicine: Principles and practice. Philadelphia: WB Saunders Co.; 1994;802.)*

tenderness along the course of the nerve and decreased grip strength of the hand.

A careful examination to assess the integrity of the ulnar collateral ligament is a necessity, particularly in throwing athletes. Disruption of the ulnar collateral ligament leads to increased force placed on the ulnar nerve during the throwing motion and subsequent ulnar neuritis. The ulnar nerve may also sublux from its position in the tunnel with increasing elbow flexion.

Because of the tremendous forces generated during the pitching motion, it is not uncommon for baseball pitchers to experience these problems. Cubital tunnel syndrome has also been described in racquet sport athletes and weight lifters.[47] Although cubital tunnel syndrome is primarily a clinical diagnosis, EMG may help detect and confirm the site of injury and typically shows slowing of the nerve conduction velocity compared to the unaffected side.

Conservative management in cubital tunnel syndrome may be instituted when there is no significant motor weakness or atrophy of the intrinsic musculature of the hand. In these cases, treatment is aimed at reducing the pressure around the ulnar nerve that occurs with direct elbow contact or with repetitive elbow flexion. In athletes, throwing, racquet sports, and weight lifting that involves elbow flexion should be limited. Ice, anti-inflammatory medications, and splinting of the elbow in approximately 45° of flexion (4 to 6 weeks) can also provide relief of symptoms. Cases that involve motor weakness, disruption of the ulnar collateral ligament, or that do not improve with conservative measures should be considered for surgical intervention.

Traumatic Elbow Injuries

Fractures about the elbow and dislocation of the elbow typically result from a single traumatic injury and can lead to significant disability. In-depth discussion of these injuries is beyond the scope of this chapter. Discussion of the general principles of diagnosis and management is warranted.

Elbow Fractures

Fractures can occur in any of the bones that constitute the elbow joint: the humerus, ulna, or the radius. In general, these fractures occur after a direct blow to the elbow. They may also be the result of an indirect force to the elbow, such as a fall onto an outstretched arm. Physical examination is likely to show swelling and limited range of motion of the elbow. Ecchymosis may also be present. At the time of presentation, care should be taken to document neurovascular status. Additionally, a thorough examination of the forearm and wrist is needed to determine the presence or absence of concurrent injury.

Radiographs of the elbow are essential in making a proper fracture diagnosis. If an associated forearm or wrist injury is suspected, additional views of these regions are indicated. The majority of fractures are easily identified on plain radiographs and a specific diagnosis can be made. In some instances, no discrete fracture line is visible but soft tissue swelling may be seen, producing either an anterior, the so-called "sail sign," or posterior fat pad sign (Fig. 3-13). The presence of these fat pad signs is a rather sensitive but relatively nonspecific indicator of a fracture to the radial head or neck.[48] The presence of a fat pad sign signals the need for further radiographic views of the elbow.

Management of elbow fractures depends on the type of fracture sustained. Fractures around the elbow include but are not limited to: radial head and neck fractures, olecrenon fractures, distal humeral fractures, supracondylar fractures, and avulsion fractures of the medial epicondyle. Classification and treatment of specific fractures require a text unto themselves and will not be covered here. In general, when treating these injuries certain rules apply. Determination of

Figure 3-13

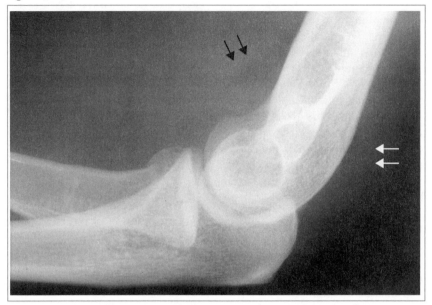

Plain radiograph demonstrating the anterior and posterior fat-pad signs (*black arrows*) in the presence of a radial head fracture (*white arrows*).

neurovascular status is crucial. Any compromise of neurovascular integrity needs to be addressed urgently and prior to treatment of the fracture. When treating the fracture, anatomic reduction is required to minimize the risk of malunion and nonunion, which can result in considerable impairment. This is particularly important to athletes who rely on being able to fully flex and extend the elbow in their athletic activities.

Elbow Dislocations

Dislocation of the elbow is a relatively rare event but poses a significant risk to the limb. The mechanism of injury in the majority of cases involves a fall onto an outstretched hand with the elbow in slight flexion. The most common type of dislocation involves the ulna being displaced posterior to the humerus. This can be a complete dislocation or the humerus may be perched on the coronoid process of the ulna.

Because associated injuries to the neurovascular structures can occur, a neurovascular evaluation before and after reduction is needed. Reduction technique involves extending the elbow, providing countertraction on the forearm, and maneuvering the olecrenon distally and anteriorly so that the coronoid process slides under the trochlea of the humerus.[49] If possible, plain radiographs should be taken before and after reduction to confirm dislocation/reduction and identify any associated fractures. Post-reduction treatment for simple dislocation involves immobilization of the elbow for 7 to 10 days followed by early range of motion. Close rehabilitation monitoring to document regaining of full extension is important, as a modest flexion contracture is not an uncommon long-term result. Dislocations with associated neurovascular injury or concurrent fracture are more complex and orthopedic surgical consultation should be obtained.

References

1. Morrey BF: Biomechanics of the elbow and forearm. In: DeLee JC, Drez D Jr (eds): *Orthopaedic Sports Medicine: Principles and Practice*. Philadelphia: WB Saunders Co: 1994;812.

2. Tullos HS, Bryan WJ: Functional anatomy of the elbow. In: Zarins B, Andrews JR, Carson WG (eds): *Injuries to the Throwing Arm*. Philadelphia: WB Saunders Co.; 1985; 191.

3. Morrey BF, An K: Articular and ligamentous contributions to the stability of the elbow joint. *Am J Sports Med* 11:315, 1983.

4. Regan WD, Korinek SL, Morrey BF, et al: Biomechanical study of ligaments around the elbow joint. *Clin Orthop* 271:170, 1991.

5. Sojbjerg JO, Ovesen J, Nielsen S: Experimental elbow instability after transection of the medial collateral ligament. *Clin Orthop* 218:186, 1987.

6. Jobe FW, Tibone JE, Perry J, et al: An EMG analysis of the shoulder in throwing and pitching. *Am J Sports Med* 11:3, 1983.

7. Fleisig GS, Andrews JR, Dillman CJ, et al: Kinetics of baseball pitching with implications about injury mechanisms. *Am J Sports Med* 23:233, 1995.

8. Pappas AM, Vitolo J: Elbow anatomy and function. In: Pappas AM (ed): *Upper Extremity Injuries in the Athlete*. New York: Churchill Livingstone; 1995; 303.

9. Pappas AM, Zawacki RM, Sullivan TJ: Biomechanics of baseball pitching. *Am J Sports Med* 13:216, 1985.

10. Sisto DJ, Jobe FW, Radovich D, et al: An electromyographic analysis of the elbow in pitching. *Am J Sports Med* 15:260, 1987.

11. King JW, Brelsford HJ, Tullos HS: Analysis of the pitching arm of the professional baseball pitcher. *Clin Orthop* 67:116, 1969.

12. Conway JE, Jobe FW, Glousman RE, et al: Medial instability of the elbow in throwing athletes. *J Bone Joint Surg* 74A:67, 1992.

13. Jobe FW, Stark H, Lombardo SJ: Reconstruction of the ulnar collateral ligament in athletes. *J Bone Joint Surg* 68:1158, 1986.

14. Rijke AM, Goitz HT, McCue FC: Stress radiography of the medial elbow ligaments. *Radiology* 191:213, 1994.

15. Lee GA, Katz SD, Lazarus MD: Elbow valgus stress radiography in an uninjured population. *Am J Sports Med* 26:425, 1998.

16. Ellenbecker TS, Mattalino AJ, Elam EA, et al: Medial elbow joint laxity in professional baseball pitchers: A bilateral comparison using stress radiography. *Am J Sports Med* 26:420, 1998.

17. Gaary EA, Potter HG, Altchek D: Medial elbow pain in the throwing athlete: MR imaging evaluation. *Am J Radiol* 168:795, 1997.

18. Timmerman LA, Schwartz ML, Andrews JR: Preoperative evaluation of the ulnar collateral ligament by magnetic resonance imaging and computed tomography arthrography. *Am J Sports Med* 22:26, 1994.

19. Morrey BF, Tanaka S, An K: Valgus stability of the elbow. *Clin Orthop* 265:187, 1991.

20. Wilson FD, Andrews JR, Blackburn TA, et al: Valgus extension overload in the pitching elbow. *Am J Sports Med* 11:83, 1983.

21. Cheng JC, Ko WM, Shen WY, et al: A new look at the sequential development of elbow-ossification centers in children. *J Ped Orthop* 18:161, 1998.

22. Brogdon BG, Crow NE: Little Leaguer's elbow. *Am J Rad* 8:671, 1960.

23. Woods GW, Tullos HS: Elbow instability and medial epicondyle fractures. *Am J Sports Med* 5:23, 1977.

24. Case SL, Hennrikus WL: Surgical treatment of displaced medial epicondyle fractures in adolescent athletes. *Am J Sports Med* 25:682, 1997.

25. Gill TJ, Micheli LJ: The immature athlete: Common injuries and overuse syndromes of the elbow and wrist. *Clin Sports Med* 15:401, 1996.

26. Bianco AJ: Osteochondritis dissecans. In: Morrey BF (ed): *The Elbow and its Disorders*. Philadelphia: WB Saunders Co.; 1985; 254.

27. Panner HI: A peculiar affection of the capitellum humeri resembling Calvé-Perthes disease of the hip. *Acta Radiol* 10:234, 1928.

28. Pappas AM: Osteochondritis dissecans. *Clin Orthop* 158:59, 1981.

29. DaSilva MF, Williams JS, Fadale PD, et al: Pediatric throwing injuries about the elbow. *Am J Orthop* 2:90, 1998.

30. Morrey BF: Osteochondritis dissecans. In: DeLee JC, Drez D Jr (eds): *Orthopaedic Sports Medicine: Principles and Practice*. Philadelphia: WB Saunders Co., 1994:908.

31. Janarv PM, Hesser U, Hirsch G: Osteochondral lesions in the radiocapitellar joint in the skeletally immature: Radiographic, MRI, and arthroscopic findings in 13 consecutive cases. *J Ped Orthop* 17:311, 1997.

32. Takahara M, Shundo M, Kondo M, et al: Early detection of osteochondritis dissecans of the capitellum in young baseball players. *J Bone Joint Surg* 80A:892, 1998.

33. Baumagarten TE, Andrews JR, Satterwhite YE: The arthroscopic classification and treatment of osteochondritis dissecans of the capitellum. *Am J Sports Med* 26:520, 1998.

34. Bauer M, Jonsson K, Josefsson PO: Osteochondritis dissecans of the elbow: A long-term follow-up study. *Clin Orthop* 284:156, 1992.

35. Bennet JB: Lateral and medial epicondylitis. *Hand Clin* 10:157, 1994.

36. Nirschl, RP, Pettrone FA: Tennis elbow. *J Bone Joint Surg* 61A:832, 1979.

37. Nirschl RP: Elbow tendinosis/tennis elbow. *Clin Sports Med* 11:851, 1992.

38. Gardner RC: Tennis elbow: Diagnosis, pathology, and treatment. *Clin Orthop* 72:248, 1970.

39. Groppel J, Nirschl RP: A biomechanical and electromyographical analysis of the effects of counter force braces on the tennis player. *Am J Sports Med* 14(3):195, 1986.

40. Morrey BF, Regan WD: Tendopathies about the elbow. In: DeLee JC, Drez D Jr (eds): *Orthopaedic Sports Medicine: Principles and Practice.* Philadelphia; WB Saunders Co; 1994;860.

41. Ho G, Tice AD: Comparison of non-septic and septic bursitis. *Arch Intern Med* 139:1269, 1979.

42. Plancher KD, Peterson RK, Steichen JB: Compressive neuropathies and tendinopathies in the athletic elbow and wrist. *Clin Sports Med* 15:331, 1996.

43. Fuss FK, Wurzl GH: Radial nerve entrapment at the elbow: Surgical anatomy. *J Hand Surg* 16A: 742, 1991.

44. Lawrence T, Mobbs P, Fortems Y, et al: Radial tunnel syndrome: A retrospective review of 30 decompressions of the radial nerve. *J Hand Surg* 20B:454, 1995.

45. Butters KP, Singer KM: Nerve lesions of the arm and elbow. In: DeLee JC, Drez D Jr (eds): *Orthopaedic Sports Medicine: Principles and Practice.* Philadelphia; WB Saunders Co.; 1994;802.

46. Hartz CR, Linscheid RL, Gramse RR, et al: Pronator teres syndrome: Compressive neuropathy of the median nerve. *J Bone Joint Surg* 63A:885, 1981.

47. Glousman RE: Ulnar nerve problems in the athletes elbow. *Clin Sports Med* 9:365, 1990.

48. Irshad F, Shaw NJ, Gregory RJ: Reliability of fat-pad sign in radial head/neck fractures of the elbow. *Injury* 28:433, 1997.

49. Hankin FM: Posterior dislocation of the elbow: A simplified method of closed reduction. *Clin Orthop* 190:254, 1985.

Philip H. Cohen
Bassil Aish

Chapter

4

The Acutely Injured Wrist

Anatomy

The wrist is a complex combination of joints that relies on a delicate balance of bony and soft tissue elements to provide it with both stability and a full range of motion. Wrist injuries in sports are exceedingly common and can be difficult to diagnose. Indeed, they are often dismissed as generic "sprains," sometimes with calamitous consequences. Proper understanding of the relevant anatomic and biomechanic features is crucial to the accurate diagnosis and management of wrist injuries. We begin with a brief overview, followed by a more detailed treatment of each area as it is involved in clinically important situations.

Bony Anatomy

The wrist is composed of the radiocarpal joint, the distal radioulnar joint (DRUJ), the intercarpal joints, and the carpometacarpal joints. The distal radius articulates with the scaphoid and lunate bones, via the scaphoid and lunate fossae, to form the radiocarpal joint. Approximately 80 percent of the axial load of the forearm goes through this joint.[1]

Normal range of motion for flexion and extension is approximately 80° and 70°, respectively. Ulnar and radial deviation are limited to 30° and 20°, respectively.[2]

DISTAL RADIOULNAR JOINT

The distal radioulnar joint (DRUJ) is formed by the articulation of the head of the ulna with the sigmoid notch of the radius. Because this articulation is typically shallow, the arc of rotation from pronation to supination is about 180 degrees.(Fig. 4-1).[3]

Maximum joint surface contact (60 percent) and stability at the DRUJ occurs when the wrist is approximately midway between pronation and supination ("neutral").[4] This is especially important when determining the position for immobilization after an injury that destabilizes the DRUJ. On average, the distal radius has an inclination of 22°, and a volar tilt of 11°. Lister's tubercle is a bony prominence on the dorsum of the distal radius, which serves as a pivot point for the tendon of extensor pollicis brevis. The radius averages about 9 mm in length greater than the ulna; this is known as negative ulnar variance.[5] Excessive negative ulnar variance is associated with an increased risk of Kienböck's disease [avascular necrosis of the lunate (AVN)]. Conversely, positive ulnar variance (when the distal ulna extends beyond the distal radius) is associated with a higher risk of triangular fibrocartilage complex (TFCC) injuries. Although the ulna does not directly articulate with the carpal bones, it, along with the TFCC, bears 20 percent of the axial load of the forearm.[1]

CARPAL BONES

There are eight carpal bones, divided into a proximal and a distal row. The largest and most radial carpal in the proximal row is the scaphoid. Named because of its skiff (boat)-like shape, it is the only carpal bone which crosses both rows, and is thus both very important to wrist stability and function AND is at increased risk of injury. The scaphoid is seated within the scaphoid fossa of the distal radius, and it articulates ulnarly with the lunate.

The lunate, named for its crescent-moon shape (when viewed laterally), articulates proximally with the radius at the lunate fossa, and ulnarly with the triquetrum. The ulnar aspect of the lunate is supported by the TFCC. The pisiform is actually a sesamoid within the substance of the flexor carpi ulnaris tendon, and is located volar to the triquetrum at the base of the hypothenar eminence. The most radial carpal in the distal row is the trapezium, which articulates proximally with the scaphoid, and ulnarly with the trapezoid. The trapezoid articulates ulnarly with the capitate. The capitate is the largest of

Figure 4-1

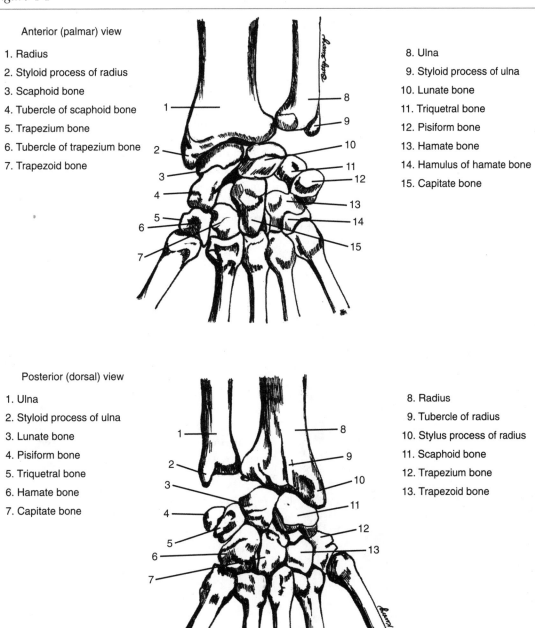

Anterior (palmar) view

1. Radius
2. Styloid process of radius
3. Scaphoid bone
4. Tubercle of scaphoid bone
5. Trapezium bone
6. Tubercle of trapezium bone
7. Trapezoid bone

8. Ulna
9. Styloid process of ulna
10. Lunate bone
11. Triquetral bone
12. Pisiform bone
13. Hamate bone
14. Hamulus of hamate bone
15. Capitate bone

Posterior (dorsal) view

1. Ulna
2. Styloid process of ulna
3. Lunate bone
4. Pisiform bone
5. Triquetral bone
6. Hamate bone
7. Capitate bone

8. Radius
9. Tubercle of radius
10. Stylus process of radius
11. Scaphoid bone
12. Trapezium bone
13. Trapezoid bone

Bony anatomy of the wrist and distal radioulnar joint. *(Illustration by Betty Kuang).*

the carpal bones and serves as the keystone of the transverse carpal arch.[6] The hamate is the ulnar-most carpal in the distal row. Its most distinctive feature is the hamulus or hook, which serves as the distal medial attachment for the transverse carpal ligament. The distal carpal row supports the carpometacarpal joints, with the trapezium forming a saddle-shaped joint under the thumb, and the trapezoid, capitate, and hamate forming supports for metacarpals two through five.

Basic Clinical Radiographic Anatomy

Several important relationships between the carpal bones can be noted on a posterior-anterior (PA) radiograph (Fig. 4-2). Using the approach devised by Gilula,[7] the examiner assesses the three carpal arcs (Gilula's lines). Arc I runs along the proximal border of the scaphoid, lunate, and triquetrum. Arc II outlines the distal border of

Figure 4-2

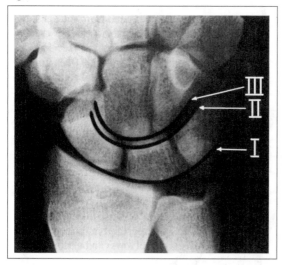

Gilula's lines. There should be three smooth arcs; any loss of congruity indicates a probable ligamentous and/or bony injury. (*Reproduced with permission from Morgan WJ: Ligamentous injuries of the wrist. In: Pappas AM (ed): Upper Extremity Injuries in the Athlete. New York: Churchill-Livingstone; 1995:415*).

these three bones. Arc III traces the proximal border of the capitate and hamate bones. Each arc should be smooth and continuous; any break in the arcs suggests ligamentous and/or bony injury. The intercarpal distances should also be consistent, averaging 2 to 3 mm; any intercarpal widening greater than this may indicate carpal instability. The radial inclination should also be noted; it ranges from 15 to 25°. Abnormality of this angle implies a distal radial fracture.[8] Finally, one should evaluate the "ulnar variance," or the length of the ulna in relation to the radius. The ulna is, on average, 9-mm shorter (negative ulnar variance) but differences in technique and forearm position may significantly impact this measurement.[7]

On a lateral radiograph of a normal wrist, one should note the linear relationship between the distal radius, lunate, capitate, and third metacarpal. The radiolunate angle is normally 0 to 30°; the normal capitolunate angle is 0 to 15°; and the normal scapholunate angle is 30 to 60°. The palmar tilt, defined as the angle between the distal radial articular surface and a line perpendicular to the long axis of the radius, is normally 10 to 25°.[7] Abnormalities in these relationships indicate various instability patterns and/or bony injuries; **however, because of interindividual variation, comparison should always be made with the unaffected wrist** (Fig. 4-3).

Ligamentous Anatomy

The ligaments of the wrist have been classified by Taleisnik[9] into the intrinsic (originate and insert on the carpals) and extrinsic (connect the carpals to the radius or metacarpals) ligaments. The volar extrinsic ligaments and the dorsal extrinsic ligaments are not addressed here.

INTRINSIC LIGAMENTS

The intrinsic ligaments consist of the interosseous ligaments and the deltoid or V ligament. The deltoid ligament runs from the capi-

Figure 4-3

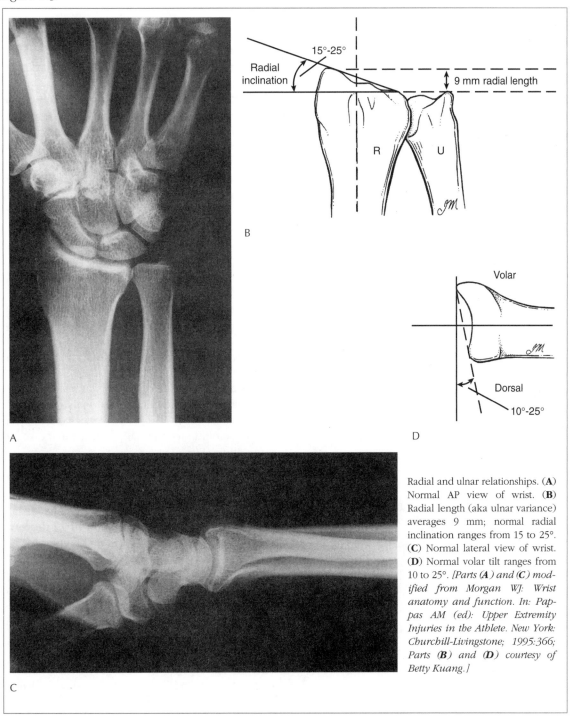

Radial and ulnar relationships. (**A**) Normal AP view of wrist. (**B**) Radial length (aka ulnar variance) averages 9 mm; normal radial inclination ranges from 15 to 25°. (**C**) Normal lateral view of wrist. (**D**) Normal volar tilt ranges from 10 to 25°. *[Parts (A) and (C) modified from Morgan WJ: Wrist anatomy and function. In: Pappas AM (ed): Upper Extremity Injuries in the Athlete. New York: Churchill-Livingstone; 1995:366; Parts (B) and (D) courtesy of Betty Kuang.]*

tate (the apex of an upside-down "V") to the scaphoid and to the triquetrum. Except for the lack of a longitudinal ligament connecting the lunate and capitate, each carpal bone is connected to its neighbors by intrinsic ligaments running radial to ulnar and proximal to distal. The distal carpal row is held together by the trapeziotrapezoidal, trapeziocapitate, and capitohamate ligaments (Fig. 4-4).

The proximal carpal row is frequently involved in injuries,[3] and is held together by the scapholunate and lunotriquetral ligaments. It has been shown[10] that these two ligaments are very strong and can withstand tensile forces of up to 45 pounds and 75 pounds, respectively, and may stretch between 50 and 100 percent before rupturing. **This has clinical importance in that a greatly stretched ligament may appear intact (i.e., on MRI) but may be severely functionally impaired.** (This may underlie the phenomenon of dynamic versus static instability.) The distal and proximal rows are spanned by the scaphotrapezial and triquetrohamate ligaments.

Figure 4-4

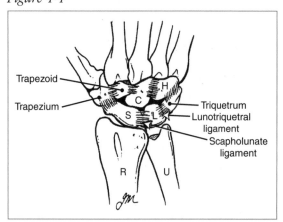

Intrinsic ligaments: *short arrow*: lunotriquetral ligament; *long arrow*: scapholunate ligament. (*Reproduced with permission from Morgan WJ: Wrist anatomy and function. In: Pappas AM (ed): Upper Extremity Injuries in the Athlete. New York: Churchill-Livingstone; 1995:369*).

TRIANGULAR FIBROCARTILAGE COMPLEX (TFCC)

The triangular fibrocartilage complex (TFCC) is the main stabilizer of the DRUJ and consists of five main stabilizing structures: the triangular fibrocartilage itself (composed of the articular disc and the volar and dorsal marginal ligaments); the ulnocarpal ligamentous complex; the infratendinous extensor retinaculum; the pronator quadratus; and the radio-ulnar interosseous membrane.

The triangular fibrocartilage originates at the ulnar border of the distal radius and inserts onto the ulnar styloid. The articular disc itself has an avascular central area, surrounded by a partially vascularized peripheral zone.[11,12] The disc itself may function to stabilize the ulnar aspect of the carpals during pronation, but it mainly functions as a shock absorber and force transducer between the ulnar carpal bones and the ulna.[11,13] Based on the work of Mikic and others,[14,15] it appears that perforations of the central part of the disc are degenerative in nature and increase with age, from 7.6 percent in the third decade up to 53 percent in the sixth decade and above. Volar and dorsal marginal ligaments surround the triangular fibrocartilage and also insert on the ulnar styloid. These ligaments confer additional stability to the DRUJ in pronation and supination (Fig. 4-5).

Extra-Articular Anatomy

It is important to note that the dorsum of the wrist is spanned by the extensor retinaculum, which runs from the radial styloid to the ulnar styloid. This structure forms the roof of the six dorsal extensor compartments of the wrist, which are fibro-osseous tunnels that admit the passage of the wrist and finger extensor tendons. On the volar aspect of the wrist lies the palmar aponeurosis (palmar carpal ligament), through which the two palmar tunnels transport the flexor tendons of the fingers and hand, and the associated neurovascular structures. The extra-articular anatomy

Figure 4-5

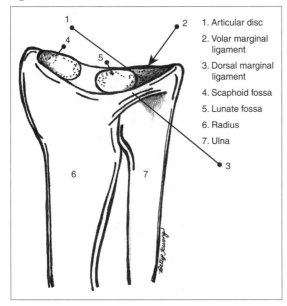

1. Articular disc	
2. Volar marginal ligament	
3. Dorsal marginal ligament	
4. Scaphoid fossa	
5. Lunate fossa	
6. Radius	
7. Ulna	

Triangular fibrocartilage complex. *(Illustration by Betty Kuang).*

of the wrist can now be divided into five clinically important zones (Fig. 4-6).[16]

Zone I is centered around the radial styloid, a frequent site of injury. Just distal to the styloid is the anatomic snuffbox. The radial border of the snuffbox is defined by the tendons of abductor pollicis longus and extensor pollicis brevis. These tendons run through the first extensor compartment, and are also frequently involved in overuse injuries (e.g., DeQuervain's tenosynovitis).

Moving ulnarly, we come to zone II, defined by the bony prominence of Lister's tubercle. Radial to Lister's tubercle, we find the second extensor compartment, which contains the tendons of extensor carpi radialis longus and extensor carpi radialis brevis. These tendons are also often involved in overuse tenosynovitis, such as intersection syndrome. The third extensor compartment is located just ulnar to Lister's tubercle, and transmits the enigmatic tendon of extensor pollicis longus. This tendon makes a 45° turn radially as it passes Lister's tubercle, crossing over the tendons of the second extensor com-

Figure 4-6

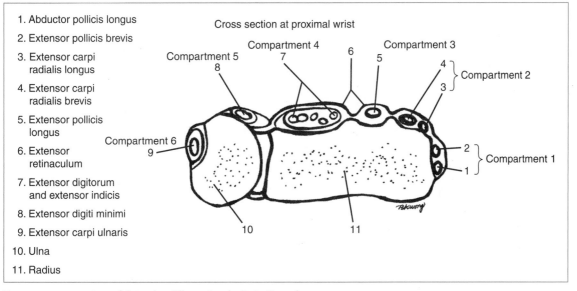

1. Abductor pollicis longus
2. Extensor pollicis brevis
3. Extensor carpi radialis longus
4. Extensor carpi radialis brevis
5. Extensor pollicis longus
6. Extensor retinaculum
7. Extensor digitorum and extensor indicis
8. Extensor digiti minimi
9. Extensor carpi ulnaris
10. Ulna
11. Radius

Cross section at proximal wrist

Extensor compartments of the wrist. *(Illustration by Betty Kuang).*

partment on its way to the thumb, forming the ulnar border of the snuffbox.

At the ulnar border of the dorsal radius lies the fourth extensor compartment, which contains the tendons of extensor digitorum communis and extensor indices (which is independent of the surrounding tendons).

Continuing ulnarly, we come to zone III, defined by the ulnar styloid process. Here, we find the fifth extensor compartment, overlying the DRUJ, and containing the extensor digiti minimi tendon, which is also capable of independent motion. The sixth extensor compartment lies in the notch between the ulnar styloid process and the ulnar head, and contains the tendon of extensor carpi ulnaris.

Moving palmarly, we come to zone IV, defined by the pisiform bone, a sesamoid contained within the substance of the flexor carpi ulnaris tendon. The flexor carpi ulnaris tendon continues distally to insert on the hamate and the base of the fifth metacarpal. The gap between the pisiform and the hook of the hamate is known as Guyon's canal (tunnel), which transmits the ulnar nerve and artery between the pisohamate ligament and the palmar aponeurosis. The ulnar nerve and artery are here subject to injury when there is trauma to the pisiform or hook of the hamate.

Zone V of the wrist is defined by the palmaris longus tendon (absent in 7 to 15 percent of the population[3,16]) and the carpal tunnel. The palmaris longus tendon runs along the midvolar aspect of the forearm, inserting into the palmar aponeurosis. The carpal tunnel is defined by four bones; the pisiform is the proximal medial border and the scaphoid tubercle is the proximal lateral border. Distally, the hook of the hamate is the medial border, and the trapezial tubercle is the lateral border. The transverse carpal ligament runs between these four bones and serves as the roof of the carpal tunnel. The floor of the carpal tunnel is formed by the carpal bones. The median nerve and the flexor tendons pass through the tunnel. Due to its bony and liga-

mentous constraints, compression of the median nerve (carpal tunnel syndrome) is a potential complication of any situation that causes swelling or mass effect within the tunnel (e.g., volar lunate dislocation). Finally, just radial to the palmaris longus tendon lies the tendon of flexor carpi radialis, which courses over the scaphoid tubercle on its way to inserting at the base of the second metacarpal (Fig. 4-7).

Vasculature

The wrist is supplied by the radial and ulnar arteries, which create three pairs of transverse arches allowing for excellent collateral flow in general. However, the tortuous nature of the overall vascular arrangement is such that the scaphoid and capitate bones (and, in some cases, the lunate) depend on the retrograde (distal to proximal) flow of a single intraosseous vessel for their entire blood supply.[17] Thus, injuries to the proximal aspects of these bones that damage this crucial retrograde flow carry a high risk for avascular necrosis or nonunion,[18] as will be seen later.

Innervation

The radial nerve supplies sensation to the dorsum of the radial side of the hand; because of extensive overlap, the purest area for sensory testing of the radial nerve is at the dorsal web-space between the thumb and index finger (Fig. 4-8). Motor branches of the radial nerve supply the wrist (C6) and finger (C7) extensors. The posterior interosseous nerve supplies sensation to the dorsum of the wrist. As it courses distally, it runs

Figure 4-7

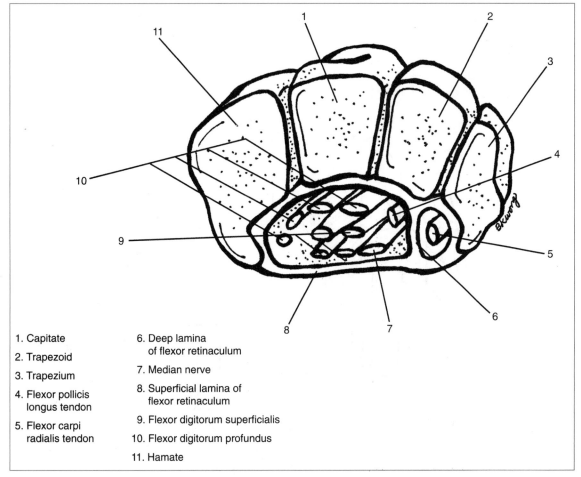

1. Capitate
2. Trapezoid
3. Trapezium
4. Flexor pollicis
   longus tendon
5. Flexor carpi
   radialis tendon

6. Deep lamina
   of flexor retinaculum
7. Median nerve
8. Superficial lamina of
   flexor retinaculum
9. Flexor digitorum superficialis
10. Flexor digitorum profundus
11. Hamate

Carpal tunnel. *(Illustration by Betty Kuang).*

between extensor pollicis longus and extensor pollicis brevis; neuropathic phenomena may occur due to entrapment at this level.

The median nerve travels through the carpal tunnel to supply sensation to the palmar surface of the thumb, index finger, middle finger, and radial aspect of the ring finger. The palmar cutaneous branch of the median nerve splits off proximal to the carpal tunnel, and gives sensation to the thenar eminence; **thus, this area may be spared in carpal tunnel syndrome**. The purest area for sensory testing of the median nerve is the palmar tip of the index finger. Motor fibers from the median nerve supply the thenar muscles and the two radial lumbricals.

The ulnar nerve supplies sensation to the ulnar one and a half fingers and the ulnar aspect of the palm and dorsum of the hand. The purest area for sensory testing of the ulnar nerve is the palmar tip of the pinky finger. Motor fibers from the ulnar nerve supply the deep head of the flexor pollicis brevis, and all the intrinsic muscles of the hand except the thenar muscles and the radial two lumbricals.[16,19–21]

Figure 4-8

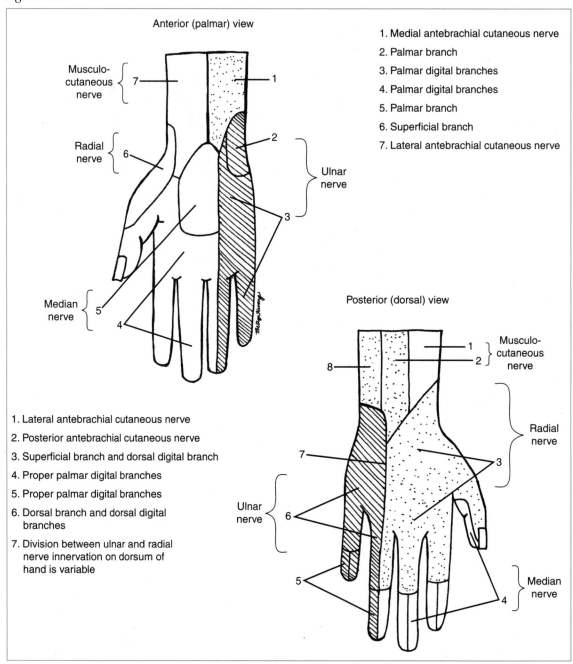

Anterior (palmar) view

Musculo-cutaneous nerve
7
1

Radial nerve
6

2

Ulnar nerve

3

Median nerve
5
4

1. Medial antebrachial cutaneous nerve
2. Palmar branch
3. Palmar digital branches
4. Palmar digital branches
5. Palmar branch
6. Superficial branch
7. Lateral antebrachial cutaneous nerve

Posterior (dorsal) view

1
2
Musculo-cutaneous nerve
8

Radial nerve

7
3

Ulnar nerve
6

5
4
Median nerve

1. Lateral antebrachial cutaneous nerve
2. Posterior antebrachial cutaneous nerve
3. Superficial branch and dorsal digital branch
4. Proper palmar digital branches
5. Proper palmar digital branches
6. Dorsal branch and dorsal digital branches
7. Division between ulnar and radial nerve innervation on dorsum of hand is variable

Wrist and hand innervation. *(Illustration by Betty Kuang).*

Mechanisms of Injury

Injuries to the wrist typically occur via four main mechanisms[2,23]: impact; twisting; weight-bearing; and throwing. Direct impact injuries may occur in racquet, club, and stick sports, such as baseball, tennis, and golf, in which the end of the implement directly injures the hook of the hamate. However, by far, the most common mechanism of acute impact injury is a Fall On an OutStretched Hand (FOOSH).[24–26] Experimental testing has revealed that with a FOOSH, loading typically occurs with the wrist in extension, ulnar deviation, and intercarpal supination.[27]

The ultimate pattern of injury that results is determined by:

1. The type of force loading
2. The magnitude and duration of the forces involved
3. The position of the hand at the time of impact
4. The biomechanic properties of the bones and ligaments involved

In the case of a FOOSH, several patterns of injury may occur. In some cases, a violent compressive force is transmitted axially, resulting in a distal radius fracture.[28] In other cases, the force follows one of several well-defined patterns, which have been investigated in detail.[24,29–31] Mayfield found that most loading injuries begin with force entering radially; consequently, the radial structures (e.g., scapholunate ligament) are the first to be injured. With increasing amounts of force, there occurs a progression of ligamentous injury around the lunate (perilunate injury pattern) ranging from a scapholunate dissociation (stage I), all the way through to a perilunate dislocation (stage III) or lunate dislocation (stage IV). In Mayfield's words, ". . . the scaphoid and distal carpal row are progressively peeled away from the lunate."[30] (Fig. 4-9).

Based on this work, two other patterns have also been described.[32] In the first pattern, force

Figure 4-9

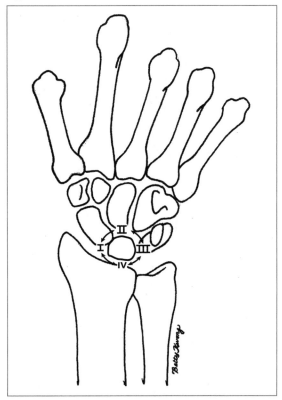

Stages of perilunate instability. With increasing amounts of energy during trauma (Stages I through IV), the scaphoid and distal carpal row are progressively peeled away from the lunate. *(Illustration by Betty Kuang).*

enters the wrist radially, travels through (possibly disrupting) the scapholunate ligament, and then exits ulnarly between the ulna and the triquetrum. In the second pattern, force enters radially and goes through the scaphoid bone itself, fracturing the scaphoid, and then travels *over* the lunate and again exits out the ulnar side between the ulna and the triquetrum.[32] Depending on the magnitude of the force and the biomechanic considerations noted previously, it is also possible that another pattern may develop, in which the force follows a greater arc and causes a complex pattern of bony and/or ligamentous destruction (Fig. 4-10).[28]

Thus, in a patient who sustains a FOOSH

Figure 4-10

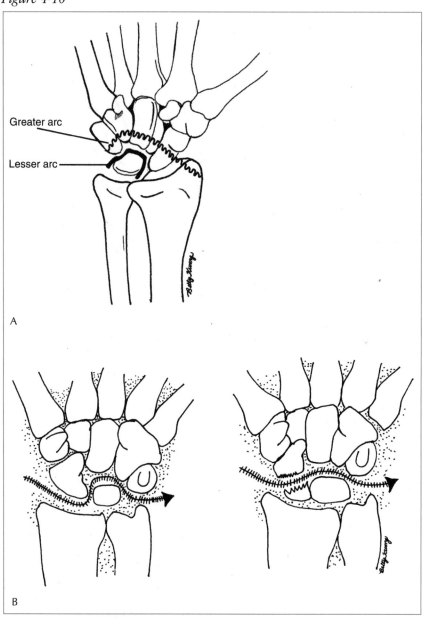

(A) Arcs of injury. Alternate patterns of force transmission through the wrist may result in purely ligamentous injuries (lesser arc) and/or complex bony injuries (e.g., greater arc trans-scaphoid, trans-capitate fractures) with associated ligamentous damage. **(B)** Variations of energy dissipation in FOOSH. Another representation of the patterns of force transmission through the wrist, resulting in injury to only the perilunar ligamentous structures *(left)* or combined damage to both osseous and ligamentous structures *(right). (Illustration by Betty Kuang).*

injury, one must automatically include six main entities at the top of the differential diagnosis:

1. Scaphoid fracture
2. Scapholunate dissociation
3. Lunate/perilunate dislocation
4. TFCC injury
5. Distal radial/ulnar fracture (or physeal injury in a skeletally immature patient)
6. Other carpal fracture or intrinsic ligament injury, including multiple injuries

Because of the various patterns and complex interplay of forces involved, one must be careful not to miss associated injuries. What appears at first blush to be an isolated carpal fracture may, in fact, be part of a complex osteoligamentous injury. Thus, a wide differential must be entertained. Naturally, this differential is modified by the appropriate history and physical examination, which is now discussed.

Key History

Obtaining a detailed and accurate history is crucial to enabling proper diagnosis and management. The following features should be keystones of the history:

1. What was the mechanism of injury (e.g., FOOSH, struck by object, twisting, etc.) and what was the magnitude of force involved (e.g., Low Force—twisting a doorknob; High Force—FOOSH from a height)? It is important to obtain specific information regarding wrist position: flexed or extended; radial versus ulnar deviation versus neutral; forearm pronated, supinated, or neutral.
2. What activity was the patient performing at the time? Many sports have high associations with specific injuries, which may help narrow one's differential(Table 4-1).[33]
3. What is the patient's age? Skeletally immature patients are much more likely to sustain a physeal injury, as the growth plates fail at a much lower load than do the other bony and ligamentous structures.
4. Can the patient localize the discomfort? If so, where is it? (Table 4-2).
5. Are there specific motions or acts that exacerbate or alleviate the patient's symptoms?
6. Was there associated swelling or deformity? If so, where and to what degree? In general, swelling and deformity increase in proportion to the magnitude of injury. However, injuries of superficial structures (such as pisi-

Table 4-1

Sports Associated with Specific Wrist Injuries

TYPE OF SPORT	COMMON INJURIES
Impact sports: Basketball, boxing, football, martial arts, rugby, skating, snowboarding.	Scaphoid fracture, triqueteral fracture, scapholunate dissociation, distal radial fracture, DRUJ dislocation.
Racquet, stick, and club sports: Badminton, racquetball, tennis, squash, baseball, softball, golf, field hockey, hockey.	Hook of hamate fracture, DRUJ dislocation, TFCC injury.
Apparatus-based sports: Weightlifting, gymnastics, rock climbing.	DRUJ dislocation, TFCC injury, impaction syndromes.

ABBREVIATIONS: DRUJ, distal radioulnar joint; TFCC, triangular fibrocartilage complex.
SOURCE: Adapted from Werner S; Plancher K. Biomechanics of wrist injuries in sports. *Clin Sports Med* 17:407, 1998.

Table 4-2

Common Acute Wrist Injuries: Identification by Location

Dorsal Wrist Pain	Volar Wrist Pain	Ulnar Sided	Radial Sided
Scaphoid fracture	Carpal instability	TFCC injury	Scaphoid fracture
Scapholunate ligament tear	Hook of hamate	ECU tendonitis	Distal radius fracture
Lunotriquetral ligament tear	fracture	Distal ulnar fracture	
Distal radius and ulna fracture		DRUJ injury	
Triquetral fracture			
Fracture and dislocation of carpus			
DRUJ injury			
Carpometacarpal dislocation			

ABBREVIATIONS: DRUJ, distal radioulnar joint; ECU, extensor carpi ulnaris; TFCC, triangular fibrocartilage.
SOURCE: Adapted from Nguyen DT, McCue FC, Urch SE: Evaluation of the injured wrist on the field and in the office. *Clin Sports Med* 17:421, 1998.

form fractures) may cause a large amount of swelling for a relatively minor injury.[34]

7. Does the patient complain of "clunking" or "clicking" sensations in the joint? This may be indicative of ligamentous instability.[35]

8. Is the patient experiencing numbness, tingling, paresthesias, or weakness? If so, one must identify the associated neurologic or vascular compromise.

Before the examiner begins the physical examination, it must be kept in mind that patients' discomfort may cause them to focus on one specific part of the wrist. However, especially in high-force injuries, it is imperative that a complete history and physical examination be performed, so as not to overlook potentially serious associated injuries.

 Physical Examination

Because the wrist is a very complex set of structures, a methodical and unhurried approach is crucial to accurate diagnosis. It is important to examine the area from at least one joint distal (e.g., the MCP joints) to one joint proximal (e.g., elbow) to the wrist, so as not to miss associated

injuries or causes of referred pain. Examination of more distant areas may be prompted by the history (e.g., pain radiating down the neck into the wrist). The uninjured wrist should always be evaluated for comparison. Another important principle is to examine the injured area last; this facilitates an accurate examination by putting the patient at ease.

The physical examination of the wrist begins with inspection, noting any swelling, hematoma, abrasion, atrophy, or deformity. Next comes palpation of the bony and soft tissue anatomy; point tenderness often signifies a fracture or ligamentous disruption. This is followed by active and passive range-of-motion testing, neurovascular examination, and finally, specific provocative testing. Examination of the uninjured wrist is helpful in that there is wide inter-individual variation in wrist functional anatomy, especially in testing of ligamentous stability.

Palpation of the wrist begins at the radial styloid process, which enters into the anatomical snuffbox. The scaphoid bone can best be palpated in the snuffbox by placing the wrist into slight ulnar deviation; this allows the proximal radial aspect of the scaphoid to slide out from behind the radial styloid.[2]

The scaphoid tubercle can be appreciated volarly at the base of the thenar eminence. Just distal to the scaphoid tubercle one can palpate the trapezial ridge. The scaphoid articulates distally with the trapezium, which in turn forms a saddle-shaped joint with the base of the first metacarpal. Flexion and extension of the thumb will make this articulation easier to appreciate.[2] Returning to the snuffbox and moving ulnarly across the dorsum of the wrist, the lunate can be palpated just distal to Lister's tubercle, in-line with the third metacarpal. Flexion of the wrist makes the lunate easier to palpate. Having found the lunate, the examiner can trace back radially to the scapholunate junction. To best appreciate this articulation and the connecting scapholunate ligament, we find that the combination of wrist flexion with radial then ulnar deviation is most helpful.

Moving distal to the lunate, the palpating finger will drop into a depression, which represents a curve in the dorsal aspect of the capitate. Just distal to the capitate is the prominent base of the third metacarpal. Detection of this normal, in-line relationship of Lister's tubercle/distal radius, lunate, capitate, and third metacarpal, is of paramount importance when assessing clinically and radiographically for instability.

Palpation continues ulnarly to the DRUJ, where the ulnar head fits into the sigmoid notch of the radius. This articulation can be identified more easily during supination and pronation, as the radius rotates about the stable ulna.[35] The TFCC should be palpated from its radial attachment at the ulnar border of the distal radius, to the ulnar styloid. Between the ulnar styloid and head, the tendon of extensor carpi ulnaris can also be noted. Distal to the ulnar styloid, the triquetrum can be palpated; radial deviation makes the triquetrum more prominent, which may be helpful in detecting such injuries as the relatively common dorsal ridge triquetral fracture.[36]

Continuing ulnarly to the volar aspect of the wrist, the pisiform can be appreciated at the base of the hypothenar eminence. The hook of the hamate should next be located; this is best accomplished by placing the volar surface of the IP joint of the examiner's thumb over the pisiform, and pointing the thumb toward the middle of the thumb/index finger web-space. This will place the tip of the examiner's thumb directly over the hook of the hamate, in line with the fourth metacarpal. Between the hook of the hamate and the pisiform is Guyon's canal, through which course the ulnar nerve and artery (Fig. 4-11).

Range-of-motion testing should begin with active motion first. This enables the examiner to note the patient's discomfort level and serves as a guide to how far and how quickly the wrist should be moved during passive testing. A patient without injury should be able to achieve an approximately 180° pronation/supination arc; 70° of extension and 80° of flexion; and about 30° of ulnar and 20° of radial deviation. Circumduction should be smooth and fluid. If there is a loss of active motion, passive testing should be performed to further delineate the magnitude and nature of the deficit; loss of passive range of motion should heighten the examiner's suspicion for a fracture of the carpals[33] or distal radius.[36]

Vascular examination should include testing of distal capillary refill, assessment of the radial and ulnar pulses, and evaluation for collateral flow (Allen's test). In this test, the radial and ulnar arteries are occluded by pressure from the examiner's fingers. The patient opens and closes his or her fist several times, until the skin of the palm blanches. Then, the examiner releases pressure from over the ulnar artery. Restoration of normal color implies a patent collateral flow via the radial artery (negative Allen's test). The test is then repeated, this time taking pressure off of the radial artery to evaluate for patency of the ulnar collateral circulation.

Neurologic testing should include evaluation of sensation at the palmar tip of the pinky (ulnar nerve), palmar tip of the index finger (median nerve), and dorsal web-space between the thumb and index finger (radial nerve). Strength testing should be performed for the wrist extensors (C6,7, radial nerve), wrist flexors (C7, C8), finger extensors (C7, radial nerve), finger flexors (C7-T1), hand intriniscs (ulnar nerve, C8, T1), thumb and index finger pinch (requires median, ulnar, and radial nerves to be intact), and thumb/pinky opposition (median nerve, C6, C7; ulnar nerve, C8).

Figure 4-11

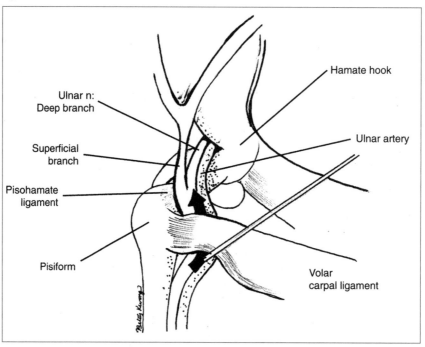

Guyon's canal. In this illustration, it can be seen how fractures of the pisiform or hamate could compromise the ulnar nerve and/or artery in Guyon's canal. *(Illustration by Betty Kuang).*

 ## Distal Radius Fractures

Fractures of the distal radius are the most common of all wrist fractures, and account for one sixth of fractures evaluated in emergency departments.[36,37] The usual mechanism of injury involves a FOOSH, with the wrist in 40 to 90° of extension.[38] The Frykman classification system divides distal radial fractures into extra-articular fractures (types I and II) and intra-articular fractures (types III through VIII)[39]:

FRYKMAN TYPE	INJURY
I	Extra-articular distal radial fracture
II	Extra-articular distal radial fracture and ulnar fractures
III	Distal radial fracture with radiocarpal joint involvement
IV	Distal radial and ulnar fractures with radiocarpal joint involvement
V	Distal radial fracture with DRUJ involvement
VI	Distal radial and ulnar fractures with DRUJ involvement
VII	Distal radial fracture with radiocarpal and DRUJ involvement
VIII	Distal radial and ulnar fractures with radiocarpal and DRUJ involvement

Types I and II are known as Colles' fractures, and are the most common type of distal radial fracture,[39] although adult athletes usually have intra-articular involvement.[40] They occur at the distal radial metaphysis, approximately 2 cm proximal to the distal radial articular surface. Sixty percent of Colles' fractures have an associated ulnar sty-

Figure 4-12

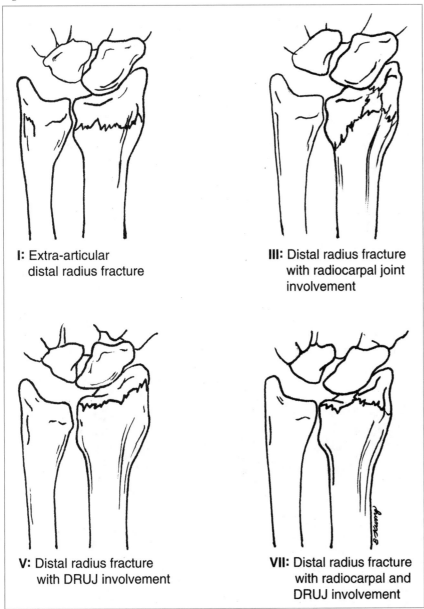

I: Extra-articular
distal radius fracture

III: Distal radius fracture
with radiocarpal joint
involvement

V: Distal radius fracture
with DRUJ involvement

VII: Distal radius fracture
with radiocarpal and
DRUJ involvement

Frykman classification of Colles' fractures. Types II, IV, VI, and VIII are the same as Types I, III, V, and VII, respectively, but also involve a fracture of the ulnar styloid/distal ulna. *(Illustration by Betty Kuang).*

loid fracture[39] and 60 percent to 70 percent of Colles' fractures occur in post-menopausal women.[41] These fractures commonly exhibit dis-placement, dorsal angulation, radial deviation, and proximal shortening, because of tension from the finger extensors (Fig. 4-12).

History and Physical Examination

Patients typically present with a history of a FOOSH and pain and swelling over the distal forearm. Examination reveals swelling and tenderness over the distal forearm, and the classic "dinner-fork" deformity[39] is often present. Traction or contusion/compression injury to the median, ulnar, or radial nerves may also occur[39,41]; thus, careful examination of these nerves, along with the vascular status, is mandatory. Colles' fractures may also be associated with carpal fractures and/or soft-tissue injuries, such as scapholunate dissociation or disruption of the DRUJ. Finally, axial force transmission may cause injury as far proximal as the elbow or even the shoulder. Therefore, a complete examination of the extremity is required.

Ancillary Tests

AP, lateral, and oblique views of the wrist should be obtained. Typically, the distal fragment is dis-

placed proximally and dorsally[41]; angulation must also be assessed. Further, the examiner must assess whether or not the fracture involves the radiocarpal joint, DRUJ, or ulna (Fig. 4-13).

Treatment

It is **vital** to understand that the deforming forces around the distal radius make these fractures **highly susceptible** to **displacement**, even after apparently successful reduction has been achieved. Thus, even with injuries that appear to be stable, a high level of vigilance and excellent follow-up is required to avoid disastrous complications!

Isolated, nondisplaced Colles' fractures with no articular involvement can be treated initially with a sugar-tong splint with the wrist in slight flexion and ulnar deviation, the forearm in neutral, and the elbow at 90°.[41] Patients should be reevaluated clinically and radiographically in 3 to 5 days; at that time, if no loss of position has occurred and swelling permits, a short-arm cast

Figure 4-13

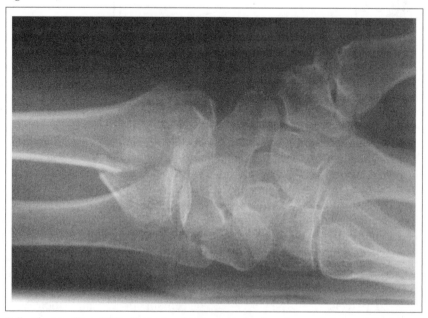

Colles' fracture (Type VIII). *(Reproduced with permission from Leanne L. Seeger, MD., Department of Radiological Sciences, UCLA School of Medicine).*

should be applied. The cast should be applied with the wrist in neutral and allow full flexion at the metacarpophalangeal joints and elbow. Immobilization should continue for 4 to 6 weeks, with repeat examination and radiographs every 1 to 2 weeks to confirm maintenance of position. Careful application of a new cast, with proper molding, is crucial to maintaining proper position.[42]

Displaced Colles' fractures may undergo closed reduction after appropriate anesthesia (regional or hematoma block). Using gentle traction (manually or with finger-traps), the physician places volarly directed pressure over the distal fragment with the thumbs, while exerting dorsally directed pressure over the proximal aspect of the forearm with the fingers. Slight flexion and ulnar deviation at the wrist are also helpful in achieving and maintaining the reduction. Post-reduction radiographs need to document excellent fragment apposition and proper realignment; **dorsal angulation, no matter how little, is NOT acceptable**.

If the reduction is successful, the patient should be placed in a sugar-tong splint. The patient needs to be reevaluated in 2 to 3 days; if positioning is good and edema allows, a long-arm cast should be meticulously applied, with the wrist in neutral to slight flexion and ulnar deviation, the forearm in neutral and the elbow at 90°. Immobilization should continue for 6 to 8 weeks, with repeat clinical and radiographic evaluation every 1 to 2 weeks. After 4 to 6 weeks, a short-arm cast may be utilized if the fracture remains in good position and radiographic evidence of some union is present.[41]

If median nerve damage is apparent at the time of injury, prompt reduction by an experienced physician may decrease the extent of nerve injury[43]; subsequently, the patient should be placed in a sugar-tong splint and urgently referred to an orthopedist for further treatment.

For distal radius fractures in general, the risk of complications, such as loss of range of motion and reflex sympathetic dystrophy, can be lessened by early institution of range-of-motion exercises for the shoulder, elbow, and fingers, and a physical/occupational therapy program after cast removal. Shorter immobilization times (e.g., 3 to 4 weeks) may also benefit older patients, who are at a much higher risk of losing range of motion.[41]

Complications

Several factors contribute to a distal radial fracture being unstable. These include significant displacement, excessive comminution, radial shortening of more than 10 mm, and dorsal angulation of more than 20°. Furthermore, up to 50 percent of distal radial fractures (especially those involving a displaced fracture of the ulnar styloid) may be complicated by rupture/avulsion of the marginal ligaments of the TFCC[44,45]; this causes significant instability of the DRUJ. Fractures characterized by any of these features, or intra-articular involvement, should be referred to an orthopedic surgeon for further care. (However, Cooney[44] states that DRUJ instability after reduction of a distal radial fracture can be treated with a long-arm cast, with the forearm in neutral to supination, for at least 3 weeks.)

Other Distal Radioulnar Joint Fractures

Smith's fracture (aka reverse Colles' fracture) is an uncommon and very unstable fracture of the distal radius, in which the distal fragment displaces volarly and proximally ("garden spade deformity"). This injury can be caused by a direct blow or by a cyclist going over the handlebars. If extra-articular, closed reduction may be attempted, but in general, due to their inherent instability, these injuries should be referred to an orthopedist.

Barton's fracture is actually a fracture-dislocation, in which the dorsal or volar aspect of the distal radial articular surface is sheared off, with disruption of the radiocarpal joint. Seventy percent of these injuries occur in male laborers or motorcyclists. These injuries are extremely unstable and require orthopedic referral for open reduction and internal fixation.

A Galeazzi fracture is a fracture of the radial shaft with associated subluxation/dislocation of the DRUJ. These injuries require open reduction with internal fixation of the fracture, along with repair and stabilization of associated TFCC and DRUJ injuries.[1,44]

Carpal Fractures

Scaphoid Fractures

The scaphoid (also known as the navicular) is the most commonly fractured carpal bone,[28,46] representing about 80 to 90 percent of all carpal fractures.[47,48] It is the second most commonly fractured wrist bone, after the distal radius,[47] and has been commonly associated with sports that involve frequent, forceful falls (e.g., football, basketball, hockey).[49] The usual mechanism of injury is a FOOSH, with hyperextension at the wrist. Frykman[50] found that scaphoid fractures were more likely with wrist hyperextension and radial deviation, whereas distal radial fractures were more likely with less loading and smaller amounts of hyperextension. Weber and Chao[38] determined that wrist extension of at least 95° and radial deviation of at least 10° was required to fracture the scaphoid. Several authors[24,51,52] have found that this position allows the unsupported waist of the scaphoid to be fractured over the dorsal rim of the radius.

Scaphoid waist fractures account for 70 to 80 percent of scaphoid fractures, with fractures of the proximal third (15 to 20 percent), distal third (4 to 10 percent), and distal tubercle (1 percent) comprising the rest.[41,53] Because the proximal aspect of the scaphoid depends entirely on retrograde flow of the distal blood supply, fractures of the waist or proximal third often interrupt this supply, greatly increasing the risk for AVN and non-union (Fig. 4-14).[41]

The mechanism of proximal scaphoid fractures requires that the scaphoid be pushed out of the scaphoid fossa before the proximal aspect is fractured by the "anvil effect" of the rim of the dorsal radius. This implies that the volar extrinsic ligaments must first be stretched or torn to allow the scaphoid to protrude from its fossa. Thus, unlike undisplaced scaphoid waist fractures, **proximal pole fractures are often associated with significant ligamentous injury.**[54] Fractures of the distal pole or tubercle are typically caused by a direct blow[29] and are rarely complicated by associated injuries.[54]

HISTORY AND PHYSICAL EXAMINATION

Patients usually present with pain in the dorsum and/or radial aspect of the wrist. Classically, anatomic snuffbox tenderness is present.

Figure 4-14

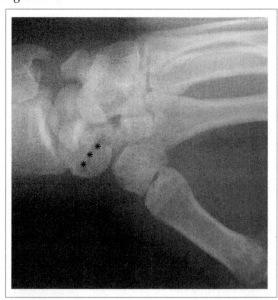

Scaphoid fracture [(see asterisk) (displaced)]. *(Reproduced with permission from Leanne L. Seeger, MD., Department of Radiological Sciences, UCLA School of Medicine).*

Swelling is usually mild,[41,49] but there is usually a decreased range of motion and decreased grip strength.[55] Because of the risk of AVN, non-union, and chronic debility from an improperly treated or overlooked scaphoid fracture, **it is imperative that a patient with a "wrist sprain" be aggressively evaluated to rule out this injury**. In addition, other injuries, such as scapholunate dissociation and fractures of the capitate or triquetrum should be sought.

ANCILLARY TESTS

Any patient complaining of wrist pain who has snuffbox tenderness should undergo a four-view radiograph series (PA with the wrist in neutral and ulnar deviation; lateral; oblique). **Initial x-rays of nondisplaced scaphoid fractures are often negative**.[49] If x-rays of a suspected scaphoid fracture are negative, the patient should be placed in a short-arm thumb spica cast (or splint, depending on swelling) and have a repeat physical and radiographic examination in 10 to 14 days. At that time, bony resorption of the fracture site should be apparent on x-rays if a fracture was present.[47] If the tenderness has resolved and no fracture is apparent, the patient may gradually return to activities as tolerated. A technetium-99m bone scan is highly sensitive within 24 h after injury, but lacks specificity.[56] MRI, ultrasonography, and computed tomography may also assist in earlier diagnosis.[55]

TREATMENT

Treatment of distal pole fractures consists of immobilization in a short-arm thumb spica cast for 8 to 12 weeks. For more proximal fractures, Gellman et al[57] showed that healing is faster when a long-arm cast is used instead of a short-arm cast for the first 6 weeks. The wrist should be maintained in slight flexion and radial deviation, to reduce stress on the fracture fragments. The thumb should be incorporated to the IP joint and, for maximum immobilization, the cast should incorporate the humeral epicondyles.[36] Middle third fractures require 6 weeks in a long-arm cast, followed by 6 to 10 weeks in a short-arm cast. Proximal third fractures require 6 weeks of immobilization in a long-arm cast, followed by 6 to 14 weeks in a short-arm cast. However, proximal pole fractures have a healing rate with immobilization alone of only 60 to 70 percent after 12 to 20 weeks[58] and nonunion may complicate up to 30 percent of these injuries. This often requires operative fixation.[41] Patients should be referred to an orthopedist for open reduction and internal fixation if the fracture is displaced greater than 1 mm, is angulated, or is associated with ligamentous instability.[36,59] Due to the prolonged periods of immobilization required, physical and/or occupational therapy is recommended after cast removal.

Lunate Fractures

Acute lunate fractures are relatively uncommon, accounting for 0.5 to 6.5 percent of carpal fractures.[60] When fractures of the lunate body do occur, they are usually the result of a powerful axial force compressing the lunate between the capitate and the distal radius in a mortar and pestle fashion, as may occur in a FOOSH.[47,61] Avulsion fractures may be caused by traction from the dorsal or volar ligaments.[47] Patients often present with dorsal wrist pain and tenderness over the lunate; axial loading along the line of the third metacarpal may also reproduce the patient's pain. Initial radiographs may not disclose the fracture; CT may help if clinical suspicion is high.[41] If the capitate appears to have displaced volarly with respect to the axis of the radius, one should strongly suspect a fracture of the volar pole of the lunate.[61]

Nondisplaced lunate fractures require immobilization until union is achieved, starting in a long-arm cast that incorporates the metacarpophalangeal joints; this greatly reduces the forces placed on the lunate by grasping. Dis-

Figure 4-15

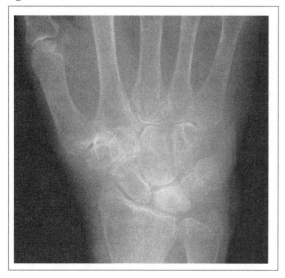

Kienböck's disease. Note the sclerotic changes in the lunate reflecting avascular necrosis. *(Reproduced with permission from Leanne L. Seeger, MD., Department of Radiological Sciences, UCLA School of Medicine).*

placed fractures require open reduction and internal fixation.[36] Kienböck's disease (AVN of the lunate) may complicate lunate fractures[62] and is more common in young men[63] and in those with negative ulnar variance.[64,65] The pathogenesis seems to involve interruption of the blood supply to the proximal fragment.[41,53] Because of the potential for such complications, early orthopedic referral is recommended (Fig. 4-15).

Triquetrum Fractures

The triquetrum is the most commonly fractured carpal on the ulnar aspect of the wrist[34] and the second most commonly fractured carpal overall.[36,42,61] The most common cause of a dorsal fracture is either (1) a FOOSH, with the wrist in extension and ulnar deviation (causing the hamate or ulnar styloid to act like a chisel on the dorsal triquetrum,[66] or (2) hyperflexion, causing

an avulsion of the dorsal triquetrum at the attachments of the dorsal radiotriquetral and scaphotriquetral ligaments.[41,61]

Patients usually present complaining of ulnar-sided wrist pain and are usually point tender over the dorsal triquetrum, 1 to 2 cm distal to the ulnar styloid. Lateral x-rays may disclose the dorsal fracture, but for optimum visualization, a partially pronated lateral will help to project the triquetrum away from the lunate and adjacent carpus.[41,61] Avulsion fractures may be treated in a short-arm cast for 4 to 6 weeks, followed by physical therapy exercises. Although local discomfort may persist for months after the injury,[61] most dorsal triquetral fractures heal with excellent results.[67] Fractures of the triquetral body are much less common, and typically occur in complex injuries such as perilunate fracture-dislocations.[61] Orthopedic referral is warranted for these complex injuries.

Pisiform Fractures

Isolated fractures of the pisiform are uncommon,[41] representing only 1 to 3 percent of all carpal fractures[61] and usually are the result of direct trauma or avulsion via the attachments of flexor carpi ulnaris or the pisohamate, pisotriquetral, or transverse carpal ligaments. Associated injuries are common, and include injury to the ulnar nerve in the adjacent canal of Guyon, as well as fractures of the hamate, triquetrum, and distal radius.[39,61] Because of the pisiform's superficial location, edema may be quite pronounced.[34] The injury is often difficult to detect with routine radiographs; a carpal tunnel view or an oblique view with 30 to 45° of supination and slight extension may allow better visualization.[41,54,61] Most pisiform fractures are nondisplaced[68] and usually heal well with 3 to 6 weeks of immobilization in a short-arm cast. In patients who develop symptomatic nonunion or posttraumatic arthritis, excision of the pisiform is curative.[41,61]

Trapezium Fractures

Trapezium fractures account for 1 to 5 percent of carpal fractures.[61] These injuries demand great care because improper healing may compromise the motions of the thumb, including opposition.[61] Vertical fractures of the trapezial body are the most common type of injury, often resulting from a fall on the outstretched thumb.[61] Fractures of the anterior trapezial ridge may be secondary to a FOOSH or to avulsion by the transverse carpal ligament. Patients usually have tenderness at the base of the thenar eminence and will have increased pain with motion or axial compression of the thumb.[39,41,61] AP views will delineate a vertical fracture, whereas ridge fractures may not be seen unless evaluated with a carpal tunnel view.[41,54,61] Nondisplaced ridge fractures are treated with immobilization in a short-arm thumb spica cast for 4 to 6 weeks.[41] Fractures with more than 1 mm of displacement, comminution, or with involvement of the first carpometacarpal joint surface require referral for operative exploration and fixation.[41,61,69]

Trapezoid Fractures

The trapezoid is the least commonly fractured carpal bone (less than 1 percent of all carpal fractures).[61] The mechanism usually involves a powerful force directed axially to the trapezoid through the base of the second metacarpal.[41,61] Because of the force required to generate this injury, it is usually accompanied by other injuries, such as dislocation of the second carpometacarpal joint.[41,47,61] Tenderness will be noted dorsally over the trapezoid near the base of the second metacarpal, but standard radiographs may be unrevealing; CT may be necessary to delineate the injury.[41] Treatment of isolated, nondisplaced fractures consists of 4 to 6 weeks of cast immobilization; displaced fractures and fracture dislocations require ortho-

pedic referral for open reduction and internal fixation.[41,61,69]

Capitate Fractures

The capitate is well protected from injury, sitting at the center of the carpus, and thus accounts for only 1 to 2 percent of all carpal fractures.[47,61] These fractures usually only occur with high-energy mechanisms, including a FOOSH; as such, they are **usually seen in conjunction with other injuries**. In the scaphocapitate syndrome,[70] a hyperextension mechanism can cause a scaphoid waist fracture and a capitate neck fracture; the proximal capitate fragment may rotate up to 180° so that the articular surface faces backwards! This injury requires open reduction and internal fixation of both the scaphoid and capitate.[61,69]

Severe ligamentous injuries can accompany these fractures, including lunate and perilunate dislocations[27,39,61]; these entities must be carefully assessed for on clinical and radiographic examination. Standard radiographs usually suffice to detect these injuries, but occasionally CT may be needed to determine displacement.

Displaced fractures require open reduction and internal fixation. Acute fractures with less than 1 mm of displacement and no associated injuries can be treated with immobilization in a short-arm thumb spica cast for 6 to 8 weeks.[39,41] However, because of the tenuous blood supply of the head and neck of the capitate, these fractures are at significant risk of developing AVN.[71] Thus, early orthopedic referral is mandatory if delayed healing is suspected.

Hamate Fractures

Hamate fractures comprise 2 to 4 percent of all carpal fractures.[61] The majority of these injuries are fractures of the hamulus, or hook, of the hamate.[34] The usual mechanism of injury involves direct trauma to the hamulus with the

Figure 4-16

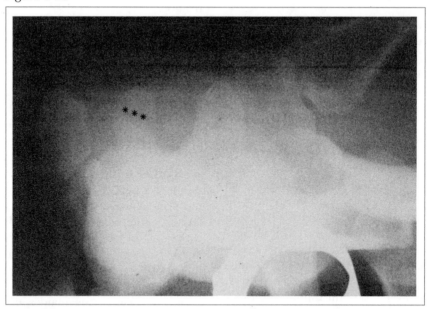

Hook of the hamate fracture (carpal tunnel view). The fracture, easily seen here (see asterisks), is often not apparent on standard views. *(Reproduced with permission from Leanne L. Seeger, MD., Department of Radiological Sciences, UCLA School of Medicine).*

handle of a racquet, bat, stick, or club, often occurring at the end of a swing.[34,36,41,72] The dominant hand (holding the racquet) is injured in racquet sports whereas the nondominant hand (closest to the handle) is usually affected in baseball, hockey, or golf.[36,73] Approximately one third of hamate fractures occur in golfers (Fig. 4-16).[74]

Radiation of pain to the dorsum of the hand is common[36] but, unlike dorsal triquetral fractures, the patient will have point tenderness over the hamulus, located at the ulnar aspect of the palm near the base of the fourth metcacarpal. The ulnar nerve, running in Guyon's canal between the pisiform and the hamulus, may be secondarily compromised; thus, ulnar sensory and motor testing is mandatory. Standard radiographs are often unrevealing but a carpal tunnel view and or oblique views will usually disclose the injury; CT may be necessary in difficult cases.[41]

Nondisplaced fractures located at the base of the hamulus, where some vascularity exists, may be treated with cast immobilization[69] for 8 to 12 weeks. It has been recommended[36] that the wrist be placed in mild flexion, the fourth and fifth metacarpophalangeal joints be placed in acute flexion, and that the base of the thumb be incorporated into the cast so as to minimize the forces transmitted to the hamulus via the surrounding musculature as well as the transverse carpal ligament. However, for fractures higher up on the hamulus, or those with any displacement, early excision is recommended to prevent nonunion and chronic pain.[36,41,47,69] Prevention of these injuries involves the use of properly sized clubs and appropriate grips. The butt of the club should be long enough so that it extends beyond the palm slightly, so that it will be less likely to be jammed into the hamate.[75]

Ligamentous and Soft Tissue Injuries of the Wrist

Scapholunate Injuries

These injuries are the most common cause of carpal instability.[76,77] The mechanism of injury is usually a FOOSH, with wrist hyperextension, pronation, ulnar deviation, and intercarpal supination.[29]

With disruption of the scapholunate ligament, the scaphoid tends to flex volarly. Because the triquetrum still exerts a pull on the lunate via the lunotriquetral ligament, these structures may both extend. If the lunate (intercalated between the distal radius and the capitate) is pulled into this extended position, this is referred to as dorsal intercalated segment instability (DISI). If not properly repaired, this will eventually lead to progressive arthritis involving the radioscaphoid and later the capitolunate joints; this is known as scapholunate dissociation with advanced collapse (SLAC) wrist.[78] Interestingly, in SLAC wrist, the radiolunate joint does **not** develop degenerative changes.[79]

HISTORY AND PHYSICAL EXAMINATION

Physical examination will usually reveal tenderness dorsally at the scapholunate interval; palpation just distal and ulnar to Lister's tubercle, with the wrist in flexion, is helpful in locating the interval.

Watson's scaphoid shift maneuver is performed by placing the examiner's index finger over the scapholunate interval dorsally and stabilizing the scaphoid volarly by placing the examiner's thumb over the scaphoid tubercle. The wrist is then passively brought from ulnar to radial deviation. Normally, the scaphoid flexes during radial deviation and can be felt to push against the examiner's thumb. But, if the scapholunate ligament is torn, this flexion will not occur. Instead, in a positive maneuver, a palpable or audible "clunk" will be noted as the wrist (with or without reproduction of the patient's symptoms) is brought into radial deviation; this represents the proximal pole of the scaphoid subluxing dorsally on the distal radius. The scaphoid shift maneuver is rather specific but lacks sensitivity; only asymmetric laxity *and* reproduction of the patient's symptoms indicate pathology (Fig. 4-17).[80,81]

ANCILLARY TESTS

Standard PA radiographs may show the scaphoid in a flexed posture; this often manifests as the "signet ring sign," created by viewing the double density of the flexed scaphoid end-on. A lateral view will reveal the flexed scaphoid and extended lunate, with an increased scapholunate angle and possibly, an increased capitolunate angle. Normally, these angles are between 30 and 60° and 0 to 30°,[82] respectively. A scapholunate angle greater than 60° implies scapholunate dissociation. A scapholunate angle greater than 70 to 80°, or a capitolunate angle greater than 30°, indicates the presence of DISI[82]; in this case, the concavity of the lunate will be tilted dorsally, marring the normal, linear relationship between the distal radius, lunate, capitate, and third metacarpal.

Widening of the normal scapholunate interval (more than 3 mm) is known as the "Terry Thomas" sign, and also implies rupture of the scapholunate ligament. This may not be apparent on standard films, but may be brought out by an AP clenched fist view or by an AP view with maximum ulnar deviation at the wrist (Fig. 4-18).[79,83,84]

As mentioned previously, comparison views of the unaffected wrist are mandatory. Partial scapholunate ligament tears may not show radiographic evidence of instability.[79] For cases that require further confirmation, other modalities, such as MRI and arthrography, may be helpful;

Figure 4-17

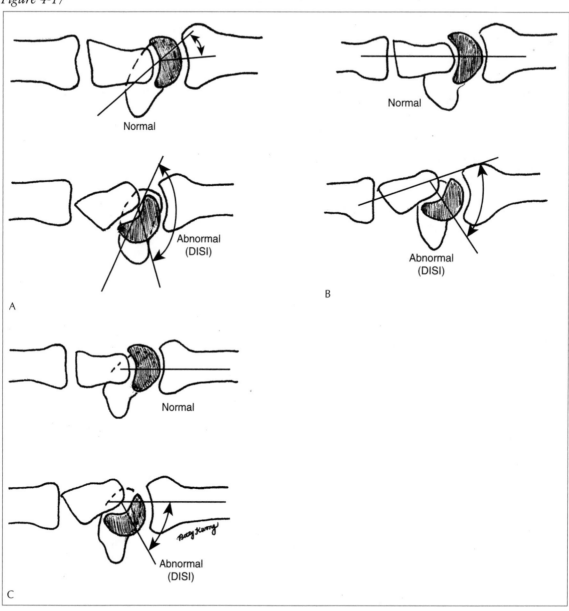

Radiographic angles. **(A)** Scapholunate angle; normal = 30° − 60°, abnormal > 65° = DISI (or < 30° = VISI). **(B)** Capitolunate angle; normal = 0° − 15°, abnormal > 15° = DISI (or < −15° = VISI). **(C)** Radiolunate angle; normal = 0° − 30°, abnormal > 30° = DISI (or < −30° = VISI). *(Illustration by Betty Kuang).*

Figure 4-18

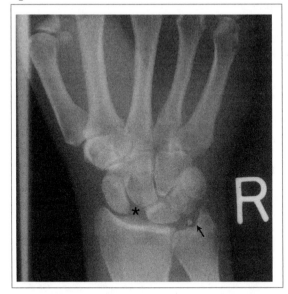

Scapholunate dissociation with "Terry Thomas Sign" (*). An incidental ossicle is present in the TFCC (*arrow*). (*Reproduced with permission from Leanne L. Seeger, MD., Department of Radiological Sciences, UCLA School of Medicine*).

however, they each have varying sensitivity and specificity.[79] Arthroscopy may be helpful in especially difficult cases.[85]

TREATMENT

Injuries to the scapholunate ligament represent a broad spectrum, from mild ligamentous stretching and traumatic synovitis[86] to complete scapholunate dissociation. Dorsal wrist syndrome may be treated conservatively, with splinting, relative rest, ice, and NSAIDs. Patients who have significant scaphoid instability with scapholunate ligament injury, as determined clinically and radiographically, should be treated with open reduction and internal fixation to reestablish stability and prevent the development of SLAC wrist. The patient should be made aware that, following surgical treatment, the wrist will require immobilization for approximately 8 weeks, and that full return to sporting activities may take 4 to 6 months.[79]

Perilunate and Lunate Dislocations

With increasing force loads, the same mechanism that produces scapholunate injury may go on to produce further injury in the perilunate pattern.[24] The type of instability has been classified into four stages.

Stage I perilunate instability (PLI) refers to scapholunate failure. Stage II PLI involves disruption of the capitolunate joint. In stage III PLI, the lunate remains in place but the ligamentous attachments between the lunate and the rest of the carpal bones have been disrupted. This leads to the rest of the carpus dislocating (usually dorsally) and is referred to as a perilunate dislocation. Less commonly, a direct strike to the dorsum of the wrist may cause a volar perilunate dislocation.

Stage IV PLI (lunate dislocation) occurs when the force of injury is so great that the dorsal radiocarpal ligaments are also disrupted. At this point, the lunate is no longer held in place and so dislocates volarly. (Rarely, a great force to the palm may disrupt all the volar radiocarpal ligaments and cause the entire carpus to dislocate dorsally) (Fig. 4-19 through Fig. 4-22).[82]

Acute perilunate injuries typically present with obvious swelling and deformity and may be associated with fractures of the distal radius, scaphoid, or capitate.[84] Patients with these injuries require a complete neurovascular examination, especially with lunate dislocations, as volar displacement of the lunate may compromise the median nerve, and an acute compartment syndrome of the carpal tunnel may also occur. Cases involving acute neurovascular compromise require emergent referral for carpal tunnel decompression and reduction/fixation. In general, perilunate and lunate dislocations are quite unstable and should be treated with open reduction and internal fixation. Full return to activities may require as long as 6 months.[84]

Figure 4-19

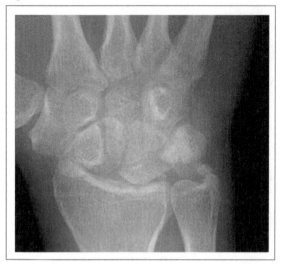

Perilunate dislocation. The disruption of Gilula's lines indicates a significant injury. Note the wedge-shaped lunate, which is pathognomonic for perilunate dislocation. *(Reproduced with permission from Leanne L. Seeger, MD., Department of Radiological Sciences, UCLA School of Medicine).*

Lunotriquetral Ligament Injuries

Injuries to the lunotriquetral ligament are the second most common intercarpal ligament injury, but are only one sixth as common as injuries to the scapholunate ligament.[87] Wrist extension with radial deviation seems to be the mechanism of injury,[88] and may result from a FOOSH or violent twisting.[89] Rupture of the lunotriquetral ligament might be expected to allow the now unopposed pull of the scaphoid to bring the lunate into flexion, with the triquetrum falling back into extension. However, the extrinsic dorsal and volar radio- and ulnocarpal ligaments tend to prevent this from happening.

HISTORY AND PHYSICAL EXAMINATION

Patients usually report ulnar-sided wrist pain, and often note a "click" with wrist loading.[79] The differential diagnosis of ulnar-sided wrist pain is broad and includes triquetral fracture, distal ulnar fracture, TFCC injury, lunotriquetral sprain, pisotriquetral sprain, and extensor carpi ulnaris tendonitis; a careful examination is necessary to distinguish among these entities.

With a lunotriquetral injury, examination reveals tenderness over the lunotriquetral joint dorsally. The most sensitive provocative test used to diagnose lunotriquetral instability is the

Figure 4-20

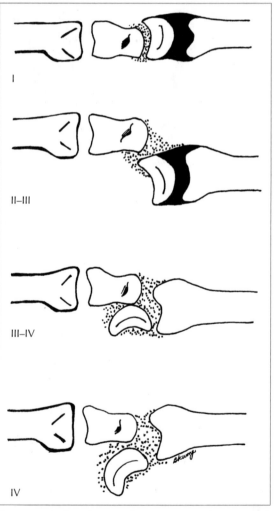

Diagrammatic lateral views of progressive perilunar instability. *(Illustration by Betty Kuang).*

Figure 4-21

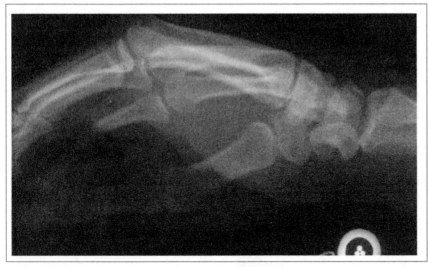

Lunate dislocation. The lunate has been "spit out" like a seed and is facing palmarly, but the rest of the carpus remains aligned. *(Reproduced with permission from Leanne L. Seeger, MD., Department of Radiological Sciences, UCLA School of Medicine).*

Figure 4-22

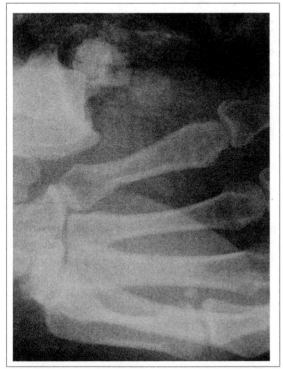

shear or ballotment test.[90] To perform this test, the examiner places his or her thumbs on the dorsum of the lunate and triquetrum, while the index fingers are placed volarly over the lunate and triquetrum (pisiform). Then, the examiner applies a shear force across the joint; a positive test results in laxity and reproduction of the patient's pain.[89] Clicking or crepitation may also occur, but this may be indicative of a more advanced state of joint injury.[34]

ANCILLARY TESTS

Plain x-rays are usually unremarkable, although there may be a small incongruity noted in the alignment between the lunate and triquetrum. If the extrinsic ligaments have also

Dramatic perilunar dislocation. At first glance, this may appear to be a complete carpus dislocation. However, other views confirmed this to be a perilunate dislocation, with the lunate still relatively seated in its fossa. *(Reproduced with permission from Leanne L. Seeger, MD., Department of Radiological Sciences, UCLA School of Medicine).*

Figure 4-23

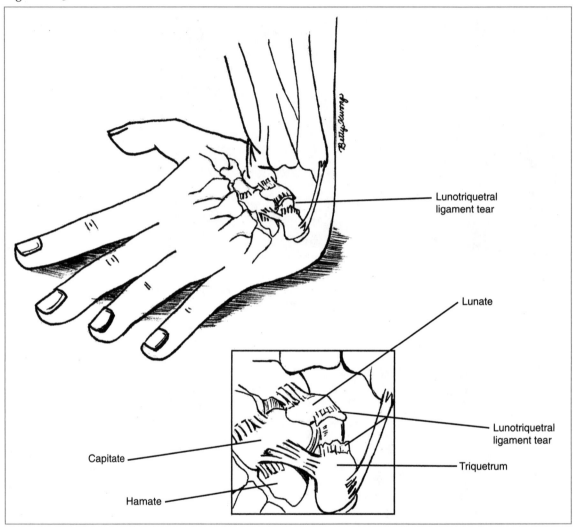

Lunotriquetral tear. *(Illustration by Betty Kuang).*

been disrupted, a pattern may appear in which the concavity of the lunate now tilts volarly. This is called a volar intercalated segment instability (VISI) and is rare (Fig. 4-23).

Arthrography may be useful, but sensitivity and specificity are less than ideal; up to 20 percent of asymptomatic individuals between ages 20 and 60 have a positive lunotriquetral dye leak.[91] MRI also has poor sensitivity and speci-

ficity (50 to 60 percent) as the ligamentous signal is very small and difficult to interpret. Arthroscopy remains the definitive tool for diagnosis in difficult cases (Fig. 4-24).[79]

TREATMENT

Eighty percent of these injuries (without VISI) will heal with conservative treatment; this usu-

Figure 4-24

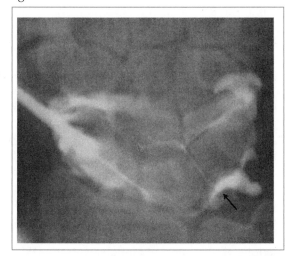

Lunotriquetral tear (three-compartment arthrogram). Note the passage of contrast between the lunate and triquetrum (*arrow*). (*Reproduced with permission from Leanne L. Seeger, MD., Department of Radiological Sciences, UCLA School of Medicine*).

ally consists of casting for 6 weeks. Again, VISI is rare, but if present, requires referral to address the associated ligamentous injuries.[79,84]

Midcarpal Injuries

Ulnar midcarpal instability occurs when there is a disruption between the ligaments that bridge the proximal to distal carpal rows. The instability is most commonly caused by damage to the triquetrohamate ligament and the associated extrinsic structures. Although less common than lunotriquetral disruptions, acute midcarpal instability may result from ulnar-sided impact along with hyperpronation.[32]

HISTORY

The patient usually presents complaining of ulnar-sided wrist pain and a "clunk" that occurs with ulnar deviation and pronation. This has been termed a "catch-up clunk"[92] and represents the abnormally flexed proximal carpal row "catching up" as it reduces into the extended position late in ulnar deviation. (Normally, the proximal row undergoes a smooth transition from slight flexion in radial deviation to extension in ulnar deviation.)

PHYSICAL EXAMINATION

On inspection, the examiner may note an indentation over the dorsal ulnar aspect of the wrist, making the ulnar head appear to be prominent. However, this actually represents sagging of the proximal carpal row into flexion, with extension of the distal row.[79] The "catch-up clunk test" can be performed by axially loading the slightly flexed and pronated wrist and then passively moving the wrist from radial to ulnar deviation, while moving from flexion to extension; reproduction of the "clunk" is a positive test.[79,93]

ANCILLARY TESTS

Radiographs may reveal a VISI pattern, but cineradiography may be the most useful technique for diagnosis. This technique allows the examiner to visualize the entire proximal carpal row moving abruptly into extension as terminal ulnar deviation is approached. Arthrography may assist in diagnosis by confirming a dye leak at the triquetrohamate joint.[84]

TREATMENT

Treatment ranges from splinting, NSAIDs, and injections to triquetrohamate arthrodesis, depending on the severity of instability and symptoms.[79,84]

Triangular Fibrocartilage Complex (TFCC) Injuries

As mentioned previously, the TFCC is both an important stabilizer of the DRUJ and also bears up to 20 percent of the compressive load through the wrist.[94] Traumatic TFCC injuries typically occur from a FOOSH or twisting injury (especially rotation with compression),[95] and tend to occur in the peripheral (better vascularized) areas of the TFCC. Degenerative lesions are associated with chronic wear and positive ulnar variance, and tend to occur in the central fibrocartilage disc region, where poor vascularity makes healing less likely.[96,97] Several classification systems for TFCC injuries exist,[97,98,99] but four main types of traumatic TFCC injury can be identified.

Type I involves a tear in the central, cartilaginous disc. Type II injuries involve an avulsion of the TFCC from the ulnar styloid. Type III injuries consist of tears in the palmar third of the TFCC, usually also involving the ulnocarpal ligaments. In type IV injuries, there is an avulsion of the TFCC from its radial attachment, and there is often an associated distal radial fracture. Injuries to the infratendinous retinaculum of the sixth extensor compartment may also produce subluxation of the extensor carpi ulnaris tendon, yet another entity that can cause "snapping" or "popping" at the ulnar aspect of the wrist.

HISTORY AND PHYSICAL EXAMINATION

Patients typically present with ulnar-sided wrist pain, which is worsened with loading or ulnar deviation.[100] Clinicians should especially suspect TFCC injury in gymnasts with ulnar-sided wrist pain, as gymnasts have a particularly high incidence of TFCC injuries.[101]

Patients who only have symptoms with pronation and supination with the wrist loaded and ulnarly deviated (as in opening a tight jar lid) are likely to have a perforation of the articular disc (type I injury). With this injury, examination usually reveals tenderness over the TFCC but no evidence of DRUJ instability. The patient's symptoms can be reproduced with the TFCC load test. In this test, the wrist is placed in ulnar deviation, axially loaded, and then passively flexed and extended.[34,35] If the TFCC load

test is negative, but there is tenderness to palpation at the ECU tendon and crepitus with active ulnar deviation, ECU tendonitis must be considered. Injection into the ECU sheath may be both diagnostic and curative in such cases.

Patients who have pain with other activities, along with a loss of their range of motion, are likely to have a more peripheral TFCC lesion (type II to IV injuries). These patients may also have a positive distal ulna ballotment test.[34] To perform this test, the examiner uses one thumb to stabilize the volar aspect of the patient's pisiform, and uses the other thumb to apply a dorsal to palmar force on the dorsum of the distal ulna. Significant displacement of the ulna is called the "piano key sign"[97] and indicates a peripheral TFCC tear and instability of the DRUJ. Because the differential diagnosis of ulnar-sided wrist pain is so complex and because TFCC tears often have associated injuries, some experts[97,102] find that injection of lidocaine into the suspected area of injury is a valuable tool in evaluating these patients.

ANCILLARY TESTS

Routine radiographs are usually not helpful unless subluxation of the distal ulna or an associated radial fracture is present. In type II injuries, an ulnar styloid avulsion fracture may be noted. Three compartment arthrograms have traditionally been considered the most effective imaging study and certainly improve sensitivity over single compartment arthrography.[97,103,104] However, arthrography does not allow identification of the exact location of the injury or provide information about injuries to the associated soft tissue structures (Fig. 4-25).

Recently, high-resolution MRI has been found to provide up to 100 percent sensitivity, 90 percent specificity, and 97 percent accuracy in the detection of TFCC tears, with excellent detail regarding location of the tear and associated injuries.[96,105–107] With continued improvements in resolution, cost, and availability, high-resolu-

Figure 4-25

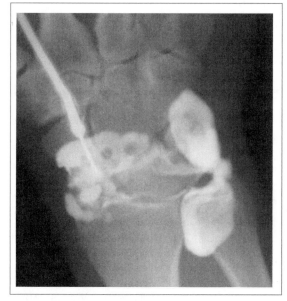

TFCC tear (three-compartment arthrogram). Contrast passing from the radiocarpal joint into the distal radioulnar joint, consistent with a TFCC tear. *(Reproduced with permission from Leanne L. Seeger, MD., Department of Radiological Sciences, UCLA School of Medicine).*

tion MRI may eventually become the imaging procedure of choice for evaluation of suspected TFCC injuries. Yet, it has been our clinical experience that high-resolution MRI is still inferior to arthrography, and that arthrography remains the radiologic diagnostic standard.

TREATMENT

Most cases of isolated TFCC injuries may be treated conservatively, with rest and splinting for 3 to 4 weeks. However, some investigators feel that long-arm cast or splint immobilization for 4 to 6 weeks, with the forearm in neutral or full supination, yields optimal results.[96,100]

For those who fail to respond (those who still have pain after a course of conservative therapy), three-compartment arthrography or high-

resolution MRI can be used to better delineate the lesion. Arthroscopy can then be utilized to perform debridement (usually in central tears) or repair (usually in peripheral tears) as needed.[96,97,100] Patients with a recalcitrant TFCC tear and positive ulnar variance should also undergo ulnar shortening along with arthroscopic debridement or repair.[96] This decompresses the TFCC and has been shown to improve outcomes.[108,109] Patients with DRUJ dislocations can be treated with closed reduction and long-arm casting in supination (for dorsal dislocations) or pronation (for volar dislocations) for 4 weeks. If closed reduction fails, or more complex injuries are present, the patient should be referred to an orthopedist for operative repair.[96]

Conclusion

The wrist is an exceedingly complex body part, which is commonly injured in athletic and nonathletic pursuits. The key to accurate diagnosis and treatment of acute wrist injuries is a thorough history and physical examination, with appropriate radiographic testing, and ancillary procedures utilized when necessary. The examiner must maintain a high index of suspicion for fractures and ligamentous disruption; simply diagnosing a generic "wrist sprain" and sending the patient off with a cock-up splint and no follow-up is UNACCEPTABLE.

Future directions in the area of acute wrist injuries include the further investigation and refinement of diagnostic techniques, such as MRI and arthroscopy, as well as continuing to apply rigorous scrutiny to our current and developing therapeutic measures. Prevention of acute wrist injuries is an emerging area of research, which merits close attention. Wrist guards have been shown to be effective in decreasing acute wrist injuries among in-line skaters[110]; however, they have also been associated with an increased risk of forearm fractures.[111] Thus, when evaluating potential means of injury prevention, we must ensure that injuries are not just being shifted to a different body part.

References

1. Werner S, Plancher K. Biomechanics of wrist injuries in sports. *Clin in Sports Med* 17:407,998.
2. Hoppenfeld S: *Physical Examination of the Spine and Extremities*. Norwalk, CT: Appleton-Century-Crofts; 1976;59.
3. Morgan WJ: Wrist anatomy and function. In: Pappas AM (ed): *Upper Extremity Injuries in the Athlete*. New York: Churchill Livingstone, Inc.; 1995;365.
4. Ekenstam F. Osseous anatomy and articular relationships about the distal ulna. *Hand Clin* 14:161, 1998.
5. Schuind F, An KN, Berglund L, et al: The distal radioulnar ligaments: A biomechanical study. *J Hand Surg* 16:1106, 1991.
6. Garcia-Elias M, An KN, Cooney WP, et al: Stability of the transverse carpal arch: An experimental study. *J Hand Surg* 14:277, 1989.
7. Gilula LA: Carpal injuries: Analytic approach and case exercises. *Am J Radiol* 133:503, 1979.
8. Totty WG, Gilula LA: Imaging of the hand and wrist. In: Gilula LA (ed): *The Traumatized Hand and Wrist: Radiographic and Anatomic Correlation*. Philadelphia: WB Saunders Co; 1992:1.
9. Taleisnik J. The ligaments of the wrist. *J Hand Surg* 1:110, 1976.
10. Lichtman DM, Schneider JR, Swafford AR, et al: Ulnar midcarpal instability: Clinical and laboratory analysis. *J Hand Surg* 6:515, 1981.
11. Garcia-Elias M: Soft tissue anatomy and relationships about the distal ulna. *Hand Clin* 14:165, 1998.
12. Bednar MS, Arnoczky SP, Weiland AJ: The microvasculature of the triangular fibrocartilage complex: Its clinical significance. *J Hand Surg* 16:1101, 1991.
13. Adams BD, Holley KA: Strains in the articular disk of the triangular fibrocartilage complex: A biomechanical study. *J Hand Surg* 18:919, 1993.
14. Mikic ZD: Age changes in the triangular fibrocar-
tilage complex of the wrist joint. *J Anat* 126:367, 1978.
15. Uchiyama S, Nakatsuchi Y: Anatomical and radiological evaluation of the triangular fibrocartilage complex of the wrist. *J Hand Surg (Br)* 19:319, 1994.
16. Hoppenfeld S. *Physical Examination of the Spine and Extremities*. Norwalk, CT: Appleton-Century-Crofts; 1976;59.
17. Gelberman RH, Gross MS: The vascularity of the wrist. *Clin Orthop* 202:42, 1986.
18. McCue FC, Bruce JF: The wrist. In: DeLee JC, Drez D (eds): *Orthopaedic Sports Medicine*. Philadelphia: WB Saunders Co; 1994;913.
19. Netter FH: *Atlas of Human Anatomy*. Cutaneous Nerves of Wrist and Hand. Plate 445, Ciba-Geigy Corporation, 1989.
20. Moore KL: *Clinically Oriented Anatomy*, 2nd ed. Baltimore: Williams & Wilkins; 1985;654, 710.
21. Rosenwasser MP, Wilson RH: The wrist. In: Scuderi GR, McCann PD, Bruno PJ (eds): *Sports Medicine: Principles of Primary Care*. St. Louis: Mosby; 1997;269.
22. Mirabello SC, Loeb PE, Andrews JR: The wrist: Field examination and treatment. *Clin Sports Med* 11:1, 1992.
23. Burton RI, Eaton RG: Common hand injuries in the athlete. *Ortho Clin North Am* 4:809,1973.
24. Mayfield JK: Mechanism of carpal injuries. *Clin Orthop* 149:45, 1980.
25. Johnson RJ: Wrist and hand: History and physical exam. In: Sallis RE, Massimino F (eds): *ACSM's Essentials of Sports Medicine*. St. Louis: Mosby; 1997;325.
26. Rettig A: Wrist injuries: Avoiding diagnostic pitfalls. *Phys Sports Med* 22:33, 1994.
27. Mayfield JK: Wrist ligament anatomy and biomechanics. In: Gilula LA (ed): *The Traumatized Hand and Wrist: Radiographic and Anatomic Correlation*. Philadelphia: WB Saunders Co; 1992;241.
28. Melone CP: Fractures of the wrist. In: Nicholas JA, Hershman EB (eds): *The Upper Extremity in Sports Medicine*. St. Louis: The CV Mosby Company; 1990;419.
29. Horii E, Garcia-Elias M, An KN: Force transmission through radiocarpal joint. In: Cooney WP, Linscheid RL, Dobyns JH (eds): *The Wrist*. St. Louis: Mosby; 1998;190.

30. Mayfield JK: Patterns of injury to carpal ligaments. *Clin Orthop* 187:36, 1984.

31. Mayfield JK: Wrist ligamentous anatomy and pathogenesis of carpal instability. *Orthop Clin North Am* 15:209, 1984.

32. Jennings JF, Peimer CA: Ligamentous injuries of the wrist in athletes, In: Nicholas JA, Hershman EB (eds): *The Upper Extremity in Sports Medicine.* St. Louis: The CV Mosby Co; 1990:457.

33. Nguyen DT, McCue FC, Urch SE: Evaluation of the injured wrist on the field and in the office. *Clin Sports Med* 17:421, 1998.

34. Raskin KB, Beldner S: Clinical examination of the distal ulna and surrounding structures. *Hand Clin* 14:177, 1998.

35. Morgan WJ: History, physical examination, and diagnostic testing of the wrist. In: Pappas AM (ed): *Upper Extremity Injuries in the Athlete.* New York: Churchill-Livingstone Inc; 1995;377.

36. Rettig ME, Dossa GL, Raskin KB, et al: Wrist fractures in the athlete. *Clin Sports Med* 17:469, 1998.

37. Jupiter JB: Current concepts review: Fractures of the distal end of the radius. *J Bone Joint Surg* 73:461, 1991.

38. Weber ER, Chao EY: An experimental approach to the mechanism of scaphoid waist fractures. *J Hand Surg* 3:142, 1978.

39. Simon RR, Koenigsknecht SJ: *Emergency Orthopedics: The Extremities*, 3rd ed. Norwalk, CT: Appleton & Lange; 1995;107.

40. Mastey RD, Weiss APC, Akelman E: Primary care of hand and wrist athletic injuries. *Clin Sports Med* 16:705, 1997.

41. Eiff MP, Hatch RL, Calmbach W: *Fracture Management for Primary Care: Carpal Fractures.* Philadelphia: WB Saunders Co; 1998;65.

42. Hunter DM: Personal communication 6/99.

43. Chapman DR, Bennett JB, BryanWJ, et al: Complications of distal radial fractures: Pins and plaster treatment. *J Hand Surg* 7:509, 1982.

44. Cooney WP: Fractures of the distal radius. In: Cooney WP, Linscheid RL, Dobyns JH (eds): *The Wrist.* St. Louis: Mosby; 1998;323.

45. Morgan W, Busconi BD: Injuries of the distal radius and distal radioulnar joint. In: Pappas AM (ed): *Upper Extremity Injuries in the Athlete.* New York: Churchill-Livingstone Inc; 1995;403.

46. Linscheid RL, Dobyns JH: Athletic injuries of the wrist. *Clin Orthop* 198:141, 1985.

47. Morgan WJ, Reardon TF: Carpal fractures of the wrist. In: Pappas AM (ed): *Upper Extremity Injuries in the Athlete.* New York: Churchill-Livingstone Inc; 1995;431.

48. Borgeskov S, Christiansen B, Kjaer A, et al: Fractures of the carpal bones. *Acta Orthop Scand* 37:276, 1966.

49. Rosenwasser MP, Wilson RH: The wrist. In: Scuderi GR, McCann PD, Bruno PJ (eds): *Sports Medicine: Principles of Primary Care.* St. Louis: Mosby; 1997:265.

50. Frykman G. Fracture of the distal radius including sequelae-shoulder-hand-finger syndrome, disturbance in the distal radio-ulnar joint and impairment of nerve function: A clinical and experimental study. *Acta Orthop Scand Suppl* 108:1, 1967.

51. Johnson RP: The acutely injured wrist and its residuals. *Clin Orthop* 149:33, 1980.

52. Weber ER: Biomechanical implications of scaphoid waist fractures. *Clin Orthop* 149:83, 1980.

53. Zemel NP: Carpal fractures. In: Strickland JW, Rettig AC (eds): *Hand Injuries in Athletes.* Philadelphia: WB Saunders Co; 1992:155.

54. Mayfield JK, Gilula LA, Totty WG: Isolated carpal fractures. In: Gilula LA (ed): *The Traumatized Hand and Wrist: Radiographic and Anatomic Correlation.* Philadelphia: WB Saunders Co; 1992;249.

55. Linscheid RL; Weber ER: Scaphoid fractures and nonunion. In: Cooney WP, Linscheid RL, Dobyns JH (eds): *The Wrist: Diagnosis and Operative Treatment.* St. Louis: Mosby; 1998;385.

56. Tiel-van Buul MM, van Beek EJ, Broekhuizen AH, et al: Radiography and scintigraphy of suspected scaphoid fracture: A long term study in 160 patients. *J Bone Joint Surg (Br)* 75:61, 1993.

57. Gellman H, Caputo RJ, Carter V, et al: Comparison of short and long thumb-spica casts for nondisplaced fractures of the carpal scaphoid. *J Bone Joint Surg Am* 71:354, 1989.

58. Cooney WP, Dobyns JH, Linscheid RL: Fractures of the scaphoid: A rational approach to management. *Clin Orthop* 149:90, 1980.

59. Brooks AA: Ligamentous injuries and fractures of the wrist. In: Baker CL (ed): *The Hughston Clinic Sports Medicine Book.* Media, PA: Williams & Wilkins; 1995;353.

60. Hindman BW, Kulik WJ, Lee G, et al: Occult fractures of the carpals and metacarpals: Demonstration by CT. *Am J Radiol* 153:529, 1989.

61. Cohen MS: Fractures of the carpal bones. *Hand Clin* 13:587, 1997.

62. Beckenbaugh RD, Shives TC, Dobyns JH: Kienböck's disease: The natural history of Kienböck's disease and consideration of lunate fractures. *Clin Orthop* 149:98, 1980.

63. Szabo RM, Greenspan A: Diagnosis and clinical findings of Kienböck's disease. *Hand Clin* 9:399 1993.

64. Hulten O: Uber anatomische Variationen den Hand-gelenkknochen. *Acta Radiol* 9:155, 1928.

65. Palmer AK, Benoit MY: Lunate fractures: Kienböck's disease. In: Cooney WP, Linscheid RL, Dobyns JH (eds): *The Wrist*. St. Louis: Mosby; 1998;471.

66. Levy M, Fischel RE, Stern GM: Chip fractures of the triquetrum: The mechanism of injury. *J Bone Joint Surg (Br)* 61:355, 1979.

67. Hocker K, Menshik A: Chip fractures of the triquetrum: Mechanism, classification, and results. *J Hand Surg (Br)* 19:584, 1994.

68. O'Brien ET: Acute fractures and dislocations of the carpus. *Orthop Clin North Am* 15:237, 1984.

69. Cooney WP: Isolated carpal fractures. In: Cooney WP, Linscheid RL, Dobyns JH (eds): *The Wrist*. St. Louis: Mosby; 1998;483.

70. Stein F, Siegel MW: Naviculocapitate syndrome: New thoughts on the mechanism of injury. *J Bone Joint Surg Am* 51:575, 1977.

71. Gelberman RH, Panagis JS, Taleisnik J, et al: The arterial anatomy of the human carpus: The extraosseous vascularity. *J Hand Surg* 8:367, 1983.

72. Metz JP: Managing golf injuries. *Phys Sports Med* 27:41, 1999.

73. Barton NJ: Sports injuries of the hand and wrist. *Br J Sports Med* 31:191, 1997.

74. Murray PM, Cooney WP: Golf-induced injuries of the wrist. *Clin Sports Med* 15:85, 1996.

75. Skolnick AA: Golfer's wrist can be a tough break to diagnose. *JAMA* 279:571, 1998.

76. Jones WA: Beware of the sprained wrist: The incidence and diagnosis of scapholunate instability. *J Bone Joint Surg* 70B:293, 1988.

77. Taleisnik J: Carpal instability: Current concepts review. *J Bone Joint Surg* 70A:1262, 1988.

78. Watson HK, Ballet FL: The SLAC wrist:

79. Cohen MS: Ligamentous injuries of the wrist in the athlete. *Clin Sports Med* 17:533, 1998.

80. Puffer JC: Personal communication, UCLA Primary Care Sports Medicine Fellows' Seminar, 5/6/99.

81. Watson HK, Weinzweig J: Physical examination of the wrist. *Hand Clin* 13:17, 1997.

82. Schreibman KL, Freeland A, Gilula LA, et al: Imaging of the hand and wrist. *Ortho Clin North Am* 28:537, 1997.

83. Honing EW: Wrist injuries: Spotting and treating troublemakers. *Phys Sports Med* 26:63, 1998.

84. Morgan, WJ: Ligamentous injuries of the wrist. In: Pappas AM (ed): *Upper Extremity Injuries in the Athlete*. New York: Churchill-Livingstone Inc; 1995, Chapter 23.

85. Cooney WP, Dobyns JH, Linscheid RL: Arthroscopy of the wrist: Anatomy and classification of carpal instability. *Arthroscopy* 6:133, 1990.

86. Watson HK, Weinzweig J, Zeppieri J: The natural progression of scaphoid instability. *Hand Clin* 13(1):39, 1997.

87. Trumble TE, Bour CJ, Smith RJ, Edward GS: Intercarpal arthrodesis for static and dynamic volar intercalated segment instability. *J Hand Surg* 13(3):384, 1988.

88. Viegas SF, Patterson RM, Peterson PD, et al: Ulnar-sided perilunate instability: An anatomic and biomechanic study. *J Hand Surg* 15A:268, 1990.

89. Reagan DS, Linscheid RL, Dobyns JH: Lunotriquetral sprains. *J Hand Surg* 9A:502, 1984.

90. Kleinman WB: The luno-triquetral shuck test. *Am Soc Surg Hand Corr News* 1985, 51.

91. Brown JA, Janzen DL, Adler BD, et al: Arthrography of the contralateral, asymptomatic wrist in patients with unilateral wrist pain. *Can Assoc Radiol J* 45:292, 1994.

92. Brown DE, Lichtman DM: Midcarpal instability. *Hand Clin* 1:135, 1987.

93. Cooney WP, Bishop AT, Linscheid RL: Physical examination of the wrist. In: Cooney WP, Linscheid RL, Dobyns JH (eds): *The Wrist*. St. Louis; Mosby; 1998;250.

94. Palmer AK, Werner FW: The triangular fibrocartilage complex of the wrist: Anatomy and function. *J Hand Surg* 6:153, 1981.

95. Rettig AC: Epidemiology of hand and wrist

injuries in sports. *Clin Sports Med* 17:401, 1998.

96. Buterbaugh GA, Brown TR, Horn PC: Ulnar-sided wrist pain in athletes. *Clin Sports Med* 17:567, 1998.

97. Cooney WP: Tears of the triangular fibrocartilage complex of the wrist. In: Cooney WP, Linscheid RL, Dobyns JH (eds): *The Wrist*. St. Louis: Mosby; 1998:711.

98. Palmer AK: Triangular fibrocartilage complex lesions: A classification. *J Hand Surg* 14A:594, 1989.

99. Bowers WH: Problems of the distal radioulnar joint. *Adv Orthop Surg* 7:289, 1984.

100. Mastey RD, Weiss APC, Akelman E: Primary care of hand and wrist athletic injuries. *Clin Sports Med* 16(4):705, 1997.

101. Dobyns JH, Gabel GT: Gymnast's wrist. *Hand Clin* 6:493, 1990.

102. Nelson DL: Additional thoughts on the physical examination of the wrist. *Hand Clin* 13(1):35, 1997.

103. Levinsohn EM, Rosen ID, Palmer AK: Wrist arthrography: value of the three-compartment injection method. *Radiology* 179:231, 1991.

104. Wilson AJ, Gilula LA, Mann FA: Unidirectional joint communications in wrist arthrography: An evaluation of 250 cases. *Am J Radiol* 157:105, 1991.

105. Potter HG, Asnis-Ernberg L, Weiland AJ, et al: The utility of high-resolution magnetic resonance imaging in the evaluation of the triangular fibrocartilage complex of the wrist. *J Bone Joint Surg Am* 79(11):1675, 1997.

106. Totterman SM, Miller RJ, McCance SE, et al: Lesions of the triangular fibrocartilage complex: MR findings with a three dimensional gradient-recalled-echo sequence. *Radiology* 199:227, 1996.

107. Oneson SR, Timins ME, Scales LM, et al: MR imaging diagnosis of triangular fibrocartilage pathology with arthroscopic correlation. *Am J Radiol* 168:1513, 1997.

108. Cooney WP, Linsheid RL, Dobyns JH: Triangular fibrocartilage tears. *J Hand Surg* 19:143, 1994.

109. Trumble TE; Gilbert M, Vedder N: Ulnar shortening combined with arthroscopic repairs in the delayed management of triangular fibrocartilage complex tears. *J Hand Surg* 22A:807, 1997.

110. Schieber RA, Branche-Dorsey C, Ryan GW, et al: Risk factors for injuries from in-line skating and the effectiveness of safety gear. *N Engl J Med* 335(22):1630, 1996.

111. Cheng SL, Rajaratnam K, Raskin KB, et al: "Splint-top" fracture of the forearm: A description of in-line skating injury associated with the use of protective wrist splints. *J Trauma Inj Infect Crit Care* 39(6):1194, 1995.

Dennis Y. Wen

Chapter 5

The Injured Finger

Introduction

Finger injuries are a common occurrence, not only during sporting and recreational activities, but also as a result of industrial and occupational accidents. Many acute finger injuries will be seen initially in an emergency department, but a large number will present to primary care physicians. Human beings, especially in our modern industrial society, have come to be very dependent on hand and finger function, not only occupationally, but also for activities of daily living and sports and leisure activities. Therefore, a seemingly minor finger injury has the potential to cause a great deal of disability, especially if optimal treatment is not rendered. Careful evaluation and treatment is necessary to minimize this potential for disability. This chapter describes the proper diagnosis and management of several common finger injuries likely to be encountered in primary care.

General Considerations

As for any other medical condition or injury, the history and physical examination are important when evaluating finger injuries. The mechanism of injury should be sought in as much detail as possible. For example, not just "I hurt my index finger playing basketball," but rather ". . . the ball hit the end of my index finger and I felt it bend backwards." History of previous injuries to the same or other fingers should be obtained. The amount of disability that the injury is causing should be elicited. This may require information on hand dominance, occupation, and sports and leisure activities.

Physical examination needs to be thorough and systematic. Neurovascular status distal to the site of injury should be documented at least

grossly. The injured finger should be compared with the same finger on the opposite hand for shape, size, range of motion, and strength. Specific examination tests are described later during discussion of specific injuries.

Seemingly innocuous injuries in the finger can potentially cause long-term morbidity and disability due to the patients' reliance on proper finger function. Especially in younger patients, such as adolescents who have not made career choices, a disabling finger injury can often preclude certain leisure or occupational pursuits. Therefore, careful evaluation and treatment of any finger injury is necessary to optimize the outcome, both for the short term and for the long term.

Digital Block Anesthesia

Many finger injuries require anesthesia for adequate examination and treatment. Pain and guarding may prohibit an adequate physical examination, or prevent easy reduction of a fracture or dislocation. Several methods of inducing anesthesia are available, of which a digital block is one that is easily performed in the office setting and effective for most finger injuries seen in primary care.

The digital nerves to each finger and thumb travel along each side, ulnar and radial, of that finger. A digital block anesthetizes the digital nerves at the web spaces of the involved finger. After prepping the dorsal side of the hand around each web space adjacent to the involved finger, a small syringe and needle (25 or 27 gauge) is used to infuse local anesthetic into each web space (Fig. 5-1). Lidocaine without epinephrine is commonly used, with or without mixing it with bupivicaine, which has a longer duration of action. The needle is moved along the entire side of the finger via the web space while infusing anesthetic, and is then removed and the procedure repeated along the other side

Figure 5-1

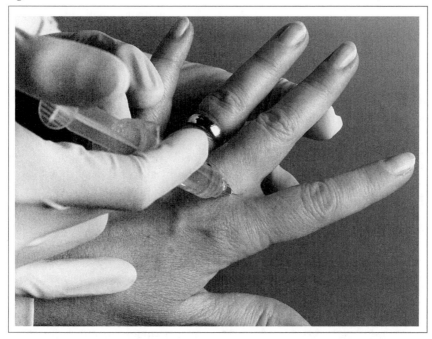

Digital block being performed between the index and middle finger web space. The needle is slowly advanced and withdrawn during injection in order to infiltrate the entire thickness of the web space. Then the procedure is repeated on the other side of the involved finger.

of the finger. Occasionally, the dorsum of the finger may also need to be infused with anesthetic. It is generally not necessary to infuse the palmar side of the finger. Adequate anesthesia following a digital block usually occurs within 5 to 15 min. A digital block will not affect motor nerve function in the finger because the nerves and muscles that control finger movement are not present in the finger itself.

Distal Phalangeal Injuries

Nail and Nailbed Injuries

Most injuries occurring to the distal phalanx involve crush-type injuries. These injuries may cause tuft fractures of the distal phalanx, injuries to the nailbed, or both. Injuries to the nailbed can result in abnormal growth of the nail, and therefore should be repaired as soon as possible following the acute injury.[1] Following digital block anesthesia (see "Digital Block Anesthesia"), the nail can be removed by blunt dissection proximally to the level of the nail matrix. The injured nailbed can then be irrigated, explored, and repaired with fine absorbable suture.

After repair is completed, a mechanical "splint" is needed under the eponychium until the new nail grows out. Otherwise this space may close, blunting new nail growth. Many different methods exist for "splinting" this space. One way is to replace the previously removed nail and suture the four corners with nonabsorbable suture. Other objects such as petroleum gauze may also be used as a "splint."

Tuft Fractures

Crush injuries to the distal finger can result in fractures of the distal phalanx. These are generally stable fractures and require no special treatment other than protection and pain relief. Tuft fractures refer to the very distal tip of the distal phalanx, and are often comminuted. Treatment involves a loose splint, which can be made from aluminum or plastic, for protection, along with elevation, local ice, and analgesics. A tight splint should be avoided because this can worsen the discomfort from soft tissue swelling. Open fractures, including nailbed injuries, should be thoroughly irrigated, perhaps after digital block anesthesia (see "Digital Block Anesthesia"). Distal phalangeal shaft fractures can usually be treated similarly to tuft fractures unless significant displacement or angulation exists.

Distal Interphalangeal (DIP) Joint Injuries

Extensor Tendon Injuries (Mallet Fingers)

The most common acute tendon injury in the finger involves the extensor tendon at the dorsum of the DIP joint. The mechanism of injury is generally forced flexion of an actively extended DIP joint. Most commonly, an axial loading force, such as a ball, an opponent, or a wall, will cause the DIP joint to acutely flex, rupturing the extensor tendon insertion at the dorsal base of the distal phalanx.

HISTORY

A detailed history should be obtained concerning the mechanism of injury. The patient will often describe a "jamming" or axially directed force, and can often recall the DIP joint being forcefully flexed.

PHYSICAL EXAMINATION

Examination will reveal a DIP joint held in some degree of flexion, hence the term "mallet finger." Tenderness and swelling may be localized over the dorsum of the DIP joint. The patient will not be able to fully extend this joint actively, and will not be able to resist a slight flexion force from the examiner. However, passive extension should be easily accomplished in a mallet finger. Over a period of time, a swan-neck deformity may occur, with not only a chronically flexed DIP joint, but also an associated hyperextended proximal interphalangeal (PIP) joint. This occurs because as patients attempt to extend the DIP joint (but are unable), the extension forces become concentrated at the PIP joint causing hyperextension.

ANCILLARY TESTS

Radiographs should be obtained in suspected mallet fingers to check for bony avulsion. The extensor tendon itself may rupture at its insertion into the base of the distal phalanx, in which case radiographs will be normal. Alternatively, a fragment of bone may be avulsed with the extensor tendon (Fig. 5-2). If this occurs, the size of the avulsed bone fragment should be noted on lateral radiographs because treatment decisions may depend on the size. Other associated bony injuries also need to be ruled out on radiographs.

TREATMENT

Treatment involves immobilization of the DIP joint in an extended position until tendon healing. For a pure tendon rupture (i.e., no bony avulsion on radiographs), the recommended period of immobilization is 6 to 8 weeks.[2] Splinting can be accomplished in several ways (Fig. 5-3). An aluminum splint can be taped onto either the dorsal or volar aspect of the finger covering the DIP joint. A splint on the dorsal aspect is probably preferred, because this will allow continued tactile sensation of the finger pad, causing less functional disability of the involved finger.

Figure 5-2

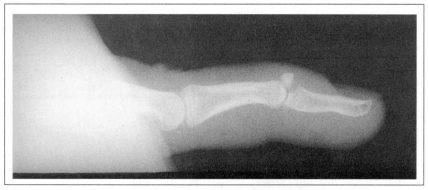

Lateral radiograph of a bony mallet finger showing a slightly displaced avulsion of the dorsal base of the distal phalanx involving approximately 30 percent of the articular surface.

Additionally, the bones are closer to the dorsal skin than to the volar skin, so more effective immobilization is accomplished with dorsal splinting. Commercially made splints are also available specifically for this type of injury.

Hyperextension of the DIP joint in the splint should be avoided because that may lead to dorsal skin necrosis. The DIP joint is the only joint that needs to be included in the splint. The PIP joint should be left free to move to avoid stiffness at the PIP and also to avoid a swan-neck deformity. Elevation, ice, and analgesics should also be recommended.

The most important instruction given to the patient is that the DIP joint needs to remain in complete extension continuously throughout the splinting period. If the DIP joint is allowed to bend, even once, the entire 6- to 8-week splinting period needs to start all over again. Therefore, if the patient chooses to remove the splint for washing or any other reason, it is best to have someone else remove it so that the patient's attention can remain focused on keeping the DIP extended. The finger should be placed flat on a table while the splint is off to avoid accidental flexion. The patient may participate in sports during the splinting period as long as the DIP is well splinted and protected to avoid re-injury.

At follow-up after 6 to 8 weeks of splinting, the splint is carefully removed and the finger is inspected for residual extensor lag. Active extension against gentle resistance can be tested. If an extensor lag still exists, or if a gentle flexion force cannot be resisted, an additional 6 weeks of continuous splinting in extension can be instituted. However, if no extension lag exists and the DIP can resist a gentle force, then continuous splinting can be discontinued. The patient should probably continue to splint the DIP in extension during sleep and during sports or any other activities that may put the finger at risk of re-injury. This sleep-time and at-risk activity splinting can be used for an additional 4 to 6 weeks.

For a bony avulsion off the dorsal lip of the distal phalanx (see Fig. 5-2), the treatment is similar to that for a pure tendon rupture if the avulsion involves only small bony fragments of less than 30 percent of the articular surface.[2] Such avulsions are considered stable and can be splinted in extension similar to the tendon rupture protocol. The only difference is that a bony avulsion may heal a little faster than a pure tendon rupture (i.e., bone heals faster than tendon). Therefore, the duration of splinting can be closer to 6 weeks, instead of closer to 8 weeks. The same precautions concerning accidental flexion apply.

For a larger bony avulsion fragment (more than 30 percent of the articular surface), the DIP

Figure 5-3

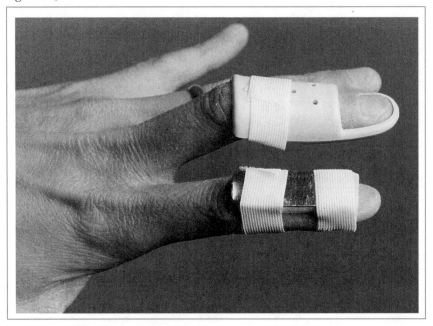

Two examples of mallet finger splints. On the index finger is a splint cut from foam-covered aluminum and taped onto the dorsum of the finger covering the DIP joint, but leaving the PIP joint free to move. On the middle finger is a commercially available plastic splint that similarly maintains the DIP joint in complete extension.

joint is potentially unstable and may require surgical treatment.[2] The collateral ligaments, which provide stability for the joint, may be attached more to the avulsion fragment than the remaining distal phalanx. If adequate closed reduction with a stable and congruent joint can be accomplished by extension, then splinting in extension as for a smaller fragment may be appropriate. A stable joint on a lateral radiograph shows no evidence of volar subluxation of the distal phalanx relative to the middle phalanx. This volar subluxation may be a very subtle finding in an unstable joint. If any question concerning stability exists, referral to a hand surgeon may be warranted.

SPECIAL SITUATIONS

In children and adolescents with open growth plates, physeal injuries may occur. Salter-Harris type I and II fractures often occur in pre-teens and early adolescents, whereas Salter-Harris type III fractures can occur in older adolescents. If a stable reduction (minimal displacement on post-reduction radiographs) can be accomplished by extension, then splinting as for adult injuries may be instituted for 4 to 6 weeks.[3] Otherwise, referral may be warranted.

The extensor pollicis longus tendon of the thumb can be ruptured similarly to the extensor tendons of the other fingers, although this is a rarer injury. Bony avulsion may similarly occur. Treatment is similar to that for the other finger extensors, with continuous splinting of the thumb interphalangeal (IP) joint in extension.

Not uncommonly, patients will present late with a chronic mallet finger. They felt that they "just jammed" their finger and that it would get better, only to realize weeks or months later that they are still unable to actively extend the DIP joint. Treatment is the same as for an acute mallet finger, but the results are not as uniformly good.[4] Prolonged, continuous splinting in extension should initially be attempted for 8 to 12 weeks, and perhaps, longer. If unsuccessful, referral may be warranted. Surgical options are available for these situations, but results are variable.

One particular injury that needs to be distinguished from a simple mallet finger is the hyperextension injury to the DIP joint. Instead of an axially directed force causing forced flexion of the DIP joint and resulting in a true mallet finger, the deforming force causes hyperextension of the DIP joint. A large (often, larger than 50 percent of the articular surface) fracture fragment occurs dorsally, mimicking an avulsion fragment. However, this is not an avulsion fragment, but is rather caused by impaction of the dorsal portion of the distal phalanx against the middle phalanx. On physical examination, a flexed DIP joint exists with inability to extend actively, similar to a true mallet finger, and attempts at passively extending the DIP joint often results in pain. As stated, on lateral radiographs a large dorsal fracture fragment is visible, and volar subluxation of the distal phalanx may be noted. For this type of injury, simple splinting in extension as for true mallet finger will not be successful. Instead, referral for possible surgical management is recommended.

Flexor Digitorum Profundus (FDP) Avulsions (Jersey Fingers)

The FDP tendon attaches to the volar base of the distal phalanx and functions to flex the DIP joint. Injury to the volarly located flexor tendons are, fortunately, rarer than extensor tendon injuries because FDP tendon avulsions tend to have more complications compared with extensor tendons. The mechanism of injury is generally a forced extension of a DIP joint that is actively flexing, such as in football when a tackler has hold of an opponent's jersey and the opponent breaks away, forcing the gripping flexed finger into extension.

HISTORY

The history often reveals a typical mechanism of injury, but at times can be vague. Usually, there will be pain at volar aspect of the DIP joint where the avulsion occurred, but this is not always the case. Pain may be diffuse, and sometimes is located proximally at the area of retraction of the ruptured tendon, rather than the rupture site itself. Unless a high index of suspicion is maintained, these injuries can, and often are, missed.

PHYSICAL EXAMINATION

The most important physical examination finding is an extended DIP joint with an inability to actively flex or to flex against any resistance. Active flexion of the DIP joint can be tested by holding the patient's PIP joint in complete extension and then asking the patient to flex the finger, first without resistance and then against gentle resistance at the finger tip (Fig. 5-4). Tenderness and swelling may be noted over the volar aspect of the DIP joint, or may be present more proximally over the flexor sheath. Sometimes the ruptured end of the tendon, with or without an attached bony avulsion fragment, may be palpated as far proximally as the palm. The findings may be subtle, again leading to frequent missed diagnoses. On history-taking, duration of the injury is important because the time-course may affect treatment decisions.

ANCILLARY TESTS

Radiographs are often normal, but may show an avulsion fracture off the volar base of the distal phalanx in the lateral view. This bony avulsion fragment is most commonly located around the level of the PIP joint, where the tendon has retracted, but may occur elsewhere along the course of the flexor sheath.

Figure 5-4

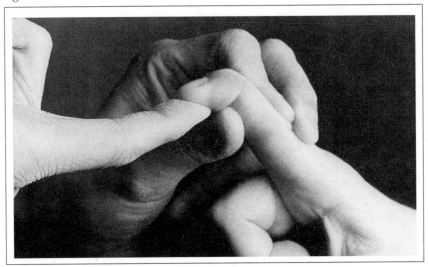

Examination of FDP function. The patient's index finger, which is being tested, is to the right in the photo. The examiner's left thumb and index finger maintain the patient's PIP joint in complete extension, while the examiner's right index finger resists an active flexion force from the patient's DIP joint.

TREATMENT

Treatment of acute FDP avulsions is early surgical repair. Splinting and/or closed reduction will not be successful and can lead to wasted time, potentially jeopardizing surgical results. The viability of the FDP tendons is maintained at the level of the finger; therefore an FDP tendon that has retracted more proximally than the finger (i.e., into the palm) degenerates rapidly. This, combined with FDP muscle contraction after tendon rupture, necessitates early referral for surgery.

Best results are obtained within the first few days; however, many hand surgeons will attempt repair up to 7 to 10 days after injury.[2] Unfortunately, many patients with FDP tendon ruptures do not present until after several days or weeks, or are originally misdiagnosed, and therefore lose their opportunity for an optimal surgical outcome. A ruptured FDP tendon that does not retract past the finger (such as with a bony avulsion to the level of the PIP joint) theoretically still has at least partial viability, and the muscle is not nearly as retracted; therefore, a more delayed surgical repair may still be possible. Nevertheless, it is probably best to make an early (within 1 to 3 days) referral to a hand surgeon for an opinion, even in these cases.

A chronic or late-presenting FDP tendon rupture is difficult to treat. In some asymptomatic cases, it can just be left alone. FDP tendon reconstruction techniques are available, but results are not uniformly optimal.

In the thumb, a similar rupture of the flexor pollicis longus (FPL) tendon can occur at the interphalangeal (IP) joint. The FPL serves to flex the IP joint of the thumb and injury can occur as with FDP ruptures of the fingers with forced extension of a flexed IP joint. Treatment is the same as for FDP ruptures with early surgical management giving the best results.

Proximal Interphalangeal (PIP) Joint Injuries

The PIP joint of the fingers is probably the most commonly injured joint in the hand. Most finger "jams" occur at this joint. An understanding of the unique anatomy of the PIP joint and a thorough history and physical examination, along with possible radiographs, are necessary to evaluate the "jammed" PIP joint to diagnose specific entities requiring more specific treatment.

Anatomy of the PIP Joint

The PIP joint is a hinge-type joint with several stabilizing structures, any of which may become injured (Fig. 5-5). The volar plate is a fibrocartilaginous structure connecting the distal volar portion of the proximal phalanx with the proximal volar base of the middle phalanx. It prevents hyperextension of the PIP joint past zero degrees. On the lateral sides of the PIP joint, the radial and ulnar collateral ligaments prevent lateral movement of the joint.

The final important structure is the dorsally located central slip of the extensor tendon. As the extensor digitorum communis tendons course distally along the proximal phalanx, each tendon divides into three parts—two lateral bands and a central slip. The two lateral bands course around the dorsal lateral portion of the PIP joint and reunite with each other and then finally insert beyond the DIP joint at the dorsal base of the distal phalanx, functioning to extend the DIP joint. This is the portion of the extensor tendon

Figure 5-5

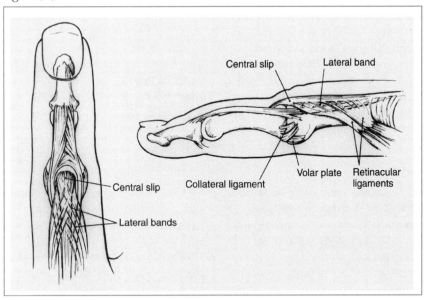

Anatomy of the proximal interphalangeal joint. (*Left*) Dorsal view: The central slip passes directly over the joint and inserts on the base of the middle phalanx. The lateral bands pass around the joint, combine with the retinacular ligaments, and unite to form the extensor tendon that attaches on the distal phalanx. (*Right*) Lateral view: Lateral motion is minimized by the collateral ligaments, and extension is limited to zero degrees by the thick volar plate. (*Reproduced with permission from Hoffman DF, Schaffer TC: Management of common finger injuries. Am Fam Physician 43(5):1594, 1991.*)

that is ruptured in mallet finger injuries. Normally, with the PIP joint in extension, the lateral bands are located dorsal to the PIP axis of rotation. Normally, with the PIP joint in flexion, the lateral bands slide volarly to allow the DIP joint to flex. The central slip of the extensor tendon inserts into the dorsal base of the middle phalanx and functions to extend the PIP joint. Flexion of the PIP joint is the function of the flexor digitorum superficialis (or sublimis), which is very rarely injured.

Central Slip Rupture (Boutonniere Deformities)

HISTORY

Rupture to the central slip of the extensor tendon at the PIP joint is in many ways analogous to a mallet finger injury at the DIP joint. The mechanism of injury is similar to that for an extensor tendon rupture at the DIP joint (mallet finger). An axial and slightly volarly directed force occurs at the PIP joint, forcing the actively extended PIP joint into flexion. The patient may describe being hit on the tip of the finger with a ball or an opponent, causing axial compression and flexion. Pain and swelling can occur at the dorsal aspect of the PIP joint.

PHYSICAL EXAMINATION

On physical examination, inspection will reveal a flexed PIP joint that the patient is unable to actively extend. A boutonniere deformity may be present with DIP joint hyperextension, PIP joint flexion, and metacarpal phalangeal (MCP) joint hyperextension. This deformity occurs because with central slip rupture and subsequent PIP joint flexion, the lateral bands slide volarly to the point that they actually become "flexors" of the PIP joint. As the patients tries to extend the PIP joint, more force is placed upon the lateral bands, causing hyperextension at the DIP joint and increased flexion at the PIP joint. More

extension force is also placed upon metacarpal phalangeal (MCP) joint, resulting in its hyperextension. Passive extension of the PIP joint should be easily accomplished. In more chronic cases, a fixed boutonniere deformity may occur with contracture of the joint.

Palpation will reveal the maximal area of tenderness over the dorsum of the PIP joint. Testing will demonstrate inability to extend the flexed PIP joint against resistance. It may be possible, however, for the patient to maintain the PIP joint in extension against resistance if the PIP joint is already in extension. This is because in extension, the lateral bands are located dorsal to the PIP joint and can act as extensors of the PIP joint in this position. However, with the PIP joint in flexion, the lateral bands are located volar to the PIP joint and cannot act as extensors. Therefore, when a central slip rupture is suspected, it is important to test resisted extension with the PIP joint in 90° of flexion.

ANCILLARY TESTS

Similar to the situation with mallet fingers at the DIP joint, lateral radiographs may reveal bony avulsion fractures with central slip avulsions off the dorsal base of the middle phalanx. If present, the size of the avulsed bone fragment should be noted.

TREATMENT

Treatment of central slip ruptures is similar to that for mallet fingers. Splinting of the PIP joint in complete extension (without hyperextension) continuously for 6 to 8 weeks is the treatment of choice.[2] An aluminum or plastic splint can be placed either dorsally or volarly over the PIP joint and taped solidly (Fig. 5-6). Dorsal splinting is preferred because the bones are closer to the dorsal surface. As with the case for mallet fingers, it is extremely important to advise patients that continuous splinting is necessary, and that a single episode of accidental flexion requires starting the 6- to 8-week splinting period all over

Figure 5-6

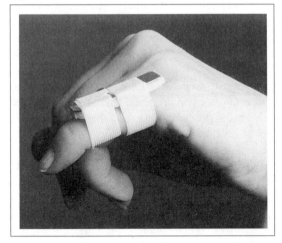

Boutonniere splint made from foam-covered aluminum. The PIP joint is immobilized in complete extension, while the DIP joint is left free to move.

again. The splint need not include the DIP or the MCP joint. In fact, it is preferable to allow motion at the DIP joint during PIP joint splinting in order to prevent scarring of the lateral bands. Sporting activities can be allowed during the splinting period as long as the PIP joint is well protected by the splint. Elevation, ice, and analgesics should also be recommended.

Following 6 to 8 weeks of continuous splinting, the splint can be removed and residual extension lag can be sought. If none exists (i.e., the PIP joint can completely extend actively without the splint), and a gentle flexion force can be resisted, then continuous splinting can be safely discontinued. As for mallet fingers, splinting at night and splinting during at-risk activities should be continued for another 4 to 6 weeks. If an extension lag persists, continuous splinting with the joint in extension can be continued for another 6- to 8-week period.

Small (less than 30 percent of the articular surface) avulsion fractures are treated the same as pure tendon ruptures, except the duration of continuous splinting may be slightly shortened (closer to 6 weeks, instead of closer to 8 weeks).

As in the situation for mallet fingers, a large (larger than 30 percent of the articular surface) avulsion fragment may cause the joint to be unstable, with subtle volar subluxation of the middle phalanx. These cases may require surgical management and referral is warranted. In children and adolescents, physeal fractures may be involved and closed reduction and splinting in extension is the preferred treatment.

SPECIAL SITUATIONS

Chronic or missed central slip ruptures can be treated with an approach similar to that used in the acute case as long as contracture at the PIP joint has not occurred. Continuous splinting in complete extension is usually successful. For a joint with a fixed deformity, dynamic splinting to maximize PIP joint extension with active DIP flexion exercises can be instituted. Referral may be warranted in these cases, because surgery may be an option if dynamic splinting is not successful.

One injury that can mimic a central slip rupture and needs to be distinguished from this rupture is known as a pseudoboutonniere injury.[2] As opposed to a flexion-induced injury to the PIP joint causing a central slip rupture, a pseudoboutonniere injury occurs as a result of hyperextension to the PIP joint rupturing the volar plate. Over time, the volar plate fibroses and contracts creating a flexion contracture at the PIP joint. The flexion contracture in a pseudoboutonniere deformity is generally fixed and rigid. Lateral radiographs may show calcification over the volar plate. Treatment can include dynamic splinting if the deformity is not severe or surgical release of the volar plate if the deformity is severe.

PIP Volar Plate Injuries

Injury to the volar plate at the PIP joint is a common entity associated with a "jammed" finger. The mechanism is generally a hyperextension

Figure 5-7

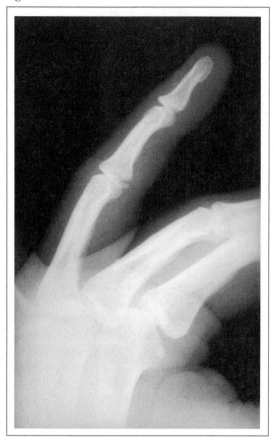

Oblique radiograph showing a ring finger PIP joint volar plate avulsion fracture. A small fragment of bone is avulsed from the volar base of the middle phalanx. Fragment sizes can vary.

injury to the PIP joint rupturing the volar plate. The entire PIP joint may be swollen and painful, but the area of maximal tenderness is generally over the volar plate. A hyperextension stress applied to the joint may provide information about stability, but usually only elicits pain. A lateral radiograph may reveal an avulsion fragment, usually off the volar base of the middle phalanx (Fig. 5-7).

Treatment involves splinting the PIP joint in slight (30°) flexion. This can be accomplished with an aluminum or plastic splint placed dorsally just over the PIP joint.[5] Alternatively, a dorsal extension block splint can be placed, allowing flexion of the PIP joint, but limiting extension to 30° (Fig. 5-8). A dorsal extension block splint can be made from aluminum, covering the PIP and MCP joints and taping to the hand and over the proximal phalanx but leaving the middle phalanx untaped, thereby allowing flexion motion at the PIP joint. Elevation, ice, and analgesics should also be recommended.

After 2 to 4 weeks of splinting in slight flexion, the finger then may be buddy-taped to an adjacent finger for an additional few weeks. Two pieces of tape are used for buddy-taping, one placed over the proximal phalanges and the other one over the middle phalanges (Fig. 5-9).

Volar plate injuries are often accompanied by collateral ligament injuries. The treatment is similar and the finger chosen to buddy-tape with the injured finger should be the one on the side of the injured collateral ligament. For relatively mild volar plate injuries, initial treatment may consist of buddy-taping.

If a large (larger than 30 percent of the articular surface) bone avulsion is noted on lateral radiographs, consideration of referral is warranted, unless stability of the joint can be confidently ascertained clinically.

PIP Collateral Ligament Injuries

Radial and ulnar collateral ligament injuries are perhaps the most common type of "jammed" PIP joints. These are generally axial-loading injuries with some degree of lateral bending force. Patients present with a history consistent with the typical mechanism of injury and complain of a swollen, painful, stiff PIP joint.

PHYSICAL EXAMINATION

Physical examination can reveal the presence of maximal swelling and tenderness over one or

Figure 5-8

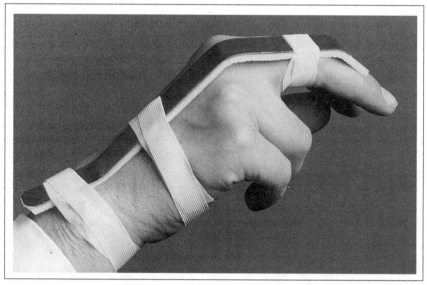

Example of a dorsal extension block splint. A foam-covered aluminum splint is fashioned to prevent PIP joint extension, but allowing flexion. The PIP joint curvature of the splint is approximately 30°, whereas the MCP joint curvature can be between 30 to 50°. Tape is applied to the wrist and/or palm to stabilize the splint, and around the proximal phalanx. No tape is applied at the distal end of the splint around the middle phalanx to allow active flexion of the PIP joint. Commercial splints are available which serve a similar function.

the other collateral ligament. However, often the swelling and tenderness can be diffuse over all sides of the joint, making diagnosis more difficult.

Associated injuries, such as to the volar plate, are often found and testing for joint laxity is warranted in suspected collateral ligament injuries. Stressing the collateral ligament in question by placing valgus or varus stress to the joint can determine the extent of damage to the collateral ligament. Stress testing can be done in two different positions, complete PIP extension and 20° of flexion of the PIP joint. Both positions are important to check. If significant laxity is present, especially compared with the same finger on the contralateral hand, a complete rupture to the collateral ligament is likely. Unfortunately, stress testing is often very painful to perform and

may need to be delayed days or weeks after the acute injury.

ANCILLARY TESTS

Radiographs may be normal, or may reveal small avulsion fragments, usually off the distal insertion of the collateral ligament into the middle phalanx. These are generally best seen on PA views.

TREATMENT

Treatment for a partial tear of a collateral ligament (no gross laxity on stress testing, either in complete extension or 20° of flexion) is buddy-taping (Fig. 5-9).[5] The injured finger should be taped to the adjacent finger on the side of the

Figure 5-9

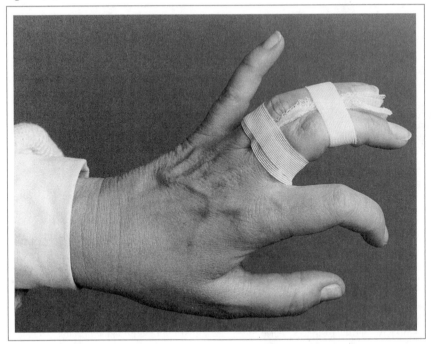

Buddy-taping of the middle and ring fingers. Tape is applied around the proximal phalanges and around the middle phalanges. Gauze or cotton can be placed between the fingers to prevent skin maceration.

injured collateral ligament. For instance, if the ulnar collateral ligament of the middle finger is injured, that middle finger would be buddy-taped to the ring finger. One piece of tape should be applied proximal to the injured PIP joint on the proximal phalanx, and a second piece applied distal to the injured PIP joint on the middle phalanx. Cotton or gauze can be placed between the fingers to prevent skin maceration. Depending on the severity of the injury, buddy-taping can be continued for 2 to 4 weeks, followed by taping just during sports and other potentially at-risk activities. Elevation, ice, and analgesics should also be recommended.

For a complete tear of a collateral ligament (gross laxity to stress testing), treatment can similarly consist of buddy-taping, but the duration may need to be prolonged. Some hand surgeons do advocate surgical treatment for complete

tears, but good results are usually obtained with conservative treatment.[6]

If an associated volar plate injury occurs, treatment can either consist of buddy-taping as for a pure collateral ligament injury, or splinting the PIP joint in slight (30°) flexion for 2 to 4 weeks followed by buddy-taping, depending on the extent of the volar plate injury.

It is often helpful to explain to patients that residual swelling and slight stiffness may persist for long periods, weeks or months or even longer, depending upon the severity of the injury, even after "healing" of the ligamentous injury.

PIP Dorsal Dislocations

The most commonly dislocated joint in the hand is the PIP joint in the fingers. The vast majority

Figure 5-10

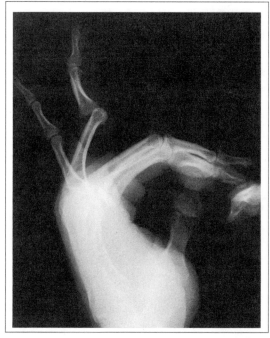

Lateral radiograph of a dorsal PIP joint dislocation of the ring finger.

of these occur in a dorsal direction (Fig. 5-10). The mechanism is generally an axial-loading force with a dorsal hyperextending component. The middle phalanx is dislocated dorsally with respect to the proximal phalanx. The volar plate is usually completely ruptured along with one or both collateral ligaments. Frequently, these have already been reduced by the patient themselves or by a bystander. A great deal of pain is often associated with dislocations, which can be partially relieved by reduction.

Radiographs can be obtained to look for avulsion fractures and to rule out other more significant fractures. These are generally done prior to attempted reduction, but in some circumstances may be delayed until after reduction.

Reduction can be attempted either with or without anesthesia. Generally, digital block anesthesia is very effective for these situations (see

"Digital Block Anesthesia"). Anesthesia can often make reductions easier for both the patient and the physician. Reduction can be accomplished with slight longitudinal traction and flexion of the middle phalanx. Often, further hyperextension of the PIP is necessary prior to flexion to dislodge the dislocated middle phalanx and allow reduction. If one or two attempted reductions are unsuccessful, immediate referral is warranted because surgical reduction is necessary in occasional cases.

Following successful reduction of a PIP dorsal dislocation, the joint can be splinted in slight (30°) flexion with an aluminum or plastic splint. Post-reduction radiographs should be obtained to check for and document satisfactory reduction. The main goals after successful reduction are to allow the volar plate and collateral ligaments to heal.[7] Elevation, ice, and analgesics should also be recommended. After 2 to 4 weeks of splinting in flexion, buddy-taping can be commenced, at first continuously, and then just with sports and other potential at-risk activities. In some cases, if stability is noted immediately after reduction, buddy-taping can be initiated right away without a period of splinting. Just as for other injuries of the PIP joint, residual swelling and stiffness may persist for months or longer after a dislocation.

PIP Volar Dislocations

Volar dislocations of the PIP joint are much more rare than dorsal dislocations but are associated with more complications. The central slip of the extensor tendon may rupture in these injuries, along with one or both collateral ligaments.[7] The volar plate may also be injured. Closed reduction may be difficult in volar dislocations because the distal portion of the proximal phalanx can be caught between the lateral bands of the extensor tendon. Traction may tighten the extensor mechanism, making reduction even more difficult. If closed reduction cannot be accomplished, referral for possible open reduction is warranted. If closed reduction is successful, and the central slip has been ruptured, then treatment is similar to that for central slip ruptures with splinting of the PIP joint in complete extension continuously for 6 to 8 weeks.

Phalangeal Shaft Fractures

Fractures of the shafts of the middle and proximal phalanges can occur from a variety of mechanisms and can often be treated by primary care physicians as long as a few basic principles are kept in mind. One of the most important principles is always to check for rotational deformity.[8] This is best assessed during the physical examination. Rotational deformity of the digits is best seen with the PIP and DIP joints in flexion, which accentuates visibility of any rotation of the shaft (Fig. 5-11). The patient is asked to show their fingernails to the examiner with the PIP and DIP joints in flexion. All four fingernails on both hands should point in a similar direction, usually toward the scaphoid bone at the radial side of the wrist. The direction of the affected finger should also be compared to the same finger on the opposite hand. While the fingers may be able to compensate for small degrees of angular (i.e., volar or dorsal) deformity, rotational deformity usually cannot be tolerated and therefore must be corrected.

Shaft fractures can be classified as transverse, oblique, or spiral, based on their radiographic appearance. Oblique or spiral fractures often result from torsional stresses such as twisting and, therefore, are prone to malrotation. Malrotation needs to be carefully sought in anyone with an oblique or spiral fracture. Malrotation should also be suspected if there appears to be shortening of the phalanx on radiographs compared with its normal length. Transverse shaft

Figure 5-11

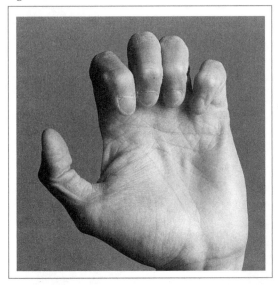

Assessing the fingers for malrotation can be done by asking the patient to flex all the finger joints. The distal phalanges and fingernails should all point towards the scaphoid bone near the thenar eminence. Flexion accentuates the degree of malrotation present in the finger bones.

fractures can be a result of direct blows and may result in angulation but are less prone to malrotation.

Treatment

Treatment of nondisplaced (meaning no angulation and no malrotation) or minimally displaced phalangeal shaft fractures involves either buddy-taping or splinting for 1 to 3 weeks followed by buddy-taping, depending on the stability of the fracture and the severity of symptoms.[8] If splinting is chosen, a malleable aluminum splint can be fashioned to include the joint above and below the involved phalanx. Alternatively, a plaster or fiberglass molded gutter splint can be used with the inclusion of an adjacent finger for additional support. The splinted DIP, PIP, or MCP joints should be placed in slight (30 to 40°) flexion. Splinting should be discontinued as early as possible with advancement to buddy-taping, and prolonged splinting should be avoided. Joint stiffness and contractures are best avoided this way, especially when the PIP joint is involved. Elevation, ice, and analgesics should also be recommended.

Treatment of displaced fractures involves reduction of the fracture, if possible, followed by protective splinting. Digital block anesthesia is generally effective for adequate pain control during reduction (see "Digital Block Anesthesia"), but in some cases reduction can be attempted without anesthesia. Longitudinal traction along with gentle manipulation of the fracture fragments reduces most fractures.[8] Often, worsening the angulation first to dislodge a bone fragment may be needed prior to applying a reduction force. Splinting with a molded aluminum splint or a molded plaster gutter splint should then be applied immediately after reduction and a post-reduction radiograph should be taken to check alignment. Again, ice, elevation, and analgesics can be recommended. After 2 to 4 weeks of splinting, advancement to buddy-taping can usually be accomplished. If there is concern about possible loss of the reduction, follow-up radiographs may be obtained 3 to 7 days after reduction to recheck alignment. If satisfactory reduction cannot be accomplished, then referral for possible surgical reduction may be necessary. Again, chronic joint stiffness and contractures are best avoided by advancement to buddy-taping and commencement of mobility as soon as possible.

A fracture that involves malrotation, with or without angulation, is often difficult to satisfactorily reduce. Angulation is much easier to reduce than malrotation. If correction of malrotation is not easily accomplished, surgical intervention is often needed.

Thumb Ulnar Collateral Ligament Injuries (Gamekeepers' Thumb; Skiers' Thumb)

A common injury to the thumb seen in primary care involves the ulnar collateral ligament (UCL). This ligament is located at the MCP joint of the thumb on the ulnar side (in the web space between the thumb and index finger). It runs from the distal portion of the thumb metacarpal, to the proximal base of the thumb proximal phalanx, and serves to stabilize this articulation and prevent excessive abduction and extension movements at the MCP joint.

History

The UCL is injured during a forced hyperabduction and/or hyperextension stress of the thumb MCP joint, generally from a fall landing onto the thumb. In skiers who fall with their thumb in an extended position, the ski pole, which is caught between the thumb and index finger, can force the MCP joint into such a hyperextended position, rupturing the UCL. This type of an injury is also common in other sports such as football, in which falls onto an outstretched hand and extended thumb happen frequently.

Physical Examination

If the history of the mechanism of injury is typical with hyperextension injury to the thumb MCP joint, a UCL injury should be suspected, especially if pain and swelling occur at the ulnar side of the MCP joint. Careful examination of the UCL should be performed, beginning with inspection for sites of local swelling and ecchymoses.

Figure 5-12

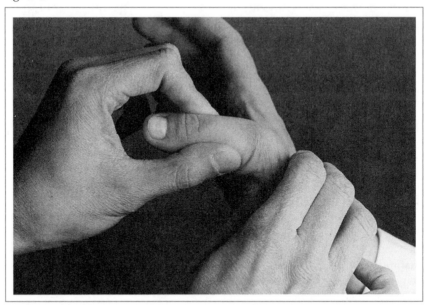

Testing for the integrity of the thumb UCL (gamekeepers'). The patient's thumb is in the center of the photo. The examiner's right hand stabilizes the patient's thumb metacarpal bone to prevent rotation during the testing procedure, while the examiner's left hand forces the proximal phalanx in a radial direction, stretching the UCL. The amount of laxity (magnitude of movement) and solidness of endpoint are noted and compared with the opposite thumb.

Palpation of the ulnar side of the MCP joint will elicit tenderness.

The rest of the thumb including other parts of the MCP joint should also be palpated to look for other injuries. Stress testing of the UCL can be performed, although some authorities recommend obtaining radiographs prior to stress testing.[9] The reason for this is that if an avulsion fracture is present that was initially non- or minimally displaced, stress testing can theoretically cause displacement of that avulsion fragment, thereby potentially altering management.

Whether stress testing is done before or after radiographs, its performance serves to determine if the UCL is partially torn or completely torn, which has important implications for management (Fig. 5-12). One hand of the examiner grasps the patient's thumb metacarpal to prevent rotation of the metacarpal during stressing. The examiner's other hand grasps the patient's thumb proximal phalanx and provides a gentle stretching force to the UCL by applying an abduction directed force. A positive test, implying a completely ruptured UCL, occurs when increased opening on the ulnar side of the MCP joint is found compared with the opposite thumb, and a "soft" endpoint is obtained. In many cases, determination of a positive versus a negative test is very difficult, and controversy surrounds more specific criteria involving actual number of degrees of joint motion that qualifies as a positive test, either in absolute terms or relative to the contralateral thumb.[10] Pain and guarding can prevent adequate stress testing. In these situations, a local anesthetic such as lidocaine can be infused into the area around the UCL with subsequent pain-free stress testing. If the stress testing is equivocal and complete rupture of the UCL is still suspected, referral may be indicated.

Ancillary Tests

Radiographs may be normal, or may show evidence of an avulsion fracture, usually located at the distal portion of the metacarpal. Stress radiography is advocated by some, but the criteria for a positive test is controversial. Other radiographic examinations including arthrography and magnetic resonance imaging (MRI) have also been used to help determine if a complete tear exists, but no consensus on the usefulness of these tests exists. If these tests are needed, the patient probably should be referred to a hand surgeon.

Treatment

Management depends upon whether the UCL ligament is partially or completely ruptured. A partially ruptured UCL ligament will generally heal satisfactorily with a course of protective splinting. This can either be done with a thumb spica cast immobilizing the MCP joint of the thumb, or with a commercially available removable thumb spica splint, which also immobilizes the thumb MCP joint. Splinting usually lasts for 2 to 6 weeks depending on the severity of the injury and severity of the symptoms. Elevation, ice, and analgesics should also be recommended. Splinting during sporting and other at-risk activities can be continued after the period of continuous splinting.

A completely ruptured UCL may or may not heal with splinting. The aponeurosis of the adductor pollicis muscle (which lies in the web space between the thumb and index finger) can become interposed between the two torn ends of the UCL This is known as a Stener lesion.[11] This interposition of the adductor aponeurosis prevents the two torn ends from meeting each other, and therefore prevents any chance of their healing to each other. Not every complete UCL tear has a Stener lesion associated with it, and if no Stener lesion is present, the UCL can theoretically heal with splinting or casting alone. However, there is no totally reliable clinical method to distinguish those complete tears with Stener lesions from those complete tears without Stener lesions. Therefore, if a complete UCL tear is suspected, an adductor aponeurosis interposition preventing the possibility of healing has to be considered likely, and referral for surgical exploration is indicated. Surgical results are generally better with early intervention rather than late intervention.[9,10] An improperly treated complete UCL rupture can result in long-term instability of the MCP joint and weakness in pinch strength.

Nondisplaced avulsion fractures can be treated similarly to partial UCL tears, with thumb spica casting or splinting. However, it must be kept in mind that a complete UCL tear can still be present with a nondisplaced avulsion fracture. Displaced avulsion fractures generally require surgery for anatomic reduction of the avulsion fragment. In children and adolescents, epiphyseal avulsion fractures can occur and if displaced, will require surgical reduction.

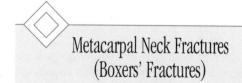

Metacarpal Neck Fractures (Boxers' Fractures)

Metacarpal neck fractures are relatively common and usually involve the fifth metacarpal, although they can certainly occur in the second, third, or fourth digits. These fractures generally occur from direct impact, as when a closed fist strikes a blunt object such as a wall. This causes fracture of the metacarpal neck or distal shaft just proximal to the metacarpal head. Despite the fact that these are commonly known as boxers' fractures, they rarely occur in boxers. Instead, they can occur quite commonly in street fights.

These fractures are often angulated, and the direction of angulation is almost always in a volar direction. This volar-directed angulation is due to the pull of the intrinsic hand muscles, specifically the palmar and dorsal interossei.[8]

Physical Examination

Physical examination of a patient with a history of blunt closed-fist trauma may reveal swelling and tenderness over the involved metacarpal neck and head. Often the fracture and the associated volar angulation can actually be palpated. With the hand in a closed-fist position with the MCP joints fully flexed, it can often be noted that the involved digit has a depressed or missing knuckle compared with the other MCP joints on the same hand and compared with the same digit on the opposite hand. This MCP knuckle depression is due the volar angulation of the fracture, but may be difficult to see on examination if significant swelling is present. As with any other fracture of the digits, malrotation needs to be assessed by checking the directions of the distal part of the fingers with the MCP, PIP, and DIP joints in flexion (see Fig. 5-11).

Ancillary Tests

Radiographic examination will show the fracture, its location, and the degree of volar angulation (Fig. 5-13). Volar angulation is best assessed on a lateral radiograph, and can be measured with a goniometer. Associated bony injuries should be ruled out on the radiographs.

Treatment

Treatment for metacarpal neck injuries is directed toward correcting potential functional deficits prior to bony healing, and then immobilization to allow bony healing. Potential functional deficits are dependent on the digit involved and the amount of angulation present. The index and middle metacarpals are not able to compensate very well for angulation at the

Figure 5-13

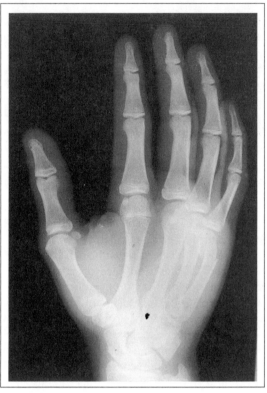

Fracture of the neck of the fifth metacarpal (boxers') in an adolescent with open growth plates. The degree of volar angulation cannot be accurately assessed on this oblique view, and a lateral view is used for that purpose.

metacarpal neck. This is due to lack of motion at the carpometacarpal (CMC) joint at the proximal base of the metacarpal. However, the ring and small finger CMC joints allow for quite a bit of motion in the sagittal plane, thereby providing much greater potential for compensation of angulation at the metacarpal neck. Therefore, the amount of acceptable residual angulation increases going from the second to the fifth metacarpal, although the exact numbers can be debated.[8] One easy method of remembering the acceptable degree of angulation is that the second can accept 10 degrees, the third can accept 20°, the fourth can accept 30°, and the fifth can accept 40°. As with the case for phalangeal fractures, no rotational deformities can be accepted. Additional considerations that need to be factored into the decision on whether to attempt a reduction of the angulation include the patient's occupation and other activities and hand dominance.

Other than a cosmetic loss of a knuckle on the dorsum of the hand, the main adverse affects of a volarly angulated metacarpal neck fracture are a prominent metacarpal head on the palm side of the hand and a slight loss of complete finger extension. This prominent "lump" in the palm may interfere with prolonged gripping activities, causing residual discomfort. Whether or not the patient will need to be performing prolonged gripping motions or fine motor movements with the fingers needs to be considered. Again, no rotational malalignment can be accepted, and those cases involving a rotational component to the deformity should be referred for possible operative treatment.

A nonangulated or minimally angulated metacarpal neck fracture can simply be splinted with an ulnar or radial gutter splint, depending on the involved digit, or casted for 4 to 6 weeks. The MCP joints should be placed in a flexed position (approximately 70 to 90°). Follow-up radiographs should be obtained early in the healing period to check for progression of the angulation before significant healing has occurred so that reduction can still be attempted if needed.

If it is determined that the angulation is more than what is acceptable (again, based on which digit is involved and functional demands), then a closed reduction will need to be attempted. Before attempting a closed reduction in the office or emergency department, the patient should be informed that even if an adequate reduction is accomplished, there is always the chance that loss of part or all of the reduction could occur over the next few days. If loss of reduction is too much (i.e., the residual angulation is no longer acceptable), closed reduction may need to be repeated. Another option should the patient desire attempted reduction but does not want to take the chance of loss of the reduction, is to refer the patient to an orthopedist for consideration of closed reduction in the operating room followed by percutaneous pinning to maintain the reduction.

Closed reduction in the office can be accomplished either with or without anesthesia. Anesthesia can be provided by a hematoma block with the local injection of lidocaine without epinephrine in and around the fracture site. Alternatively, if the ring or small digits are involved, an ulnar nerve block at the wrist can be used. Lidocaine without epinephrine can be infused around the ulnar nerve at the volar side of the wrist, carefully avoiding the ulnar artery, along with infusion around the ulnar side of the wrist. An additional injection along the dorsal ulnar side of the wrist ensures maximal anesthesia. Again, some reductions can be performed without anesthesia depending on the patient's desires.

Cast padding should be applied prior to reduction so the actual splint or cast can be applied immediately following the reduction. The actual reduction can be performed in a number of ways, but one simple method is to apply dorsally directed force on the PIP joint that is flexed 90° with the MCP joint also flexed 90° (Fig. 5-14). The operator's other hand should stabilize the proximal portion of the involved metacarpal while this dorsally applied force is being exerted upon the distal metacarpal.[8] Usually, the reduction can be palpated and when finished, the operator should continue to hold the reduction while a helper applies the splint or cast. A plaster splint or cast is more desirable in these situation than a fiberglass one because the plaster tends to mold more finely and therefore may prevent loss of reduction better. The operator should continue to hold and maintain the reduction until the splint or cast dries. Post-reduction radiographs should then be taken to document the reduction.

Figure 5-14

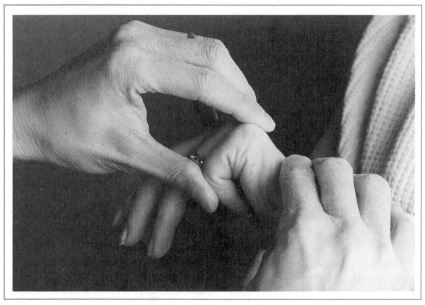

Reduction of boxers' fracture. The patient's fifth digit is in the center of the photo. The examiner's right hand stabilizes the proximal portion of the fifth metacarpal with a slight palmarly directed force (with respect to the patient), while the examiner's left hand and thumb push in a dorsal direction against the proximal phalanx to accomplish the reduction. The patient's MCP joint is held in 90° of flexion. Stockinette and cast padding can be applied prior to reduction (not shown), so that a cast or splint can be placed immediately after successful reduction.

Post-reduction care involves early (3 to 7 days) and frequent repeat radiographs to check for loss of reduction because loss of reduction is a frequent occurrence. The options should loss of reduction occur are to: (1) leave the angulation alone and continue splinting or casting for 4 to 6 weeks to allow healing in this angulated position; (2) attempt another closed reduction followed by splinting or casting, knowing that loss of the new reduction is a possibility; or (3) referral for consideration of operative closed reduction followed by percutaneous pinning to maintain the reduction. As with the decision concerning the first reduction, decisions concerning a second reduction should take into account the digit involved, the degree of angulation, and the patient's functional demands.

Fractures of the distal metacarpal shaft slightly more proximal than the neck can be treated sim-ilarly to neck fractures, except that the degrees of acceptable angulation for the various digits becomes less as the fracture site becomes more proximal along the shaft. This is due to less compensatory ability at the CMC joints as the fracture site becomes more proximal.

Thumb Metacarpal Fractures (Bennett's and Rolando Fractures)

Fractures of the thumb metacarpal neck or shaft occur rarely. Instead, most fractures involving

Figure 5-15

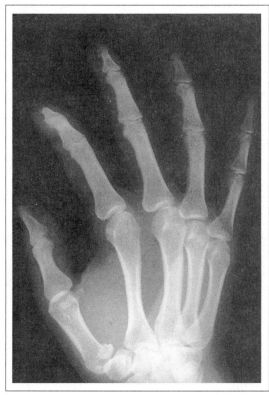

Bennett's fracture. Avulsion fragment at ulnar base of the thumb metacarpal with radial subluxation of the metacarpal itself.

the thumb metacarpal occur at the base where it articulates with the trapezium bone.

A Bennett's fracture usually occurs with an axial load injury to the thumb and is characterized by a small avulsion fragment along the ulnar base of the metacarpal (Fig. 5-15).[12] Although this fracture can appear benign on radiographs, significant morbidity can result if not recognized. The thumb metacarpal is maintained in its proper location articulation with the trapezium by a volar ulnar ligament at its base. With a Bennett's fracture, this volar ulnar ligament remains attached to the small avulsion fragment, and therefore the rest of the metacarpal has no remaining stabilizing ligaments. The ten-

don of the abductor pollicis longus, which attaches to the radial base of the thumb metacarpal, tends to pull and sublux the metacarpal in a radial direction, making closed treatment difficult or impossible. Referral for operative treatment is necessary for all Bennett's fractures.[7,9]

Rolando fractures have a similar pathology as Bennett's fractures, but are more comminuted, forming a "T" or a "Y" shape.[13] These also require referral for operative treatment.[7,9]

References

1. Abbase EA, Tadjalli HE, Shenaq SM: Fingertip and nail bed injuries: Repair techniques for optimum outcome. *Postgrad Med* 98:217, 1995.
2. Aronowitz ER, Leddy JP: Closed tendon injuries of the hand and wrist in athletes. *Clin Sports Med* 17:449, 1998.
3. Markiewitz AD, Andrish JT: Hand and wrist injuries in the preadolescent and adolescent athlete. *Clin Sports Med* 11:203, 1992.
4. Geyman JP, Fink K, Sullivan SD: Conservative versus surgical treatment of mallet finger: A pooled quantitative literature evaluation. *J Am Fam Prac* 11:382, 1998.
5. Kahler DM, McCue FC: Metacarpophalangeal and proximal interphalangeal joint injuries of the hand, including the thumb. *Clin Sports Med* 11:57, 1992.
6. Liss FE, Green SM: Capsular injuries of the proximal interphalangeal joint. *Hand Clin* 8:755, 1992.
7. Palmer RE: Joint injuries of the hand in athletes. *Clin Sports Med* 17:513, 1998.
8. Capo JT, Hastings II H: Matacarpal and phalangeal fractures in athletes. *Clin Sports Med* 17:491, 1998.
9. Langford SA, Whitaker JH, Toby EB: Thumb injuries in the athlete. *Clin Sports Med* 17:553, 1998.
10. Newland CC: Gamekeeper's thumb. *Orthopedic Clin North Am* 23:41, 1992.
11. Stener B: Displacement of the ruptured ulnar collateral ligament of the metacarpal phalangeal joint of the thumb: A clinical and anatomical study. *J Bone Joint Surg [Br]* 44:869, 1962.

12. Bennett EH: Fractures of the metacarpal bone of the thumb. *BMJ* 2:12, 1886.

13. Rolando S: Fracture de la base du premier métacarpien et principalement sur une variété non encore décrite. *Presse Med* 33:303, 1910.

Lower Extremity
Problems

Jeffrey A. Housner

Chapter

6

Hip Pain

Pediatric Hip Disorders	*Slipped Capital Femoral*
Muscle Strain	*Epiphysis*
Avulsion Fracture	*Septic Arthritis*
Apophysitis	*Transient Synovitis*
Legg-Calvé-Perthes' Disease	**Conclusion**

Introduction

The evaluation of the patient who presents with the complaint of sports-related hip pain can often be quite complex. It is, therefore, imperative that the primary care clinician develop a systematic approach to this problem.

The initial point to recognize is that a patient's perception of "hip" pain may not necessarily involve the hip joint itself. The problem may actually be in the groin, lateral thigh, buttock, pelvis, or lower abdomen. It is also important to know that many hip complaints may originate from the lumbrosacral spine. See Chap. 19 for a comprehensive evaluation of the back. In those patients who may have referred pain from the lumbar spine, a general survey of the lower back should be conducted, including specific tests for a lumbar radiculopathy.

This chapter begins by outlining a clinical approach (anatomy, history, physical examination, laboratory tests, and imaging studies) that

Figure 6-1

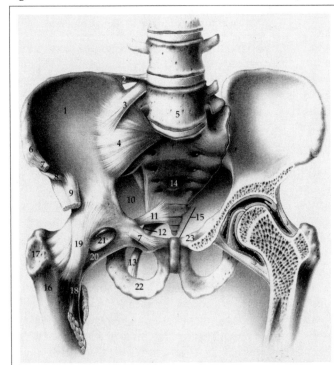

BONES & LIGAMENTS OF THE PELVIS & HIP JOINT
1 Ischium
2 Superior band of iliolumbar ligament
3 Inferior band of iliolumbar ligament
4 Ventral sacroiliac ligament
5 5th lumbar vertebra
6 Anterior superior iliac spine
7 Inguinal ligament (cut)
8 Anterior inferior iliac spine
9 Rectus femoris tendon
10 Greater sciatic foramen
11 Sacrospinous ligament
12 Lesser sciatic foramen
13 Sacrotuberous ligament
14 Sacrum
15 Coccyx
16 Femur
17 Greater trochanter
18 Lesser trochanter
19 Ileofemoral ligament
20 Pubofemoral ligament
21 Ileopectineal bursa
22 Ischial tuberosity
23 Superior ramus of pubis

Bones and ligaments of the pelvis and hip joint.

helps the clinician tackle a broad differential diagnosis for hip pain. This is followed by a brief synopsis of each diagnosis, covering the salient clinical features, treatment options, and referral guidelines. A fairly comprehensive list of diagnoses is covered, including both sports- and nonsports-related causes of hip pain.

Anatomy

Bones

The bones and ligaments of the hip and pelvis are illustrated in Fig. 6-1. The pelvis consists of three paired bones (ilium, ischium, and pubis) that interconnect to form the innomiate bones, or os coxae. They meet anteriorly in the midline at the pubic symphysis and posteriorly with the sacrum at the sacroiliac joints, thereby completing the make-up of the "pelvic girdle."

The hip joint consists of the acetabulum (formed by the triradiate junction of the ilium, ischium, and pubis) and proximal femur. This ball-and-socket joint is reinforced by a strong fibrocartilaginous labral rim and capsule-ligamentous complex providing a high degree of stability.[1] Readily palpable landmarks include the iliac crest, anterior superior iliac spine (ASIS), posterior superior iliac spine (PSIS), greater trochanter, and ischial tuberosity.

Muscles

The muscles of the hip and upper thigh are illustrated in Fig. 6-2.

Range of Motion

Average hip motion consists of 45° of external rotation, 40° of internal rotation, 45° of abduction, 20° of adduction, 135° of flexion, and 30° of extension.[2]

Figure 6-2

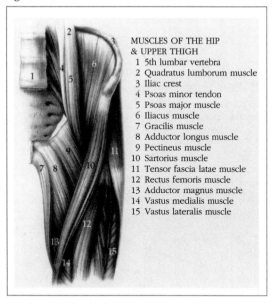

MUSCLES OF THE HIP & UPPER THIGH
1 5th lumbar vertebra
2 Quadratus lumborum muscle
3 Iliac crest
4 Psoas minor tendon
5 Psoas major muscle
6 Iliacus muscle
7 Gracilis muscle
8 Adductor longus muscle
9 Pectineus muscle
10 Sartorius muscle
11 Tensor fascia latae muscle
12 Rectus femoris muscle
13 Adductor magnus muscle
14 Vastus medialis muscle
15 Vastus lateralis muscle

Muscles of the hip and upper thigh.

Clinical Approach

There are many ways to approach the presenting complaint of hip pain. The approach should include a focused history and physical examination that elicits enough information to answer the following questions: (1) What is the working diagnosis (or diagnoses)? (2) Which, if any, imaging studies or laboratory tests are indicated? (3) Does the patient need to be referred to a specialist and, if so, is an emergent, urgent, or routine referral indicated? (4) What treatment plan should be prescribed, including specific rehabilitation instructions?

History

One common way of organizing the extensive differential diagnosis is to establish three

Figure 6-3

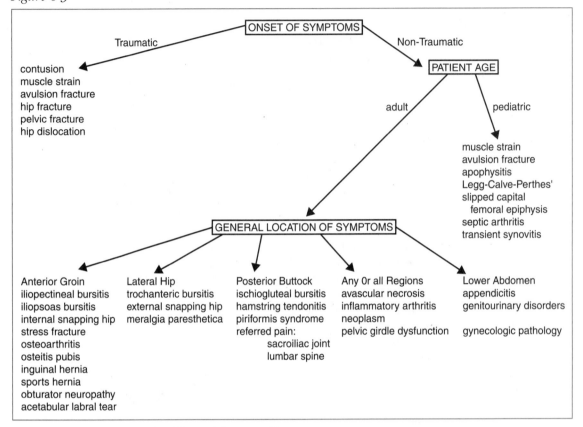

Basic algorithm for organizing the differential diagnosis of hip pain.

fundamental features from the patient's history (Fig. 6-3). This approach involves determining the onset of symptoms (traumatic versus non-traumatic), the age of the patient, and the general location of symptoms (anterior groin, lateral hip, posterior buttock, or lower abdomen). There are two potential drawbacks to this clinical approach: (1) patients sometimes find it difficult to localize their symptoms, and (2) some diagnoses are not exclusive to only one category. However, this method does provide an organizational framework on which to guide the remainder of the history. For example, this approach should include the following questions, each of which should be asked when appropriate depending on the patient presentation:

- What was the exact mechanism of injury?
- What is the quality, severity, and timing of the pain?
- Are there any exacerbating or alleviating factors?
- What is the relationship of symptoms to exercise, athletic performance, or occupational duties?
- What is the type, duration, frequency, and intensity of exercise or occupational activity?
- Is there a history of hip problems and, if so, how were they treated and what was the outcome?
- Is there a history of menstrual irregularities or disordered eating?
- Is there a history of stress fractures?
- Is there a history of inflammatory arthritis?

- Is there a history of drug or alcohol abuse, or corticosteroid use?
- Are constitutional symptoms present? (i.e., fever, chills, night sweats, weight loss, malaise, etc.)

It should be noted that complaints other than pain, such as clicking, snapping, restriction of motion, weakness, and limping may also cause the patient to come in for evaluation.

Physical Examination

The sequence of physical examination tests and maneuvers for a complete hip evaluation is variable and may be adapted according to the history. The hip examination, as described here, is presented in a systematic, logical manner.

The physical examination begins with general observation. With the patient standing, the examiner should look for posture abnormalities such as asymmetry of pelvic landmarks; abnormal hip, knee, or foot position; lower extremity rotation; muscle atrophy; and skin changes. Swelling in and around the hip is difficult to detect.

In the event of an "on-site" evaluation following a traumatic injury, note the position of the patient's leg. If shortened and externally rotated, a fractured femoral neck is the provisional diagnosis; if flexed, internally rotated, and adducted, a posterior hip dislocation should be suspected.[3] Active, passive, and resisted hip extension are tested with the patient prone. The primary assessment may also include a detailed neurologic, vascular, abdominal, genitourinary, and/or gynecologic evaluation if indicated by the patient's history.

PALPATION

Pinpointing the involved anatomical structure by palpation is extremely helpful in establishing the diagnosis. Palpation of the lateral and posterior structures is easily performed while the patient is standing. Palpation of the anterior region is facilitated with the patient lying supine.

LEG LENGTH

When the patient is placed in the supine position, true leg lengths are measured from the ASIS to the medial malleolus. Differences of more than 1 cm can usually be detected reliably by this method, but lesser discrepancies are difficult to record.[2] True leg lengths that are unequal should raise suspicion of hip disease on the shorter side.

Apparent leg length discrepancy is measured from the umbilicus to the medial malleolus. Unequal apparent lengths usually indicates pelvic tilt, adductor contractures, or hip capsule tightness.[3]

RANGE OF MOTION

Range of motion of the hip that is symmetric and painless virtually rules out intra-articular disease. Subjective measurements and side-to-side comparisons should be made. More accurate rotational angles can be measured with a goniometer. Passive hip flexion, adduction, abduction, and internal/external rotation can be assessed in the supine position. (Note, however, internal rotation (Fig. 6-4) and external rotation (Fig. 6-5) can be more accurately measured with the patient sitting or prone, both with the knees flexed 90°.) Strength testing of the hip flexors (iliopsoas, rectus femoris), hip abductors (gluteus medius and minimus), and hip adductors (adductor longus, adductor brevis, adductor magnus, pectineus, and gracilis) is recorded.

TRENDELENBURG'S TEST

Trendelenburg's test is performed to evaluate the strength and proper function of the abductor muscles, principally the gluteus medius. The test is performed with the patient standing in front of and facing away from the examiner. The patient is asked to stand on one leg (supported side) and flex the opposite hip (unsupported side). Normally, the pelvis on the unsupported side elevates slightly, indicating that the gluteus medius muscle on the supported side is func-

Figure 6-4

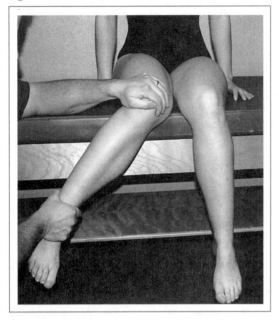

Passive internal rotation of the hip.

tioning properly (Fig. 6-6A). This normal action is a negative Trendelenburg's sign. If the pelvis on the unsupported side drops or stays in position, it indicates a positive Trendelenburg sign (Fig. 6-6B). A positive Trendelenburg test alerts the clinician to the possibility of underlying intra-articular pathology or gluteus medius weakness of the supported side.

STANDING FLEXION AND ONE-LEGGED STORK TEST

The standing flexion test and one-legged stork test are used as screening tests for pelvic girdle dysfunction.[4] For the standing flexion test, the examiner sits behind the patient and uses the thumbs to palpate both the right and left posterior superior iliac spine (PSIS). As the patient bends forward in a smooth fashion, excursion of each PSIS is followed. The test is positive on the side in which the PSIS appears to move more cephalad (Fig. 6-7).

For the stork test, the examiner is seated

behind the patient with right thumb on the right PSIS and left thumb on the sacral crest at the same level. The patient flexes the right hip. A normal response is for the thumb on the PSIS to move caudad in relation to the thumb on the sacrum. A positive response finds the thumb on the PSIS moving more cephalad (Fig. 6-8). Comparison is made to the opposite side.

GAIT OBSERVATION

A brief observation of the patient's gait is helpful. An abductor or gluteus medius lurch (Trendelenburg gait) is manifested by a lateral shift of the body to the weight-bearing side with ambulation. This abnormal gait is often associated with a positive Trendelenburg's sign, described previously. An antalgic (painful) gait is manifested by a shortened stance phase, which gives the appearance of a short hop as the

Figure 6-5

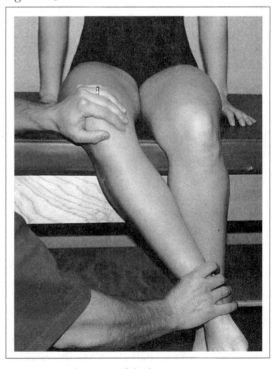

Passive external rotation of the hip.

Figure 6-6

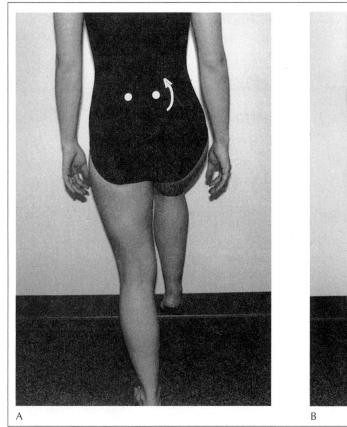 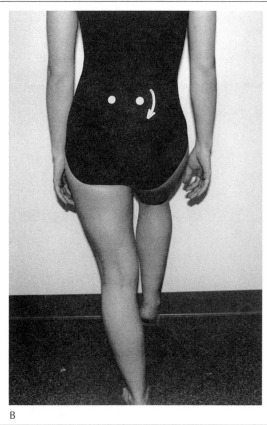

A   B

Trendelenburg's test. **(A)** Negative, **(B)** Positive.

patient attempts to unload the painful extremity. Both of these gait abnormalities usually indicate significant intra-articular joint problems.

THOMAS' TEST

Thomas' test is a specific test to assess hip flexion contracture (the most common contracture of the hip) and can be incorporated into the testing of passive hip flexion.[5] The examiner flexes one of the patient's hips, bringing the knee to the chest to flatten out the lumbar spine. The patient is then asked to hold the thigh in a maximally flexed position. If a hip flexion contracture is present, the knee of the contralateral leg will flex (Fig. 6-9A). If no contracture is

present, the knee will remain fully extended (Fig. 6-9B).

To further assess hip flexion contracture due to a tight rectus femoris muscle, the patient is positioned on the table so that the knees are bent over the edge. The patient again maximally flexes the hip holding one knee onto the chest. The test is positive for a tight rectus femoris on the opposite leg if the opposite knee extends (Fig. 6-10A). The opposite knee should normally remain at 90° (Fig. 6-10B).

HAMSTRING FLEXIBILITY

One of the many ways to assess hamstring flexibility begins with the patient's hip and knee

Figure 6-7

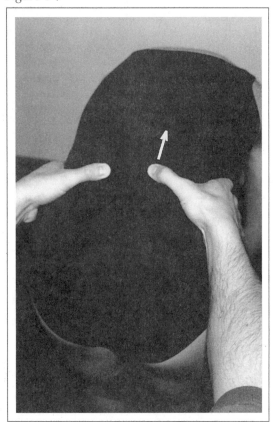

Standing flexion test, demonstrating a positive response on the right.

flexed 90°. The knee is then passively extended. When no further extension can be achieved, the angle short of full extension is recorded (Fig. 6-11A). Full extension is desirable (Fig. 6-11B). If a lumbar radiculopathy is suspected, a passive straight-leg raising test can be performed at this juncture.

PATRICK TEST

The Patrick, or FABER, test can be performed to evaluate both the hip and sacroiliac joint. With the patient lying supine, the foot of the involved leg is placed on the contralateral knee, anteriorly. The flexed leg is then slowly lowered into abduction. The hip is now *f*lexed, *ab*ducted,

and *externally* rotated (*FABER*). Pain may be noted in the hip or ipsilateral sacroiliac joint. If the leg does not lower to an almost parallel position, there is a possible contracture at the hip or protective iliopsoas spasm. Pressure on the knee and counterpressure on the opposite pelvic brim may elicit pain at the hip or sacroiliac joint (Fig. 6-12).

OBER'S TEST

When the patient is in the lateral decubitus position, Ober's test for contracture of the iliotibial band of the "up" leg can be performed. The knee is passively flexed to 90° while the leg is abducted away from the table as far as possible. The examiner then releases the abducted leg

Figure 6-8

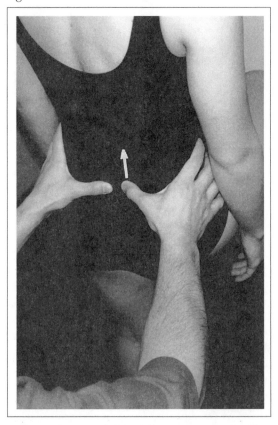

Stork test, demonstrating a positive response on the right.

Figure 6-9

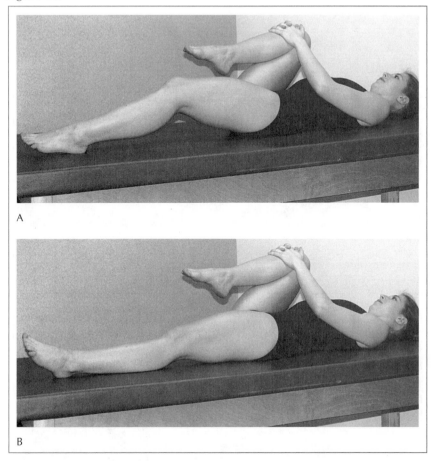

Thomas's test. **(A)** Positive. **(B)** Negative.

while maintaining support of the abducted foot. If there is a contracture of the iliotibial band, the thigh remains abducted when the leg is released (Fig. 6-13A); if the iliotibial band is normal, the thigh should drop to an adducted position (Fig. 6-13B).

Ancillary Tests

BLOOD TESTS

Blood tests are rarely helpful in the evaluation of hip pain. If infection is suspected, the patient should be evaluated immediately by an orthope-

dic surgeon. A complete blood count (CBC) with differential and erythrocyte sedimentation rate (ESR) may be considered. Rheumatoid factor, CBC, acute phase reactants (ESR, C-reactive protein), and antinuclear antibody (ANA) tests may be helpful if inflammatory arthritis is suspected.[5]

Imaging Studies

Unless the diagnosis is readily reached via the history and physical examination, imaging studies are usually needed. If any imaging is contemplated, standard radiographs of the hip and

Figure 6-10

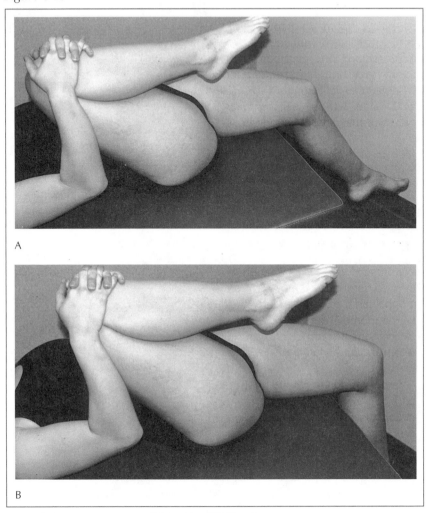

Rectus femoris contracture test. **(A)** Positive, **(B)** Negative.

pelvis should be obtained before any other imaging studies are considered. This includes an anterior-posterior (AP) view of the pelvis and hip along with a frog-leg or true lateral view of the involved side. Generally, a frog-leg lateral is ordered in the nontraumatic setting. A true lateral is obtained when complete evaluation of injuries to the proximal femur is needed.

Bone scans are sensitive in detecting stress fractures, avascular necrosis, osseous neoplasms, and infection. However, the specificity of the bone scan in identifying these problems is low.

Computed tomography (CT) is the preferred modality for assessment of the osseous-based abnormalities of the hip.[6] Magnetic resonance imaging (MRI) can image osseous and soft tissue structures including the hip capsule, the labrum, fluid-filled bursae, articular surfaces, muscles, and tendons. It has proved to be both sensitive and specific for the detection of stress reactions, stress fractures, occult fractures, musculoskeletal tumors, marrow replacement processes, and

Figure 6-11

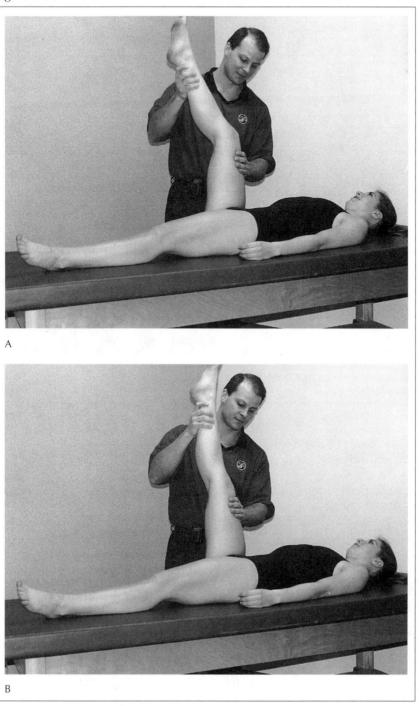

Hamstring flexibility test. **(A)** decreased flexibility, **(B)** normal

Figure 6-12

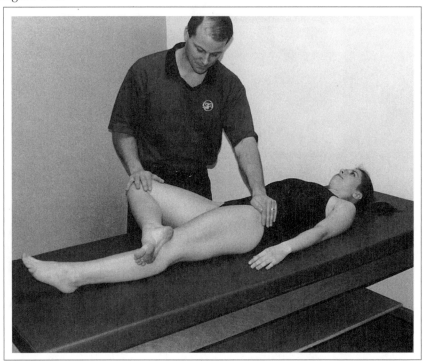

Patrick's or FABER test. Positive test indicated by pain in the hip or sacroiliac joint.

osteomyelitis.[6] MRI is the definitive test for evaluation of avascular necrosis.[7] Its major disadvantage is relatively high cost and limited availability.

Imaging of the lumbar spine (see Chap. 19) should be considered if this site is the suspected source of referred pain to the hip.

 The Diagnostic Challenge

When using the diagnostic tests just described, the primary care clinician is equipped to approach the complaint of hip pain. The following sections provide a synopsis of each diagnosis listed in Fig. 6-3, grouped in a similar manner. This format can be used as a general reference in the clinical setting when presented with a patient who has hip pain.

Traumatic Causes

CONTUSION

A direct blow to the hip or pelvis may cause a contusion. The most common site is the iliac crest, usually referred to as a "hip pointer." There is well-localized pain over the injured site without evidence of intra-articular injury. If a hematoma develops, aspiration followed by local lidocaine injection may be considered. Further treatment consists of rest, ice, and non-steroidal anti-inflammatory drugs (NSAIDs) or cyclooxygenase-2 (COX-2) inhibitors. Begin stretching and strengthening exercises when pain, ecchymosis, and swelling subside.

Figure 6-13

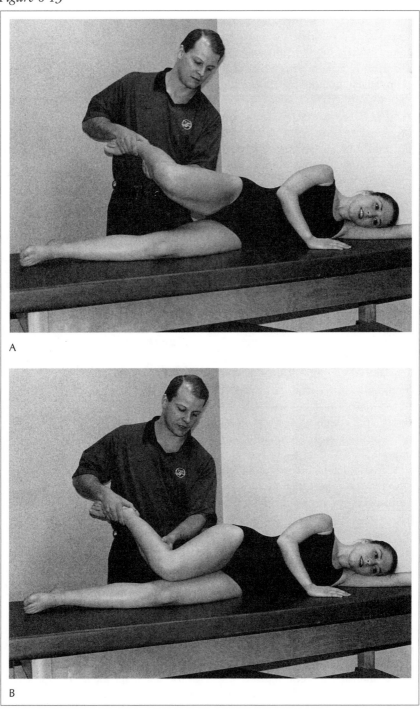

A

B

Ober's test. **(A)** Positive, **(B)** Negative.

MUSCLE STRAIN

Muscle strains are common injuries in sports that are often caused by sudden changes in direction. The injury occurs when a muscle violently contracts during a forceful stretch. Commonly involved muscles include the *adductor longus, adductor magnus, pectineus, rectus femoris, iliopsoas,* and *sartorius.* Examination findings include localized tenderness of the involved muscle, pain with passive stretch, and pain with muscle resistance testing. Initial treatment involves relative rest, ice, and NSAIDs. This is followed by a physical therapy program that involves gentle stretching and gradual strengthening.

AVULSION FRACTURE

Avulsion fractures have many similarities with muscle strains (see Chap. 18). The primary difference is that they occur in the young adolescent with open apophyses (the growth center at the site of tendon insertion). Commonly involved apophyseal/*muscle tendon* sites about the hip include the ASIS/*sartorius*, AIIS/*rectus femoris*, iliac crest/*abdominal muscles*, lesser trochanter/*iliopsoas*, and ischial tuberosity/*hamstrings*. The history and physical examination are similar to the muscle strains. X-rays confirm the avulsion fracture. Treatment is the same as for muscle strains. Orthopedic referral should be considered for those injuries resulting in significant disability, and/or fracture displacement of more than 2 cm.[8]

HIP FRACTURE

Hip fractures are a common problem among the elderly, especially women with osteoporosis. With increasing physical activity among older individuals, the rate of hip fracture may increase. The fracture generally involves either the femoral neck or the intertrochanteric region.

Most patients report a fall followed by the inability to walk. The classic presenting position in a patient with a femoral neck or an intertrochanteric fracture is an externally rotated, abducted, and shortened limb.[5] Plain films are usually adequate to confirm the diagnosis. Bone scan, CT, or MRI may detect occult fractures. Emergent orthopedic consultation should be made in most cases.

PELVIC FRACTURE

Pelvic fractures are classified as minor or major. Minor pelvic fractures include fracture of a single pubic ramus, fracture of the wing of the ilium, or fracture of the ischium.[2] Major pelvic fractures involve more than one break in the pelvic ring. They are rare outside of motor vehicle accidents or high-speed sports such as skiing or cycling. X-rays are usually adequate to confirm the diagnosis. Major pelvic fractures constitute an **orthopedic emergency**.

HIP DISLOCATION

A hip dislocation is also an **orthopedic emergency**. This condition is seen almost exclusively in young adults subjected to high-impact trauma. Patients will have pain and will be unable to move the lower extremity. Posterior hip dislocations are most common.[5] The classic presentation is severe pain with the hip in a fixed position of flexion, internal rotation, and adduction.[5] X-rays confirm the diagnosis. Emergent orthopedic consultation should be made.

Nontraumatic Causes

SYMPTOMS LOCALIZED TO THE ANTERIOR GROIN

ILIOPECTINEAL BURSITIS/ILIOPSOAS TENDONITIS   These conditions are difficult to distinguish clinically, and may be related to the "internal snapping hip," described as follows. The iliopsoas tendon is formed from the convergence of muscle fibers of the iliacus and psoas muscles. The tendon crosses the hip capsule, separated from it by the iliopectineal bursa (see Fig. 6-1), and inserts on the lesser trochanter of the femur (see Fig. 6-1). The bursa is aggravated by repetitive hip flexion. There is exquisite point tenderness of the tendon and/or bursa, localized to an area just below the inguinal ligament and lateral to the femoral artery.[9] Palpation is facilitated with the hip and knee flexed to about 40°, externally rotated, and supported on a pillow.[2] Pain may be aggravated with resisted hip flexion. Treatment consists of rest, NSAIDs, and hip flexor stretches, followed by gradual strengthening. A corticosteroid injection performed by an experienced physician may be considered.[10]

INTERNAL SNAPPING HIP   As stated previously, this condition may be related to chronic iliopectineal bursitis. The primary cause of internal snapping hip is the iliopsoas tendon snapping over the iliopectineal eminence. Patients report pain or snapping with hip flexion. Symptoms may be reproduced as the patient extends the hip from a flexed, abducted, and externally rotated position, or when rising from a chair. Most patients respond to stretching of the hip flexors. If pain is absent, reassurance may be all that is needed.

STRESS FRACTURE   Stress fractures of the femoral neck or superior pubic ramus (see Chap. 20) are a cause of pain in the anterior groin. Although these stress fractures are uncommon, they have a high complication rate if the diagnosis is missed or the patient is improperly treated.

The primary presenting complaint is pain that is exacerbated with weight-bearing or physical activity. Historical features may include an increase in duration, frequency, and/or intensity of weight-bearing exercises or a change in exercise terrain or shoes. Low bone mineral density, which may be caused by disordered eating behavior or menstrual irregularities (see Chap. 12), is a known risk factor. On physical examination, the patient may have an antalgic gait. Bony tenderness is difficult to elicit because

of the overlying soft tissue. Hip motion, especially internal rotation, may be painful or limited.

Plain radiographs may demonstrate the fracture if it has been present for 2 to 4 weeks. However, bone scintigraphy is effective in detecting stress fractures with virtually 100 percent sensitivity before they become evident on plain films.[11] MRI has comparative sensitivity to radionuclide techniques for the detection of stress injury to bone, and typically allows depiction of abnormalities several weeks prior to the development of radiographic alterations.[12]

Femoral neck stress fractures are classified as compression or distraction. Compression-type fractures occur at the lower medial margin of the femoral neck. Nondisplaced, incomplete, compression-type stress fractures are usually treated by rest until the patient is free of pain and the hip regains full motion. Nonweight-bearing ambulation with crutches is maintained until radiographic healing is complete. Distraction fractures occur at the superior margin, or tension side, of the femoral neck. All patients with distraction-type fractures and any compression-type fracture that is complete should be referred for emergent orthopedic consultation.[11]

Stress fractures can also occur along the superior pubic ramus, causing pain in the anterior groin. These fractures can be treated conservatively with relative rest. A rehabilitation program that includes range-of-motion exercises and gradual strengthening should be prescribed.

OSTEOARTHRITIS   Osteoarthritis is characterized by a loss of articular cartilage. Onset is usually after age 50, with gradual onset of pain deep in the groin (occasionally located in the lateral thigh or buttock). The earliest physical sign is loss of internal rotation.[5] Gradually, as the arthritis worsens, patients will lose flexion and extension.[5] An antalgic or Trendelenburg gait may develop. Classic radiologic features are joint space narrowing, osteophytes, cyst formation, and subchondral sclerosis.[5] Treatment begins with acetaminophen, NSAIDs or COX-2 inhibitors, and physical therapy to improve strength and range of motion. Patients who have exhausted all conservative measures and/or have significant disability may be considered for total hip arthroplasty.

OSTEITIS PUBIS Osteitis pubis (pubic symphysitis) is a poorly understood inflammation of the symphysis pubis. In the athletic population, it appears to be an overuse injury associated with excessive kicking or abdominal muscle contraction.[13] It may also be seen in women following vaginal delivery.

Pain is dull and aching, localized to the groin. The characteristic finding on examination is tenderness over the pubic symphysis. X-rays may reveal sclerosis and erosion of the pubic symphysis.[13] Pubic instability may be demonstrated on "flamingo" views (standing on one leg). Bone scan may be helpful if the diagnosis is in question. This condition is difficult to treat.

Management consists of NSAIDs or COX-2 inhibitors and avoidance of pain-provoking activities. A corticosteroid injection by an experienced clinician may be valuable in recalcitrant cases.

INGUINAL HERNIA Inguinal hernias (direct or indirect) can masquerade themselves as a cause of "hip" pain. Symptoms may include a dragging sensation of the lower abdomen aggravated by increased intra-abdominal pressure. Examination may reveal an obvious swelling or palpable cough impulse. Treatment consists of surgical correction.

SPORTS HERNIA A sports hernia is a disruption of the inguinal canal, characterized by three surgical findings:[14] (1) a torn external oblique aponeurosis causing dilatation of the superficial inguinal ring, (2) a torn conjoined tendon, and (3) a dehiscence between the torn conjoined tendon and inguinal ligament. Athletes who participate in sports that require repetitive twisting and turning at speed, such as soccer or ice hockey, are at risk. The predominant complaint is groin pain that may radiate to the adductor region or testicles.

Examination may reveal a dilated superficial inguinal ring, or local tenderness over the conjoined tendon and inguinal canal.[14] However, **a true hernia is not clinically detectable**. Radiographic studies may be helpful to exclude coexisting pathologic conditions.

Although conservative management is rarely effective for a sports hernia, it may help in patients who have coexisting conditions causing functional disability. Surgical repair, followed by a structured rehabilitation program, is the preferred treatment.[14]

OBTURATOR NEUROPATHY Obturator neuropathy, as described by Brukner and colleagues,[15] is a rare cause of exercise-related anterior groin pain. Athletes who play sports that involve a lot of running, twisting, turning, and kicking are at risk. Symptoms include pain that begins insidiously at the adductor origin and worsens with exercise. Physical examination diagnosis includes a pectineus muscle stretch done immediately after exercise. To perform this test, the patient stands in a partial "lunge" position with the unaffected extremity forward. The affected hip is then extended, externally rotated, and abducted.[15] This maneuver will induce diagnostic pain in the groin. Imaging studies do not play a significant role in confirming the diagnosis. Surgical release of the anterior branch of the obturator nerve is the preferred treatment.

ACETABULAR LABRAL TEAR Although rare, the fibrocartilaginous labrum of the acetabular fossa may develop tears. Symptoms may or may not follow a traumatic event. Patients report deep anterior groin pain usually associated with clicking or a catching sensation. Pain may be ilicited with internal rotation and extension. Radiography and CT are not able to detect labral tears. Similarly, MRI will usually miss these lesions. If a labral tear is suspected, magnetic resonance arthrography using intra-articular gadopentetate dimeglumine enhancement is the most useful diagnostic imaging study.[7] Hip arthoscopy is currently the gold standard for the diagnosis of acetabular labral tears, as well as the preferred treatment.[7]

LOCALIZED TO THE LATERAL HIP

TROCHANTERIC BURSITIS Trochanteric bursitis is characterized by pain and tenderness over the greater trochanter. It is seen frequently in runners, ballet dancers, and cross-country skiers. In addition to point tenderness over the greater trochanter, patients may exhibit a positive Ober's test, indicating a tight iliotibial band. Treatment consists of rest, ice, NSAIDs, and an iliotibial band-stretching program. Recalcitrant cases may respond to bursal injection with local anesthetic and corticosteroid.

EXTERNAL SNAPPING HIP The most common cause of external snapping hip is the iliotibial band snapping over the greater trochanter. The symptomatic snap may be reproduced by extending the knee and hip in adduction and then flexing the hip.[16] Because many patients may insist that the hip is "dislocating," reassurance may be all that is needed. If pain is also present, treatment is the same as for trochanteric bursitis.

MERALGIA PARESTHETICA Meralgia paresthetica is caused by entrapment of the lateral femoral cutaneous nerve as it exits the pelvis near the ASIS. Causative factors may include obesity, tight clothing or belts, pregnancy, or trauma (e.g., a direct blow to the ASIS, nerve stretch secondary to extreme hip extension, or repetitive trauma to the nerve). Symptoms include pain and dysethesia in the anterolateral thigh. Examination reveals hypoesthesia in the distribution of the lateral femoral cutaneous nerve (Fig. 6-14). Removing the source of nerve compression forms the primary basis of treatment. If other conservative measures, such as ultrasound and NSAIDs, fail to relieve the symptoms, a corticosteroid injection in the area just lateral to the ASIS may be considered.[2]

SYMPTOMS LOCALIZED TO THE POSTERIOR BUTTOCK

ISCHIOGLUTEAL BURSITIS/HAMSTRING TENDONITIS Clinically, it is difficult to distinguish between ischiogluteal bursitis and hamstring tendonitis. Each condition may occur suddenly after violent muscle contraction or, insidiously, after overuse. Both may be aggravated with sitting or sprinting. Both are associated with localized tenderness of the hamstring insertion. Pain is reproduced with resisted muscle contraction. Treatment consists of rest, ice, NSAIDs, and deep friction massage. A corticosteroid injection by an experienced clinician may be considered.[13]

Figure 6-14

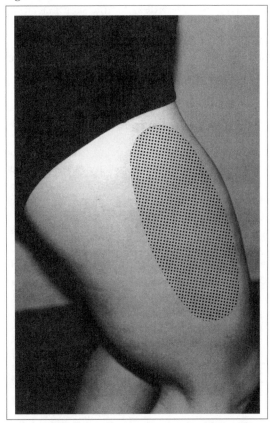

Sensory distribution of the lateral femoral cutaneous nerve.

STRESS FRACTURE Stress fractures can occur along the ischium and inferior pubic ramus. See Chap. 20 for in-depth discussion of evaluation for stress fractures. Treatment is usually conservative, with cessation of impact activities. A gradual return to all activities may be initiated when the patient becomes pain free.

PIRIFORMIS SYNDROME The piriformis syndrome results from pressure on the sciatic nerve as it courses through or below the piriformis muscle. This can present with local and referred pain to the posterior buttock. On examination, there may be tenderness in the belly of the piriformis muscle. Pain may be reproduced with voluntary hip flexion, adduction, and internal rotation.[17] Treatment involves stretching the piriformis muscle and soft tissue therapy.

REFERRED PAIN Disorders of the sacroiliac joint and lumbar spine may refer pain to the posterior buttock. Common causes are sacroiliitis secondary to a spondyloarthopathy and radicular pain from lumbar nerve root impingement (see Chap. 19).

SYMPTOMS LOCALIZED TO ANY OR ALL REGIONS

AVASCULAR NECROSIS Avascular necrosis, or osteonecrosis, involves death of living elements of bone. The biologic process that initiates the pathologic phenomenon is unknown. Trauma (i.e., femoral neck fracture, hip dislocation) is the most common cause. Other causes include excessive alcohol intake, systemic corticosteroid intake, and rheumatologic disorders. Pain is poorly localized and usually gradual in onset. Decreased range of motion and an antalgic gait develop as degenerative changes progress. Radiologic changes may lag several months behind the vascular insult. MRI is the best technique for the early diagnosis of osteonecrosis of the femoral head.[18] Urgent orthopedic consultation should be made if avascular necrosis is demonstrated.

INFLAMMATORY ARTHRITIS Many systemic inflammatory conditions, including ankylosing spon-

dylitis, calcium pyrophosphate deposition disease, gout, Reiter's syndrome, and systemic lupus erythematosus, may involve the hip joint.[5] Dull, aching pain may be localized to the groin, lateral thigh, and/or buttock. Pain is episodic and worse in the morning. The patient may have systemic manifestations of the disease. Examination reveals an antalgic gait and painful range of motion. X-rays confirm the diagnosis. Laboratory tests (e.g., CBC, ESR, RF, ANA) may be helpful. Treatment depends on the specific diagnosis. Initial treatment involves anti-inflammatory medications (nonsteroidal, steroidal, or COX-2 inhibitors) and physical therapy. Orthopedic and/or rheumatologic referral should be considered early in the course of the disease.

NEOPLASM Bone tumors can be classified as either primary or metastatic. Primary bone tumors are further characterized as either benign or malignant. Patients with bone tumors may present with unusual pain syndromes or with constitutional symptoms such as fever, chills, night sweats, or weight loss. A work-up for metastatic bone disease is imperative in the patient with bone pain who was previously diagnosed with a cancer known to metastasize to bone. X-rays may show a destructive lesion. Bone scan, CT, and MRI are sensitive tests for the early detection of bone tumors. Orthopedic and/or oncology consultation is indicated.

PELVIC GIRDLE DYSFUNCTION The evaluation and treatment of pelvic girdle dysfunction is complex.[4] Abnormalities can occur within the joints of the pelvic girdle (symphysis pubis, sacroiliac, iliosacral) as well as imbalance or weakness of the surrounding pelvic muscles. Complaints of pain and/or weakness are experienced anywhere around the hip (anterior, lateral, or posterior). For screening purposes, the evaluator looks for abnormal gait patterns, asymmetry of paired anatomic landmarks and altered range of motion (by the standing flexion test and stork test).[4] Manual medicine (i.e., manipulation) techniques are the cornerstone of therapy.

Pediatric Hip Disorders

MUSCLE STRAIN (PREVIOUSLY DISCUSSED)

AVULSION FRACTURE (PREVIOUSLY DISCUSSED IN THIS CHAPTER; ALSO SEE CHAP. 18)

APOPHYSITIS

Apophysitis (see Chap. 17) is inflammation of the apophyseal growth centers secondary to repetitive microtrauma. It can occur at any of the muscular attachment sites about the hip. Common sites include the iliac crest and posterior superior iliac spine. Poor flexibility coupled with chronic stress is the cause. The discomfort begins insidiously, eventually progressing to pain with activity. Pain is well localized at the involved site. X-rays are negative for avulsion fracture but may show slight widening of the physis.[19] Treatment consists of rest and ice, followed by a gradual stretching and strengthening program.

LEGG-CALVÉ-PERTHES' DISEASE

Legg-Calvé-Perthes disease is idiopathic osteonecrosis of the femoral head. It typically affects children between the ages of 5 and 10 years. It is 3 to 5 times more common in boys. The affected child limps, and may have pain in the anterior thigh or referred pain to the **knee**. X-rays confirm the diagnosis. Urgent orthopedic referral is indicated.

SLIPPED CAPITAL FEMORAL EPIPHYSIS

Slipped capital femoral epiphysis is literally a slippage of the femoral head off the femoral neck. It occurs most often in obese males aged 9 to 15 years. Typically, the patient presents with a limp and aching pain in the medial knee, thigh, or groin. Almost 20 percent of patients have medial knee pain alone.[20] Examination reveals restricted hip motion, particularly loss of internal rotation.[20] X-rays confirm the diagnosis. Immediate cessation of weight-bearing and emergent orthopedic consultation are indicated.

SEPTIC ARTHRITIS

Although acute bacterial infections of the hip can occur at any age, they are most frequently seen between 1 to 2 years of age. Children with septic arthritis usually have a rapid onset of limping or refuse to walk. Commonly, there is a history of fever and irritability. Examination reveals limited and painful range of motion. Fever, leukocytosis with a left shift, and an elevated ESR are characteristic laboratory findings. X-rays may be normal (early stage) or reveal erosions (late stage). Bone scan or MRI may be helpful to localize the disease. Arthrocentesis is diagnostic. If septic arthritis is suspected, emergent orthopedic referral is indicated.

TRANSIENT SYNOVITIS

Transient synovitis is a sterile effusion of the hip that resolves without therapy or sequelae.[21] It is the most common cause of pediatric hip pain, typically affecting boys 3 to 7 years of age.[20] The child usually presents with a limp. If present, pain may be localized to the groin, medial thigh, or **knee**. Examination reveals mild restriction of motion, particularly abduction.[21] The CBC, ESR, and x-rays are usually normal.

Most children can be treated by bed rest, with close observation for systemic signs. Emergent orthopedic referral is indicated in those cases with signs or symptoms suggestive of septic arthritis.

Conclusion

Although the evaluation of the patient who presents with the chief complaint of hip pain may sometimes seem overwhelming, the clinical approach outlined in the chapter can make this task more manageable. Hopefully, the clinician used to dreading seeing "hip pain" on his or her clinic schedule will now take on this diagnostic challenge with more enthusiasm.

References

1. Sutton WR: Functional anatomy of the pelvis and hip. In: Baker CL (ed): *The Hughston Clinic Sports Medicine Book*. Philadelphia: Williams & Wilkins: 1995;379.
2. Reid DC: Problems of the hip, pelvis, and sacroiliac joint. *Sports Injury Assessment and Rehabilitation*. New York: Churchill Livingstone; 1992;601.
3. Murtagh J: Hip and buttock pain in adults. *Aust Fam Physician* 21:848, 1996.
4. Greenman PE: Pelvic girdle dysfunction. *Principles of Manual Medicine*. Philadelphia: Williams & Wilkins; 1996;305.
5. Liebermann JR: Hip and thigh. In: Snider RK (ed): *Essentials of Musculoskeletal Care*. American Academy of Orthopedic Surgeons, 1997;265.
6. Conway WF, Totty WG, McEnery KW: CT and MR imaging of the hip. *Radiology* 198:297, 1996.
7. O'Kane JW: Anterior hip pain. *Am Fam Physician* 60:1687, 1999.
8. Weiker GG: How I manage hip and pelvis injuries in adolescents. *Phys Sport Med* 21:72, 1993.
9. Toohey AK, LaSalle TL, Martinez S, et al: Iliopsoas bursitis: clinical features, radiographic findings and disease associations. *Semin Arthrit Rheumat* 20:41, 1997.
10. Weiker GG: Selected hip and pelvis injuries. *Phys Sport Med* 22:96, 1994.
11. Boden BP, Speer KF: Femoral stress fractures. *Clin Sports Med* 16:3077, 1997.
12. Deutsch AL, Coel MN, Mink JH: Imaging of stress injuries to bone: Radiography, scintigraphy and MR imaging. *Clin Sports Med* 16:275, 1997.
13. Brukner PD, Khan KM: *Clinical Sports Medicine*. Sydney: McGraw-Hill; 1993.
14. Kemp S, Batt ME: The "sports hernia": A common cause of groin pain. *Phys Sport Med* 26:36, 1998.
15. Brukner PD, Bradshaw C, McCrory P: Obturator neuropathy: A cause of exercise-related groin pain. *Phys Sport Med* 27:62, 1999.
16. Kahler DM: Overuse injuries of the hip. In: Baker CL (ed): *The Hughston Clinic Sports Medicine Book*. Philadelphia: Williams & Wilkins; 1995;401.
17. Housner JA, Schwenk TL: Musculoskeletal injuries: ten principles of rehabilitation. *Consultant* 37:1777, 1997.
18. Plancher KD, Razi A: Management of osteonecrosis of the femoral head. *Orthop Clin North Am* 28:461, 1997.
19. Dyment PG: Apophyseal injuries. *Pediatr Ann* 26:28, 1997.
20. Lewis DP: Evaluation of the limping child. *Fam Prac Recert* 20:15, 1998.
21. Greene W: Pediatric orthopaedics. In: Snider RK (ed): *Essentials of Musculoskeletal Care*. American Academy of Orthopedic Surgeons, 1997;548.

Harry L. Galanty

Anterior Knee Pain

Introduction

Anterior knee pain is one of the most common musculoskeletal complaints seen in both sports medicine and primary care. Despite its frequent occurrence, this problem remains somewhat enigmatic. Not only are the exact causes of anterior knee pain debated, but therapy, although usually effective, has long been inconsistent.

Anterior knee pain has been recognized as a clinical entity since the early 1900s. As our understanding of this problem has progressed, its name has been changed and broadened to reflect the variety of entities that may cause this pain. Referred to as chondromalacia patella, patellofemoral pain syndrome, excessive lateral pressure syndrome, and anterior knee pain, these names reflect changes in how this entity has been conceptualized.

The demands placed on the knee during physical activity make anterior knee pain prevalent in the athletic population. In fact, studies show that this problem represents up to 10 percent of all sports medicine visits.[1] Reported to be the most common complaint among runners and especially prevalent in adolescent athletes, anterior knee pain represents the most common overuse injury in sports medicine.[2,3]

The term chondromalacia patellae was introduced in the literature by Koenig in 1924.[4] Since that time, it has commonly been used to describe the clinical entity of anterior knee pain. By definition, chondromalacia refers to softening of the articular cartilage of the posterior patella, a diagnosis that can only be made by direct observation at surgery. The pain syndrome associated with anterior knee pain, however, may or may not correlate specifically with changes found on the patella. In fact, up to half of patients with anterior knee pain have normal patellar cartilage on surgical examination.[5] From these general inconsistencies, the need arises to understand the concepts of patellar alignment and the biomechanics of the patellofemoral unit that play a major role in the cause, diagnosis, and treatment of anterior knee pain.

History

Early literature postulated that in chondromalacia patellae, degenerative cartilage changes were the cause of anterior knee pain. In addition, it was initially believed to be a precursor for the subsequent development of osteoarthritis. Outerbridge described a classification, still used today, of the four grades of severity for chondromalacia patellae from observations during open meniscectomies.[6] He theorized that the medial ridge of the patella succumbed to repetitive compression during knee flexion and subsequent injury led to breakdown of this cartilage. In contrast, Hughston believed that injury to the medial facet was related to repetitive subluxing of the patella against the lateral trochlea of the femur, thus initiating the concept of subluxation as one of the important causes of patellofemoral pain.[7] Ficat and Hungerford described the more popular belief that tight lateral retinacular tissues would produce lateral pressure on the patella with the chronic stress leading to cartilaginous injury and pain.[8] Advancing this theory, Insall proposed that certain anatomic variations and alignment patterns may accentuate these symptoms.[9] Although each of these explanations represents a distinct theory as to a cause for this pain, an underlying theme in all of these theories is a disturbance to the natural alignment of the patella and how it tracks throughout motion in the femoral trochlea.

Anatomy

The patellofemoral joint is made up of the patella and the femoral trochlea, a shallow groove through which the patella glides. The patella is a sesamoid bone and, as such, it lies within the quadriceps tendon. Its main function is to act as a fulcrum to increase the lever arm of the quadriceps muscle in knee extension. The articular surface of the patella is covered with smooth hyaline cartilage. This cartilage varies between 4 and 5 mm in thickness, making it the thickest portion of hyaline cartilage in the body; it is responsible for protection of the knee during load bearing. Being both insensate and avascular, sensation in the region arises in the subchondral bone and peripatellar soft tissues.[10]

Survival of the cartilage is dependent on the pressures exerted on it through motion and activity.[2] These pressures force articular fluid into the cartilage, thus providing nourishment for the cartilage. It is interesting to note that not only can excessive pressure lead to degradation and breakdown of the articular surface, but also that the lack of pressure may lead to death of the cartilagenous tissue from insufficient nutrition.

The posterior patella has a medial and lateral facet forming a convex shape to conform with the trochlear groove of the femur. The patella moves (or tracks) through this femoral articular surface during knee extension and flexion. At full extension, the patella sits superior to the trochlea and as flexion progresses, the patella initiates its contact. Initial contact of the patella occurs at its distal pole as the knee reaches 20° of flexion.[11] As further flexion continues, the contact area of the patella with the femur moves proximally, while also increasing its area. By 90° of flexion, the contact area, which is now maximal, has reached the superior aspect of the patella. Beyond 90° this contact area diminishes

slightly, with only the lateral and medial edges of the patellar facets touching the articular surface of the femur.[11] This increased contact area is extremely important as it disperses patellofemoral forces, maintaining a constant load on the joint even when the total load continues to rise with greater flexion.

Patellar tracking describes the appropriate motion of the patella within the femoral trochlea. Any abnormalities in tracking will lead to changes in patellofemoral forces, disrupting their normal dispersion by the articular surface. The normal contact area is thus altered, which creates higher than normal loads on the joint and thereby leads to injury.

The greatest control for tracking comes from both the dynamic and static stabilizers of the patella (Fig. 7-1). The main dynamic stabilizers for the patellofemoral joint are the surrounding muscles, including the quadriceps mechanism and iliotibial band. As the only muscle providing a medial force, the vastus medialis oblique (VMO) muscle of the quadriceps mechanism plays an important role in stabilizing the patella. Each of the other muscles of the quadriceps provide a lateral pull. The static stabilizers of the patellofemoral joint include the articular capsule, the retinaculum surrounding the patellofemoral joint, and the patellofemoral ligaments. It appears that the medial patellofemoral ligament is the major static restraint to lateral displacement of the patella contributing greater than 50 percent of support on testing.[12]

A great deal of force is borne by the patella during weight-bearing activities. It is estimated that the pressure exerted by the patella on the femur during walking is about one-third of body weight. With stair climbing and full squatting, the forces can be up to three times and seven times that of body weight, respectively.[2] Athletic activities can increase these forces even further. The patella must be able to continually absorb these forces so that the athlete can perform with-

Figure 7-1

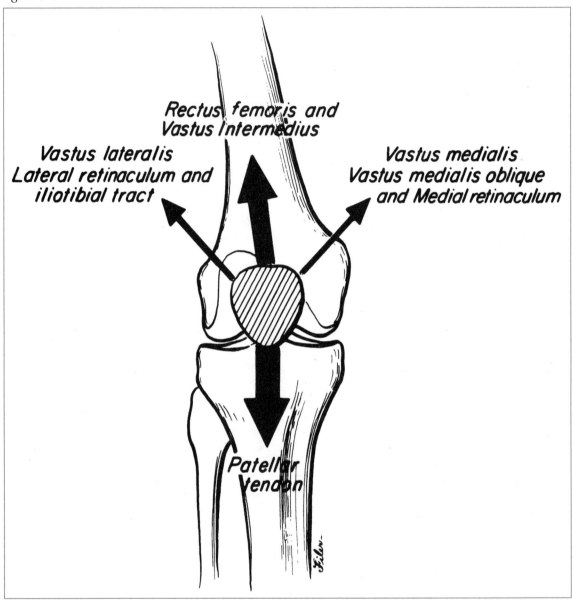

Forces acting on the patella. *(Adapted with permission from Fu FH, Seel MJ, Berger RA: Patellofemoral biomechanics. In: Fox J, Del Pizzo W (eds). The Patellofemoral Joint. Blue Ridge Summit, PA: McGraw-Hill, Inc.; 1993:49).*

out any loss of function. Any imbalances that occur in the relationship between the body and its alignment can influence the patellofemoral joint and the resultant reaction forces.

Causes of Pain

It is very difficult to explain exactly why pain develops under and around the patella. Considerable documentation of the poor association between softened patellar articular cartilage and pain in the anterior knee exists, but it is known that no nerve endings exist in the articular cartilage.[13] In fact, the largest number of nerve fibers is found in the retinaculum and capsule surrounding the joint.[14] Fulkerson has shown that pain often exists around the retinacular regions. In addition, he identified small nerve injuries at these locations in patients with anterior knee pain.[15] It has been hypothesized, therefore, that abnormal stress or stretching of these tissues may be associated with the increased sensation of pain. Dye even exposed himself to pain testing during unanesthetized arthroscopy, reporting the most significant pain to be located in the peripatellar regions.[16] These highly innervated tissues likely play a large role in the development of knee pain, with exacerbation occurring from stretching or imbalances that take place during knee motion.

Clinical History

The most common complaint seen in athletes with patellofemoral problems is pain, but it is often generalized and difficult to pinpoint to an exact location. Some will state that the pain is directly beneath the patella, whereas others will complain that it is in the peripatellar regions. In some instances, pain may be referred to the posterior or popliteal region of the knee. Quite often, patients place their hands completely over the anterior aspect of their knee in describing the location of their pain. The quality of the pain is typically nagging, yet some will describe it as an ice pick or sharp pain around the kneecap. It is rarely constant, seldom inhibiting the patient from walking or performing most routine activities.

The pain is accentuated in those activities that increase patellofemoral forces, including sports, climbing or descending stairs, squatting, crawling, or kneeling. It is important to ask about traumatic injuries, as in certain instances a fall on the knee can lead to retinacular injury and the development of anterior knee pain. Patients may also report episodes of subluxation or dislocation of the patella. With subluxation, they may describe a feeling of giving way or a popping of the knee joint, leading one to suspect that instability may be an underlying cause of their patellofemoral symptoms.

The theater sign, in which the patient complains of patellar pain after prolonged sitting (such as in a movie theater), may be present in patients with patellofemoral symptoms. Giving way, which is sometimes reported, is not caused by true instability of the knee joint but is likely due to a pain inhibition response. The clinician should also question the patient as to other activities that they perform, because overuse secondary to sports may increase the likelihood of knee pain. Any changes in activity, such as increased practice or running mileage, can exacerbate symptoms.

Physical Examination

Malalignment

Observation is the initial step in the physical examination, and the examiner should observe

Figure 7-2

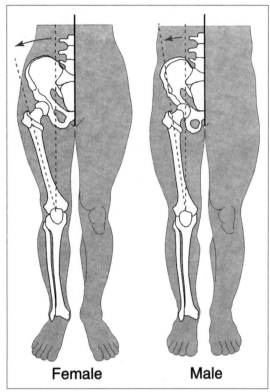

Female   **Male**

Factors causing malalignment: femoral anteversion and increased Q angle. *(Reprinted with permission from Arendt EA, Teitz CC: The lower extremities. In: Teitz CC (ed). The Female Athlete. Rosemont, IL: American Academy Orthopaedic Surgeons; 1997:45).*

the patient in the standing, seated, and lying positions, looking for signs of malalignment. Malalignment refers to those anatomic factors that influence the stabilizers, causing the patella to pull or rotate laterally with knee motion. The majority of patients do not have signs of malalignment; however, if they are present, malalignment has been reported to increase the likelihood of improper tracking.[10,17,18]

Factors causing malalignment include anteversion of the femoral neck and external tibial torsion (Fig. 7-2). Both of these factors can increase the Q angle, a measurement to detect abnormal alignment. To measure the Q angle, the patient must lie in the supine position. Lines

are extended from the anterior superior iliac spine to the center of the patella and then from the tibial tubercle through the center of the patella.[19] The normal measurement for the Q angle is less than 10° in males and 15° in females, with angles greater than 20° considered abnormal. The greater the Q angle, the greater the likelihood of abnormal tracking. Pes planus can cause further lateral rotation of the lower extremities, increasing the Q angle and leading to malalignment.

Range of Motion and Crepitus

Once the examiner has observed the general alignment of the patients' lower extremities, it is important to evaluate the patella and its surrounding structures. The clinician must assess range of motion of the knee; those with patellofemoral pain rarely have limitations to motion. Then, the hand should be placed on the patella to palpate for crepitus. In many instances, crepitus does not cause pain and, therefore, it is unlikely that patellar cartilage breakdown is the cause of the problem. However, the clinician must be concerned about the possibility of articular cartilage injury if crepitus is painful.[20]

Palpation

An assessment is then made to locate the site of the patellar pain. The patella is palpated under both the medial and lateral facets, insertion site of the quadriceps and patellar tendon, and the surrounding peripatellar regions. Retinacular structures are also palpated medially and laterally for any specific areas of tenderness.

The patella itself is compressed with the knee in extension and in flexion of at least 30°. Compression in these positions often recreates the symptoms in someone suffering anterior knee pain.

The quadriceps compression test is also a sensitive test for anterior knee pain. In this test, the clinician will place an inferiorly directed force

Figure 7-3

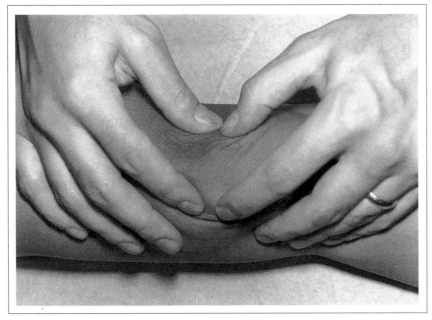

Testing patellar mobility.

along the patella as the quadriceps is contracted. Contraction most likely stresses the painful structures, thereby recreating the specific symptoms and elucidating the diagnosis.

Patellar Position and Mobility

Examination should include a close inspection of the patellar position in relation to the peripatellar tissues. The patella should be mobilized to evaluate whether these tissues are overly tight, causing possible tracking abnormalities and even pain (Fig. 7-3). Lateral displacement and tilt are the most common tracking abnormalities.

With the patient supine, the clinician may grasp the patella with the thumb and forefingers and attempt to elevate the lateral aspect of the patella and feel its lateral undersurface. Inability to palpate this lateral articular surface is consistent with tight lateral structures. If pain is also elicited, this tightness is the likely instigator.

A glide test may also be performed to evaluate the structures supporting the patella.[19] This test involves placing the knee in 20 to 30° of flexion, with the examiner measuring how many quadrants the patella may be passively moved in both the medial and lateral directions. The patella is divided into four quadrants and should easily displace two quadrants in both directions. If the examiner is unable to displace the patella medially more than one quadrant, then once again, the patient has excessive tightness of the lateral retinaculum.

In certain instances, a patella can be so mobile that it moves three or more quadrants. This is seen in two circumstances: (1) the patient with prior injury to the supporting structures and (2) the patient with generalized ligamentous laxity. This laxity is more likely painful with lateral displacement of the patella in the previously injured knee. If it causes a sense of instability, it is referred to as apprehension. The patient may actually have symptomatology of subluxation, which is another suggestion of patellar instability and poor tracking. Observation may detect a

Figure 7-4

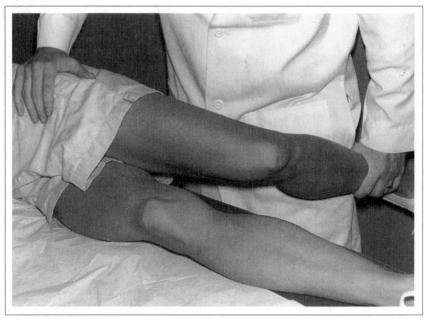

Ober's test is performed by hyperextending and internally rotating the hip.

patella that moves to an excessively lateral position as full extension is reached. This is known as the "J" sign, pathognomonic for subluxation.

Quadriceps

The physician should also inspect the musculature of the quadriceps, specifically that of the VMO. Tenderness may occur in this region, but atrophy is more common. A weak VMO denotes a tracking problem because this muscle creates the only force dynamically that can help resist the lateral pull on the patella. The longer the symptoms have been present, the more likely a significant amount of atrophy will be present.

Flexibility

Lower extremity flexibility must be assessed with special attention paid to the iliotibial band. Ober's test best assesses its flexibility. By placing the patient on his or her side with the injured leg being examined closest to the physician, the hip is then hyperextended and internally rotated (Fig. 7-4). If excessive tightness or pain is exhibited along the lateral structures of the thigh, then the test is positive and this inflexibility must be considered as causing or contributing to pain.

Other Structures

It is also important to note that anterior knee pain need not be specifically related to the patellofemoral region. The clinician should examine the patellar tendon and its attachments for pain to assess for signs of apophysitis, tendinitis, or bursitis. In examining younger patients, sometimes hip and back pain radiate to the knee. A full lower extremity examination will rule out any significant underlying hip or back pathology that may be causing so-called knee pain. Legg-Calvé-Perthes disease and slipped capital femoral epiphysis are reported causes of referred knee pain that can cause significant disability if they are not diagnosed and treated.

Ancillary Tests

X-Rays

Radiographic studies are an important part of the clinical examination of patients with patellofemoral pathology. X-rays should include standard anterior-posterior, lateral, and axial views of the knee. To visualize the patella, most experts suggest using the Merchant axial view. This view is obtained with the patient lying supine, knees flexed between 30 and 45°, with the film shot from the superior to the inferior direction along the line of the patella.[21] The AP and lateral views can help rule out associated serious bony conditions, such as tumors and infections, as well as detect bony loose bodies within the knee joint. A lateral radiograph of the knee can also help in the assessment of patella alta or baja. The Merchant view will demonstrate malalignment and also portray the shape of the patella and the femoral condyles, assisting in the assessment of femoral or patellar dysplasias.[21]

Certain measurements have been extrapolated from the Merchant view, such as the patellofemoral index and the congruence angles.[22] These measurements designate distances between the femoral condyles and facets of the patella, quantifying the amount of patellar angulation. Although they are helpful in deciding the severity of patellar tilt, and assist with preoperative planning, these measurements are not necessarily needed as part of the general evaluation for anterior knee pain.

Other Imaging Studies

Although not indicated in the routine study of anterior knee pain, computed tomography (CT) can be useful in defining the presence and amount of malalignment. Images are taken repeatedly at varying degrees of knee flexion (extension, 15°, 30°, 45°, and 60°) and patellar tracking is noted at each of these different angles of flexion.[10] CT evaluation is beneficial in the analysis of extreme cases of patellar tilt unresponsive to normal therapeutic options. In addition, this assessment can help plan surgical treatment.

Magnetic resonance imaging (MRI) is helpful in the evaluation of articular cartilage and soft tissue structures. Thus, it is helpful in detecting patellar or femoral osteochondritis dissecans and can further define those tendon injuries not seen on other radiographic imaging studies. MRI is, however, less useful in evaluating patellofemoral malalignment than CT.

Technetium bone scan is rarely needed for the patients with anterior knee pain. However, it may be selectively useful in identifying occult injuries such as fractures or other pathology that may escape detection with other imaging tests.

Other Testing

Blood testing is almost never required in the evaluation of anterior knee pain. However, for those patients in whom infection or a rheumatologic disorder is suspected, blood tests such as a CBC, ESR, and ANA may help determine the diagnosis.

Differential Diagnosis

Following a complete history and physical examination, the clinician should create a differential diagnosis consistent with the data accumulated. Generally, the clinician can expect that the majority of cases will represent the classic anterior knee pain syndrome that has been described. However, a number of entities exist that can be similar to anterior knee pain and must, therefore, be considered. This section discusses those diagnoses and provides some specific treatment options.

Patellar Instability/Subluxation

Although complaints and symptomatology will be very similar to those of anterior knee pain, patients with patellar instability/subluxation may report recurrent lateral dislocation of the patella or episodes of slipping and catching of the patella with certain maneuvers. In those who have had acute episodes, medial retinacular structures may be most tender and possibly have some swelling. Patellar apprehension will be present with lateral pressure, although pain and apprehension are less common in patients with more subtle instabilities. If the patella moves three or more quadrants laterally and subluxation episodes have been experienced, one can be reasonably confident that underlying instability exists. Radiographs and CT scan may be beneficial to confirm these patellar instabilities.

In the majority of cases, patellar instability can be treated in the same fashion as anterior knee pain. However, if instability episodes continue to limit routine or athletic activities and do not respond to the recommended programs, surgical treatment for stabilization of the patella may become necessary.

Posttraumatic Patellofemoral Pain

This condition occurs following a blow directly to the patella from a fall on the knee or a car dashboard injury. In these instances, the degree of damage to the articular cartilage often determines the severity of injury. Pain will usually be posterior to the patella and patellar compression can be exquisitely painful. Effusions are more common in this situation as well. Most episodes of posttraumatic anterior knee pain will respond to a rehabilitation program but in some in-

stances, posttraumatic patellofemoral pain may persist longer than the other types of knee pain. It is important to recognize that damage to the articular cartilage can complicate the symptomatology. If longstanding pain exists, which is unresponsive to treatment, MRI and potentially arthroscopy may be beneficial to confirm the severity of the damage and allow for more aggressive therapeutic intervention, such as debridement or resection of the offending area of cartilage.

Patellar Arthrosis

This diagnosis is more likely found in the older patient, and is often a result of old patellar fractures, longstanding severe patellar tilt, or idiopathic degeneration of the patellar articular surface.[18] Most of the pain is found directly posterior to the patella, and crepitus is common and in most cases, will be painful. Malalignment is an unlikely finding in this disorder. Radiographs of the patellofemoral joint will demonstrate this arthrosis, and when found, patients will respond better with a reduction of stress-related activities performed by the knee.

Formal exercise programs can be beneficial, and nonsteroidal anti-inflammatory agents can also control pain. Unfortunately, conservative treatment programs cannot reverse articular damage that has already taken place; they can only control symptoms.

Osteochondritis Dissecans (OCD)

OCD is a form of avascular necrosis that tangentially affects the articular surface. Although the majority of OCD lesions are found in the femoral condyles, this condition can also affect the articular surface of the patella. A history of antecedent trauma is usually not elicited, but pain is found directly posterior to the patella and tenderness can be appreciated with patellar compression. Swelling is more common with activities. Radiographic studies, such as patellofemoral radiographs or MRI, can be diagnostic. Osteochondritis dissecans of the patella can be an extremely difficult problem to correct. A large number of these cases will fail conservative treatment (usually joint rest) and are likely to require arthroscopic evaluation and possibly, debridement or drilling of the osteochondral defect.[10]

Patellar Tendinitis

This should be easily distinguished from other types of anterior knee pain by the physical examination. Pain will be found directly over the patellar tendon, which is inferior to the patella. Pain can be elicited with resisted quadriceps extensions and squatting activities. This entity is more likely seen in athletes who perform jumping activities such as basketball and volleyball. While plain radiographs are rarely helpful, MRI can delineate the soft tissue inflammatory changes and breakdown that can occur in chronic episodes of tendinitis. Patellar tendinitis can be difficult to treat, especially with athletes who continue to participate in their sport. Periods of rest with formal physical therapy and strengthening programs can be quite beneficial. Often the use of an infrapatellar strap or band can relieve some of the pressure and allow continued participation in activities. Surgical exploration and debridement of the tendon may be helpful in those cases unresponsive to any conservative treatment options.

Bursitis

There are many bursae surrounding the anterior aspect of the knee and inflammation in these bursae can mimic anterior knee pain. The most common bursitis encountered is prepatellar bursitis. The prepatellar bursa sits anterior to the patella and inflammation of this bursa can occur after a direct blow to the patella, or in patients, such as carpet layers, who perform prolonged kneeling activities. Pain is typically evident only if there is inflammation or infection to this bursa. Most cases will present with a soft swollen area directly over the patella and thickening of the skin may be present due to repetitive trauma. The typical patellar malalignment examination will be normal, with no tilt or patellar compression pain.

Rest, ice, anti-inflammatory medications, and avoidance of offending activities are the mainstay of treatment. If infected, antibiotics should be prescribed. Aspiration of the bursae is sometimes recommended, yet in many cases following this procedure, the inflammatory fluid will just reaccumulate.

Plica

The plical bands are synovial folds or redundancies situated in the peripatellar regions, most often in proximity to the medial retinaculum. These become symptomatic following overuse. If a thickened, inflamed plica can be palpated on examination and doing so recreates the patient's pain, the diagnosis is likely. Treatment includes patellofemoral training and reduction of inflammation with occasional corticosteroid injections. This can provide relief to the symptomatic tissue. If no improvement occurs with these treatments, arthroscopic resection of the plica may be indicated.

Apophysitis

The most common cause for anterior knee pain between the ages of 9 and 12 is Osgood-Schlatter disease. Physical examination will demonstrate tenderness, swelling, and inflammation at the tibial tubercle, not under or around the patella itself. These patients respond well to modified activities and symptom-related treatments. Symptoms rarely occur following skeletal maturity. Apophysitis is discussed in more detail in Chap. 17.

Management

Although it has been stressed that the exact cause of anterior knee pain can be truly difficult to diagnose, the fact that most patients with this disorder respond extremely well to specific conservative treatment techniques makes understanding of these treatment options especially important.[23–26] In many instances, a clinician seeing a patient with patellofemoral symptoms will immediately send the patient to the therapist stating "evaluate and treat." All of the treatment options are then left to the therapist, hoping that the therapist is well versed in those techniques most beneficial to the patient. Ideally, however, the sports medicine clinician should be in charge of the specific care and rehabilitation of the patient with anterior knee pain. If the clinician keeps up with the treatment programs and closely follows the athlete's progress or lack thereof, treatment can be modified to assure further improvement expeditiously.

Rehabilitation Theories

Several theories underlie the overall rehabilitation program that is performed for anterior knee pain. Keeping these in mind will allow the clinician to understand how the therapy program addresses patellofemoral pain.

THEORY 1

Initially during a therapy program, attempts should be made to keep patellofemoral contact forces at a minimum. In this way the pressure, which can be destructive to the articular surface of the patellofemoral joint, can be controlled. Knowing that patellofemoral contact force is greatest between 60 and 110° of knee flexion, most exercises should be performed at less than

45° of knee flexion.[12] By limiting exercise-related pain, the rehabilitation programs progress more quickly to functional activities.

THEORY 2

Stabilization and medialization of the patella are extremely important components of the program. Tight lateral structures, including the retinaculum, must be stretched to help centralize patellar tracking and eliminate pain. Taping and soft tissue techniques will also correct this problem.

THEORY 3

Muscular endurance is more important than strength. Muscle fatigue, specifically of the VMO, is thought to play a role in the lack of ability of the patella to maintain central tracking. As a result of pain or lack of use from injury, this muscle can become quite weak. If this muscle is unable to maintain consistent strength and provide stability during repetitive activities that can often exacerbate anterior knee pain, poor tracking and pain can develop. A good rehabilitation program will stress this endurance factor to enhance and extend performance.

THEORY 4

Because a lot of the pain appears to originate from fibers in the peripatellar retinaculum, the mainstay of a successful treatment program is the cessation of these painful stimuli. Successful techniques include taping and stretching of lateral structures, which will decrease activity in the sensation fibers around the patella. Although specific scientific data does not exist to explain how pain is completely relieved, it is likely that these techniques improve reflex inhibition, improve proprioceptive sense, and inhibit pain.[13,20]

Physical Therapy Program

FLEXIBILITY

Improved flexibility is a cornerstone in patellofemoral rehabilitation. Patellofemoral contact forces, which are increased during activity, can be lessened if the contracting muscles around the joint are more flexible. Stretching of the quadriceps is the most important way to improve muscle flexibility and can be done easily with the patient in the prone position with the heel pulled toward the buttock. One may facilitate this stretch by using a towel wrapped around the ankle. The athlete's progress can be assessed easily by measuring the distance between the heel and buttock.

Hamstring flexibility also affects patellofemoral contact pressure, especially during knee extension. Suggested exercises include standing toe touches or hurdler's stretches. The gastrocnemius is stretched in coordination with hamstring maneuvers by dorsiflexing the foot. Finally, the lateral structures, namely the lateral retinaculum and the iliotibial band, should be mobilized. The lateral retinacular structures can be stretched passively by the therapist, and then patients are taught to continue these stretches on their own. For the iliotibial band, cross adduction of the hip will accentuate the tendon's flexibility.

STRENGTHENING

Strengthening of the entire lower extremity is important and will benefit the patient with patellofemoral pain, but emphasis should be placed on strengthening the quadriceps and specifically the VMO.[1,26,27] For many years, the typical strength program for patellofemoral pain has included straight leg raises and quadriceps extension exercises. Some studies now show that this approach may actually aggravate patellofemoral compression as well as worsen the patellar alignment.[28] Steinkamp noted that

leg press exercises, or closed chain exercises from 0 to 30° of knee flexion, will stimulate quadriceps strengthening and decrease patellofemoral joint reaction forces in comparison to knee extensions.[29] Thus, it may be more beneficial to perform leg presses in the earlier stages of rehabilitation as they may limit pain by lowering these forces (Fig. 7-5).

It is logical that the most beneficial therapy program would be one that could either isolate the VMO during exercise or strengthen it preferentially. Unfortunately, at this point it does not appear that most strengthening exercises can specifically work the VMO preferentially over the other muscles of the quadriceps mechanism.[30] Most of the strengthening exercises recommended during therapy will strengthen the quadriceps diffusely; however, those exercises creating the greatest preference for strengthening the VMO are isometric knee extensions at 15° of flexion.

Another approach to selectively strengthen the VMO is biofeedback training.[24] By facilitating selective muscular timing and training to encourage the VMO to contract earlier in the gait cycle or in flexion activities, the patella is theoretically stabilized earlier.

A strengthening program should also involve a majority of closed chain exercises. Exercises are considered closed chain if the athlete keeps the foot in contact with the floor while exercise occurs. Squats and leg presses are good examples of these exercises. Patterned to be similar to their athletic maneuvers, closed chain exercises teach the athlete how to perform correct VMO contractions. Over the course of treatment, the activities will be increased with an emphasis on endurance. Each exercise is continued until the athlete reaches fatigue as long as pain does not interfere. Another important point is that as strength improves, the program should be molded to recreate activities of daily living and the athlete's specific functional activities. The clinician should want to emphasize those flexed

Figure 7-5

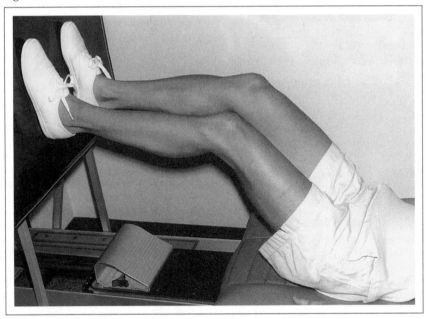

Leg presses: an example of a closed chain exercise.

knee positions commonly maintained during sports and strengthen similarly during therapy (Fig. 7-6). With restoration of the proper motor patterns, the patient will develop further muscle memory and endurance strength, both of which are protective during activity. Our progressive strengthening program is shown in Table 7-1. As the patient continues to show progress, both an increased number of repetitions and progressive resistance may be added to these exercises. If the patient develops pain, then the exercises are limited and repetitions decreased until pain is well controlled.

With most of our athletes, it is not only imperative that they perform these exercises while under the therapist's supervision, they must also continue to perform them on their own. By teaching and reinforcing a good program to be performed daily, the patients build confidence in the program, allowing them to be more easily weaned from the formal therapy program.

PATELLAR TAPING

Patellar taping, the newest treatment approach to anterior knee pain, has been successful based on limited reports. The most widely used program, recommended by McConnell, involves mobilizing the patella by altering its position through surface tape.[31] Tape is pulled across the patella, causing changes of pressures and correcting the position of the patella at rest and through motion.

The therapist initially evaluates the position of the patella relative to the femoral condyles. Patellar malalignment may occur in four directions: laterally positioned (glide), tilted laterally, tilted in the anterior/posterior plane, or rotated. Multiple abnormalities may exist concomitantly. Following an assessment, the tape is placed over the patella pulling it to a more central position and controlling its abnormal motion. With a successful taping program, the pain encountered during exercise and activity is substantially and

Figure 7-6

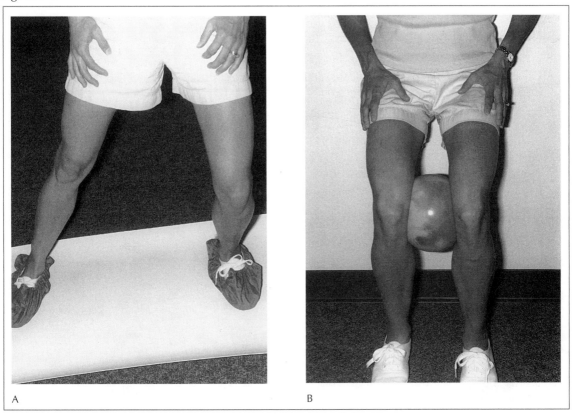

Progression of quadriceps training. **(A)** Slide board. **(B)**. Partial squats with ball between knees to accentuate adduction.

almost immediately reduced. This program allows for early and more aggressive exercises with minimal pain.

One test the author has found helpful in deciding if patellar taping may be beneficial uses various patellar manipulations during resisted knee extensions. If correcting tilts or glides during this motion causes a decrease in the symptoms, then there is a much better likelihood that patellar taping will provide benefit during rehabilitation (Fig. 7-7).

If the taping is successful, patients are taught to perform the taping on their own and should continue to wear the tape during offending activities. Once improvement in symptomatology and

quadriceps strength has occurred, they can be weaned from the tape. However, if certain activities continue to cause pain, there is little disadvantage to long-term taping for specific sports activities.

Even though it has been hypothesized that taping leads to improved patellar tracking, studies do not seem to support this theory. In fact with aggressive exercise, tape has been unable to hold any changes in patellar tracking.[32,33] Even though one cannot find consistent patellar stabilization through taping, the most consistent finding of this taping program is reduction in pain.[20] Pain alleviation is likely related to subtle changes in patellofemoral pressures and

Table 7-1

Patellofemoral Syndrome: Rehabilitation Progression

TREATMENT PROGRESSION*
Isometrics
Quad sets, Hamstring sets, Quad sets with adduction (electrical stimulation with quad sets may
help strengthen quads)
Straight leg raise (SLR) with quad sets
Straight SLR
Add external rotation of foot 45° when SLR pain free
Isometric closed chain exercise
Partial squat, hold at comfortable knee angle
Progress to balance board as strength improves
Low amplitude dynamic leg extension
Rocker board low amplitude side to side movement
Stairs with low amplitude steps, progress step height as tolerated
Leg press bilateral
Start with low weights and quarter squats
Progress weight and squat depth as pain-free range improves
Leg press with adduction
Add ball or pillow between knees
Progress weight and squat depth as pain-free range improves
Stairs
Progress step height, resistance, and time
Unilateral leg press
Add as tolerated

*Patient must be able to tolerate each level without increased pain as they progress.

decrease in the pain efferent fiber stimulation. It is important to note, however, that the only prospective study assessing the use of tape in therapy found no benefit over a standard strengthening program.[34]

MALALIGNMENT

Correction of malalignment has a place in anterior knee pain treatment, especially if the treatment regimen just presented is not successful. The most common method for correcting lower extremity malalignment is the use of orthoses for pes planus and foot pronation. The use of over-the-counter or custom-molded orthoses for these conditions can help decrease internal rotation of the lower extremities, thus correcting an increased Q angle that contributes to anterior knee pain.

OTHER MODALITIES

ICE AND ULTRASOUND   Ice is the most commonly used modality for pain and inflammation control. Following a completed therapy session, patients apply ice as a massage over the tender areas of the patellofemoral region. Other modalities, such as ultrasound and electrical stimulation, may be included when significant pain in the early

Figure 7-7

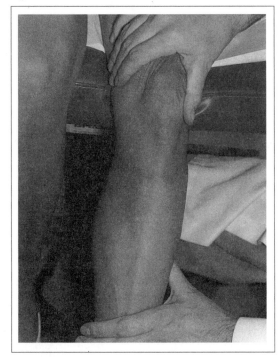

Correction of glide during a resisted knee extension: if knee pain improves, patellar taping may be beneficial.

stages of rehabilitation prevents even the mildest of quadriceps strengthening activities.

BRACES

Although bracing alone is not an appropriate therapy, patellofemoral bracing can have a role in treatment of anterior knee pain. There are many braces available, all of which attempt to buttress the lateral aspect of the patella and prevent it from subluxing laterally. No clinical studies have shown that these braces perform these functions; however, it is likely that they provide feedback similar to that of taping, making patients aware of mild pressure changes and improving proprioception.[35] Bracing alone is not appropriate.

ACTIVITY MODIFICATION

When symptoms are severe, the athlete must be withdrawn from athletic participation. In these situations, it is best to suggest a short period of relative rest for the injured knee, but allow limited aerobic activities to keep the athlete as fit as possible. In these instances, a short course of nonsteroidal anti-inflammatory medications may be indicated as well. Fortunately, few athletes complain of this much pain, so removal from sports participation is rarely needed.

Conditions to Refer

The mainstay of treatment is nonoperative, yet a small subset of patients exist who do not respond at all to a nonsurgical approach. Such patients will have undergone 4 to 6 months of physical therapy without substantial improvement. These patients should be referred to an orthopedic surgeon, who may suggest procedures to abate the patients' symptoms. Such operations include arthroscopic debridement, particularly for those with true chondromalacia or patellar arthrosis.[36,37] For those with diagnosed patellofemoral malalignment, recommended procedures include lateral releases and bony realignment procedures. Both of these surgeries decrease patellar forces by shifting the patella itself, or by moving the tibial tubercle either medially or anteriorly. Each of these procedures has been reported in the literature to improve symptomology if done appropriately.[10,19]

References

1. Natri A, Kannus P, Jarvinen M: Which factors predict the long-term outcome in chronic patellofemoral pain syndrome? A 7-yr prospective

follow-up study. *Med Sci Sports Exerc* 30:1572, 1998.

2. Percy ED, Strother RT: Patellalgia. *Physician Sportsmed* 13:43, 1985.

3. Galanty H, Matthews C, Hergenroeder AC: Anterior knee pain in adolescents. *Clin J Sports Med* 4:176, 1994.

4. Kelly MA, Insall JN: Historical perspectives of chondromalacia patellae. In: Scuderi GR (ed): *The Orthopedic Clinics of North America*. Philadelphia: WB Saunders Co; 1992;517.

5. Hughston JC, Walsh WM, Puddu G: *Patellar Subluxation and Dislocation*. Philadelphia: WB Saunders Co; 1984.

6. Outerbridge RE: The etiology of chondromalacia patellae. *J Bone Joint Surg* 43-B:752, 1961.

7. Hughston JC: Subluxation of the patella. *J Bone Joint Surg* 50(A):1003, 1968.

8. Ficat RP, Hungerford DS: *Disorders of the patellofemoral joint*. Baltimore: Williams & Wilkins; 1977.

9. Insall J: Chondromalacia patellae. Patellar malalignment syndrome. *Orthop Clin North Am* 10:117, 1979.

10. Fulkerson JP: *Disorders of the Patellofemoral Joint*, 3rd ed. Baltimore: Williams & Wilkins; 1997.

11. Fu FH, Seel MJ, Berger RA: Patellofemoral biomechanics. In: Fox J, Del Pizzo W (eds): *The Patellofemoral Joint*. Blue Ridge Summit, PA: McGraw-Hill, Inc.: 1993;49.

12. Ho SSW, Jaureguito JW: Functional anatomy and biomechanics of the patellofemoral joint. *Operative Techniques Sports Med* 2:238, 1994.

13. Dye SF, Staubli HU, Biedert FM, et al: The mosaic of pathophysiology causing patellofemoral pain: Therapeutic implications. *Operative Techniques Sports Med* 7:46, 1999.

14. Biedert RM, Stauffer E, Friederich NF: Occurrence of free nerve endings in the soft tissue of the knee joint. *Am J Sports Med* 20:430, 1992.

15. Fulkerson JP: Patellofemoral pain disorders: Evaluation and management. *J Am Acad Orthop Surg* 2:124, 1994.

16. Dye SF, Vaupel GL, Dye CC: Conscious neurosensory mapping of the internal structures of the human knee without intraarticular anesthesia. *Am J Sports Med* 26:773, 1998.

17. Tria AJ, Palumbo RC, Alicea JA: Conservative care for patellofemoral pain. In: Scuderi GR (ed): *The Orthopedic Clinics of North America*. Philadelphia: WB Saunders Co; 1992;545.

18. Shea KP: Clinical evaluation of patellofemoral pain and instability. *Operative Techniques Sports Med* 2:248, 1994.

19. Boden BP, Pearsall AW, Garrett Jr WE, et al: Patellofemoral instability: Evaluation and management. *J Am Acad Orthop Surg* 5:47, 1997.

20. Post, WR: Patellofemoral pain. *Physician Sportsmed* 26:68, 1998.

21. Ghelman B, Hodge JC: Imaging of the patellofemoral joint. In: Scuderi GR (ed): *The Orthopedic Clinics of North America*. Philadelphia: WB Saunders Co; 1992;523.

22. Fulkerson JP, Shea KP: Current concepts review disorders of patellofemoral alignment. *J Bone Joint Surg* 72:1424, 1990.

23. Douchette SA, Boble EM: The effect of exercise on patellar tracking in lateral patellar compression syndrome. *Am J Sports Med* 20:434, 1992.

24. Gray D: Physical therapy techniques for conservative treatment of patellar pain and instability. *Operative Techniques Sports Med* 2:263, 1994.

25. Henry JH: The patellofemoral joint. In: Nicholas JA, Hershman EB (eds): *The Lower Extremity & Spine*, 2nd ed. St. Louis; Mosby; 1995;935.

26. O'Neill DB, Micheli LF, Warner JP: Patellofemoral stress: A prospective analysis of exercise treatment in adolescents and adults. *Am J Sports Med* 20:151, 1992.

27. Messier SP, Davis SE, Walton WC, et al: Etiologic factors associated with patellofemoral pain in runners. *Med Sci Sports Exerc* 23:1008, 1991.

28. Ingersoll CD, Knight KL: Patellar location changes following EMG biofeedback or progressive resistive exercises. *Med Sci Sports Exerc* 23:1122, 1991.

29. Steinkamp LA, Dillingham MF, Markel MD, et al: Biomechanical considerations in patellofemoral joint rehabilitation. *Am J Sports Med* 21:438, 1993.

30. Mirzabeigi E, Jordan C, Gronley JK, et al: Isolation of the vastus medialis oblique muscle during exercise. *Am J Sports Med* 27:50, 1999.

31. McConnell J: The management of chondromalacia patellae: A long term solution. *Aust J Physiotherapy* 32:215, 1986.

32. Bockrath K, Wooden C, Worrell T, et al: Effects of patella taping on patella position and perceived pain. *Med Sci Sports Exerc* 9:989, 1993.

33. Larsen B, Andreasen E, Urfer A, et al: Patellar tap-

ing: A radiographic examination of the medial glide technique. *Am J Sports Med* 23:465, 1995.

34. Kowall MG, Kolk G, Nuber GW, et al: Patellar taping in the treatment of patellofemoral pain: A prospective randomized study. *Am J Sports Med* 24:61, 1996.

35. Muhle C, Brinkmann G, Skaf A, et al: Effect of a patellar realignment brace on patients with patellar subluxation and dislocation: Evaluation with kinematic magnetic resonance imaging. *Am J Sports Med* 27:350, 1999.

36. Federico DJ, Reider G: Results of isolated patellar debridement for patellofemoral pain in patients with normal patellar alignment. *Am J Sports Med* 25:663, 1997.

37. Greenfield MA, Scott WN: Arthroscopic evaluation and treatment of the patellofemoral joint. In Scuderi GR (ed): *The Orthopedic Clinics of North America.* Philadelphia; WB Saunders Co; 1992; 587.

Bryan W. Smith

The Acutely Injured Knee

Introduction

Knee injuries are common, particularly in sports that place a substantial pivoting force on the knee. For many athletes, an acute knee injury is the most dreaded injury of all due to the frequent need for surgical intervention. As interest in sports medicine has grown over the past decade, an increasing number of primary care physicians have become involved in the management of acute knee injuries. Proper diagnosis requires knowledge of the anatomy and biomechanics of the knee. Accurate assessment, use of a thorough history and physical examination, and judicious use of radiographic and imaging studies facilitates proper management and return to activity.

Anatomy and Biomechanics

Bone

The knee joint proper (Figs. 8-1 and 8-2) is comprised of the femur, tibia, and patella. These bones comprise two joints, the tibiofemoral and patellofemoral. The fibula has evolved in humans such that it only articulates with the tibia and this tibiofibular joint is not felt to be part of the knee.[1] The distal femur is composed of two femoral condyles with an intercondylar notch in between. The anterior aspect of the condyles articulates with the patella. The posterior aspect of the condyles articulates with the tibia and is the weight-bearing portion of the femur. The medial joint compartment bears more weight and acts as a pivot point. The more mobile lateral compartment allows the femur to rotate.

The knee's bony architecture of two femoral condyles that articulate on two tibial plateaus

allows for the complete motions that distinguish this complex hinge joint from a simple one. These complex motions can be described as translation (anteroposterior, mediolateral, and proximodistal) and rotation (flexion-extension, internal-external, and varus-valgus).[2] In the last 15 to 20 degrees of extension, the femur internally rotates on the tibia. This is called the screw-home mechanism and stabilizes the knee in extension.

Menisci

Between the condyles and plateaus are two semilunar-shaped disks of fibrocartilage called menisci. These menisci are considered extensions of the tibial surfaces.[3] The medial meniscus is more C-shaped whereas the lateral meniscus is more circular. The outer edge of both is thick and convex and the inner edge is thin and concave. A transverse ligament connects the anterior horns of the medial and lateral menisci. Both menisci are attached anteriorly and posteriorly to the tibia.

The entire outer periphery of the medial meniscus is attached to the joint capsule. The posteromedial capsule is thickened by the tendon sheath of the semimembranosus muscle.[3] At the midpoint of the meniscus, there is an attachment to the deep portion of the medial collateral ligament.

The lateral meniscus has a looser attachment to the joint capsule and no attachment to the lateral collateral ligament. At the posterior horn, the lateral meniscus can be attached by meniscofemoral ligaments either anteriorly (ligament of Humphry) or posteriorly (ligament of Winsberg) to the posterior cruciate ligament. Posterolaterally, the meniscus is grooved by the tendon of popliteus muscle, with an aponeurotic attachment.[3]

The vascular anatomy of the menisci changes with age as vascularity decreases from 50 percent in newborns to less than 20 percent by the age of 40.[4] The outer third of the meniscus

Figure 8-1

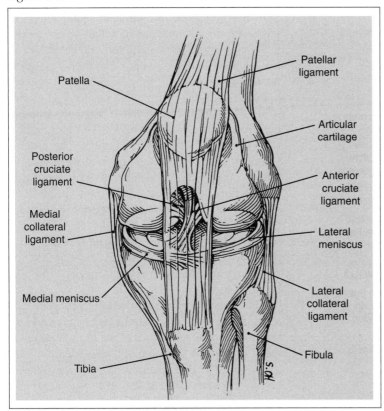

Anatomy of the anterior knee. *(Reproduced with permission from Smith BW, Green GA: Am Fam Physician 51:615, 1995.)*

retains vascularity and will mount a healing response when injured. The inner, avascular portion receives nutrition from synovial fluid via diffusion or mechanical pumping through microchannels.[3]

Biomechanically, the menisci are responsible for enhancing the articulation between the femur and the tibia, thereby augmenting joint stability and distributing the compressive load more uniformly across the joint. The menisci are shock absorbers protecting articular cartilage and subchondral bone. The medial meniscus is more often damaged due to its greater load and its decreased mobility. Levy, Torailli, and Warren found that the medial meniscus also provides anteroposterior stability in the ACL-deficient knee.[5] Both menisci move in an anteroposterior plane, which limits extremes of the joint in flexion and extension.

Ligaments

Ligaments along with the joint capsule provide stabilization to the joint, guide joint motion, and prevent excessive motion. They are not completely static but elongate prior to failure. In the knee, ligaments can be divided into three groups: extracapsular (lateral collateral ligament, superficial medial collateral ligament), capsular (deep medial collateral ligament), and intracapsular (anterior and posterior cruciate ligaments).

Figure 8-2

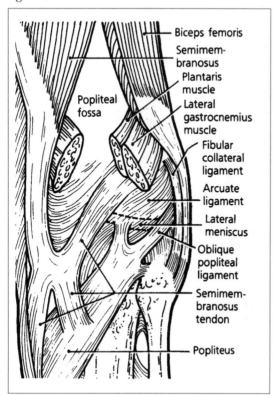

Biceps femoris

Semimem-
branosus

Plantaris
muscle

Lateral
gastrocnemius
muscle

Fibular
collateral
ligament

Arcuate
ligament

Lateral
meniscus

Oblique
popliteal
ligament

Semimem-
branosus
tendon

Popliteus

Popliteal
fossa

Anatomy of the posterior knee. *(Reproduced with permission from Hunter-Griffin LY: Athletic Training and Sports Medicine, 2nd ed. Park Ridge, IL: AAOS; 1991: 314.)*

ANTERIOR CRUCIATE LIGAMENT

The anterior cruciate ligament (ACL) is made up of bundles of longitudinal fascicles that pass in lateral spiral rotation from femur to tibia. The femoral attachment on the medial surface of the lateral femoral condyle is a circular area tilted slightly forward from the vertical.[3] The tibial attachment is in front and bilateral to the anterior tibial spine. The ACL is the primary restraint to anterior translation of the tibia on the femur and provides secondary stabilization to varus/valgus rotation and internal/external rotation of the knee. A portion of the ACL, the posterolateral bulk, limits hyperextension.

POSTERIOR CRUCIATE LIGAMENT

The larger posterior cruciate ligament (PCL) has a broad femoral semicircular origin at the lateral surface of the medial femoral condyle and passes posteriorly, laterally, and distally to insert posterior to the ACL in a depression approximately 1 cm below the tibial surface.[6] The construct of the PCL is that of two bundles of fibers: anterolateral and posteromedial proper, along with the meniscofemoral ligaments. The anterolateral bundle is twice the size and sizably stiffer and stronger than the posteromedial bundle.[7,8] The anterolateral bundle is taut in flexion whereas the posteromedial bundle is taut in extension. The variable meniscofemoral ligaments are stronger than the posteromedial bundle and have been recently recognized as providing an important secondary posterior stabilizer role.[7–9]

The PCL is the primary restraint to posterior tibial translation on the femur and is a secondary stabilizer to external rotation. Functioning is most evident at 90° of flexion and least in full extension. The deep portion of the posterolateral corner appears to assist the PCL in maintaining posterior knee stability.[7,8] Anatomy of the posterolateral corner varies with authors. It has been described as a layered structure with deep contributions from the posterior third of the joint capsule, popliteus tendon, arcuate ligament, popliteal aponeurosis to the lateral meniscus, popliteofibular ligament, and the lateral collateral ligament.[1,7,10]

MEDIAL COLLATERAL LIGAMENT

The medial collateral ligament (MCL) is composed of superficial and deep layers. The extracapsular, superficial MCL originates just distal to adductor tubercle on the medial epicondyle of the femur and extends distally and obliquely to insert just posterior and deep to the pes anserinus tendons on the anteromedial tibia. The deep MCL is entwined in the joint capsule. Beneath the superficial MCL, this portion of the MCL is situated more posterior and is attached to the medial meniscus at its mid portion.[3] As the deep MCL moves toward its insertion, it may either merge with the superficial MCL or insert on the tibia slightly distal to the superficial MCL.[1]

The positioning of the MCL results in different strands of tensioning at varying degrees as the knee moves. The superficial MCL is the primary restraint to valgus stress. This is most noted at 30 to 40° of flexion. The superficial MCL also plays a major role in limiting tibial external rotation. Finally, the superficial MCL acts as a secondary restraint to anterior tibial translation in the absence of an ACL. The deep MCL functional role as a static stabilizer is minor at best.

LATERAL COLLATERAL LIGAMENT

The lateral collateral ligament (LCL) originates at the lateral femoral condyle and terminates at the proximal lateral point of the fibular head. The LCL has been commonly believed to be the primary restraint to varus rotation; however, its role is actually small. When the LCL, popliteus tendon, and arcuate ligament are viewed as a complex (posterolateral complex), this complex has a major role in not only restraining varus rotation but in controlling external rotation, too. The posterolateral complex contributes to limiting posterior tibial translation at varying degrees of knee flexion.

Patellofemoral (Extensor Mechanism) Complex

The patellofemoral complex is responsible for knee extension. The patella is a sesmoid bone imbedded in tendon. The patella has the thickest amount of articular cartilage of any bone in the body. The superior patella is the point of attachment for the quadriceps tendon. The patellar tendon moves inferiorly from the patella to insert on the tibial tuberosity.

Medial and lateral to the patellar are retinacula, which function as extensions of the quadriceps tendon. They attach the patella to the joint capsule and to the femoral condyles. Static stabilization of the patellofemoral joint primarily involves the shape and positioning of the patella and the intercondylar notch of the femur. The shape and positioning of both the patella and the intercondylar notch are extremely variable.

PLICAE

These represent synovial folds that persist from fetal life. They can be located infrapatellar, suprapatellar, and mediopatellar. Approximately 20 percent of the population have one.[11]

BURSAE

There are numerous bursae located in the knee proper. Bursae are closed sacs or cystic spaces that are lined with synovium.

MUSCLE

Anteriorly, the quadriceps pull the knee into extension. Posteriorly, the popliteus muscle runs from the tibia to lateral femoral condyle. With weight-bearing, the popliteus externally rotates the tibia and assists in knee flexion. In non-weight-bearing, the popliteus internally rotates the tibia and assists in knee flexion.

The gastrocnemius and plantaris muscles originate on the femur and assist in knee flexion. Medially, the sartorius, semitendinosus, and gracillis commonly insert on the tibia at the pes anserinus. The semimembranosus has been described to insert in as many as five locations medially.

Laterally, the biceps femoris' two heads combine near the styloid process of the fibula and form a broad insertion on the styloid process of the fibula to Gerdy's tubercle on the tibia. The semitendinosus, semimembranosus, gracillis, and biceps femoris are commonly referred to as the hamstrings and are the prime knee flexors.

The iliotibial band is the distal extension of the tensor fascia lata. This fascial band passes superficially over the lateral aspect of the knee anterior to the fibula to insert onto Gerdy's tubercle on the tibia.

NEUROVASCULAR

Posteriorly, the popliteal artery and vein along with the tibial nerve lie in the popliteal fossa. The common peroneal nerve comes off the tibial nerve and wraps around the fibular neck distal and posterior to the biceps femoris muscle.[1]

Injury History

No technological advance can replace a thorough history and physical examination in the evaluation of an acute knee injury. The history can provide important details regarding the extent, the severity, and, most importantly, the mechanism of injury. The history should cover the following points: (1) the type of activity in which the patient was involved at the time of injury; (2) the position of the knee, lower leg, and foot at the time of injury; (3) the mechanism of injury (e.g., direct blow from contact with another person or from contact with an object); (4) the surface played on; (5) whether a "snap" or "pop" was heard at the time of injury; (6) the location of pain; (7) whether any locking, catching, or giving way occurred post-injury; (8) how soon after the injury did swelling develop; (9) whether the patient was able to continue activity following the injury; and (10) previous history of injury to the injured knee or contralateral knee.

Physical Examination

The physical examination should be performed in a relaxed manner to minimize patient guarding. For the sake of comparison, both knees should be examined. The uninjured knee should be examined first. Waiting to examine the injured area of the knee last may instill confidence in the patient and reduce the amount of guarding.

Ideally, the knee should be examined as soon after the injury as possible because subsequent development of a joint effusion can cause pain and limited range of motion. Acutely, pain and apprehension in the patient may hinder a meaningful examination. If this situation occurs, the knee should be elevated and an ice pack applied for 10 to 15 min. By such time, the patient is usually more calm and cooperative, and the ice will have provided a degree of mild analgesia.

When the examination is performed "in the field," it should focus on the injured knee before the patient has had time to become apprehensive. In the office, the examination should begin with an inspection of both legs, from the hips to the toes, to assess symmetry. Edema, ecchymoses, and muscle atrophy should be noted. Edema should be identified as either extra-articular (edema from a bursa or a sprain of the superficial fibers of the medial collateral ligament) or intra-articular (edema associated with a cruciate ligament tear and/or meniscal tear). Small effusions are often appreciated by the patient as posterior knee pain limiting extension and flexion. Patellar ballottement can be helpful in detecting effusion. It can be useful in differentiating free fluid from soft tissue edema.

Range of Motion

Functional testing of the knee should begin with passive and active assessment of the range of motion, and any decreased motion should be noted. The usual range of motion of the knee is 135 to 145° for flexion and 0° for extension, although some patients may normally exhibit recurvatum or hyperflexion. Signs of dysfunction in static patellar location and/or active patellar tracking can be assessed during the evaluation of the range of motion.

Palpation

Palpation of the knee should follow range-of-motion assessment. The intent of palpation is to identify structures that are tender and therefore likely to be injured.

If edema does not permit adequate flexion of the knee, palpation should be performed with the patient seated or with the knee in 30° of flexion. Starting from the tibial tuberosity, palpation is performed up the patellar tendon to the inferopatellar border, then circumferentially around the patella to evaluate the retinaculae. Various bursae are then palpated, noting any tenderness or warmth. Vascular integrity should also be assessed, particularly if dislocation has occurred or the examiner suspects that multiple structures have been injured.

The joint line spaces are palpated next, beginning with the uninjured knee. Flexion of the knee enhances palpation of the anterior half of each meniscus. If the leg is internally rotated, the medial meniscus is more easily palpated.[12] Alternatively, external rotation allows improved palpation of the lateral meniscus.[12] If signs of joint line tenderness are elicited, palpation superiorly and inferiorly along the collateral ligaments is helpful in differentiating between a collateral ligament sprain and a meniscal tear. In the latter, tenderness is limited to the joint line. Tenderness elicited when palpating either the posterolateral or posteromedial corners may suggest damage to multiple structures.

Tenderness that extends superiorly from the anteromedial joint line may be caused by inflammation of the retinacular tissue secondary to dysfunctional patellar tracking or a symptomatic synovial plica. A plica may be detected by moving the fingers along this area and noting a mobile, soft tissue mass.[11]

On the lateral side of the knee, the iliotibial band should be palpated superiorly from its insertion while the knee is actively extended. Any symptomatic snapping of the band over the femoral condyle should be noted.

Patellofemoral Mechanism

To evaluate the patellofemoral mechanism begin by measuring the Q angle, which is an angle formed by the intersection of a line from the anterior superior iliac spine to the patella and a line from the patella to the tibial tuberosity. Q angles greater than 15° are associated with patellar subluxation. Patellar mobility should also be assessed. Increased passive glide of the patella beyond the midline (3+ to 4+) or increased patellar tilt increase the likelihood of patellar instability.[13]

A high-riding patella, called patella alta, is also associated with patellar instability and is seen with a prominent infrapatellar fat pad. A lateral view of a knee with patella alta gives one the impression of two humps and is called the camelback sign.[14]

Patellofemoral dysfunction, another cause of knee pain, is extremely common, but not an acute traumatic injury. It is discussed in the chapter on anterior knee pain (see Chap. 7).

Acute patellar instability that results from recurrent subluxation or dislocation can be determined by the patellar apprehension test (Fig. 8-3). This test is performed by attempting to laterally displace the patella while the knee is extended and noting whether the patient is apprehensive. This test may be performed with the knee in 30° of flexion to full extension.

Figure 8-3

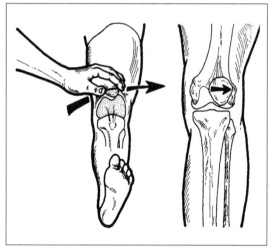

Patellar apprehension test. *(Reproduced with permission from Hunter-Griffin LY: Athletic Training and Sports Medicine, 2nd ed. Park Ridge, IL: AAOS; 1991: 314.)*

Specific Maneuvers

Valgus and varus stress testing (Fig. 8-4) provide assessment of the integrity of the medial and lateral collateral ligaments and their capsular components. With the knee in 30° of flexion, the collateral ligaments can be isolated. Laxity in extension suggests accompanying damage to the capsular components and/or the cruciate ligaments.

Three tests have commonly been employed to evaluate the anterior cruciate ligament; the Lachman test (Fig. 8-5), the pivot shift test (Fig. 8-6), and the anterior drawer test, which is essentially the Lachman test performed with the knee in 90° of flexion. The predictive value of these three tests in assessing cruciate ligament integrity has been evaluated in a study that compared the physical findings with the findings of arthroscopy performed within 2 weeks of the injury.[15] While all three tests demonstrated a specificity greater than 95 percent for excluding anterior cruciate ligament disruption, the sensitivity of the anterior drawer test was only 22 per-

cent for anterior cruciate ligament disruption.[15] The Lachman test was 78 percent sensitive and the pivot shift test was 89 percent sensitive.[15] While the pivot shift test may be more sensitive than the Lachman test, particularly in the first hour post-injury, subsequent muscle spasm, edema, and pain can make this test difficult to perform and increase the likelihood of a false-negative result.[16] Therefore, the Lachman test is the test of choice to determine the presence of an anterior cruciate ligament disruption.

Grading of the anterior drawer test and the Lachman test is the same in terms of degree of tibial displacement. The scale is 0 to 4+ with 1+ signifying 5 mm, 2+ signifying 10 mm, 3+ signifying 15 mm, and 4+ signifying 20 mm of displacement. It is important with the Lachman test to evaluate the endpoint of the tibial displacement. This endpoint is characterized as firm, soft, or none. The usual minimum diagnostic criteria for a torn ACL is a 1+ Lachman test with a soft endpoint.

Although the anterior drawer tests is a poor choice for evaluating the integrity of the ACL alone, performing the test with the foot externally rotated will test for anteromedial rotatory instability, which is increased with injury to the MCL or the medial meniscus. Anterolateral rotatory instability can be tested with the anterior drawer test with the foot internally rotated, but the pivot shift test is a better test. If secondary stabilizers, such as the lateral meniscus or posterolateral corner are injured, these tests will be more pronounced.

Because the larger anterolateral bundle of the PCL is maximally taut at 90°, the posterior drawer test (Fig. 8-7) is the preferred test to evaluate PCL integrity.[6–8,17] Another test for PCL integrity is the tibial sag test, in which the knee is flexed to 90°; in the presence of a ruptured posterior cruciate ligament, the tibia is displaced posteriorly on the femur (Fig. 8-8). A companion test is the quadriceps active test in which the patient performs the tibial sag test and then actively contracts the quadriceps, which results

Figure 8-4

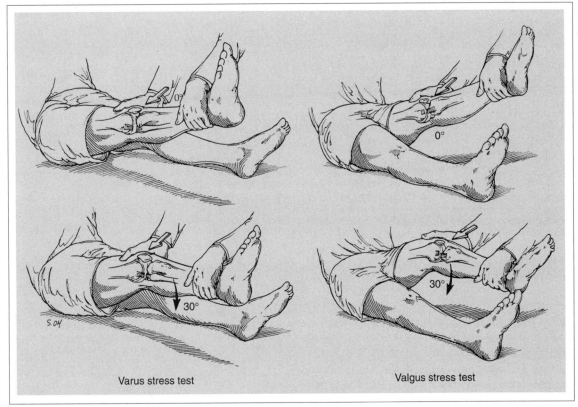

Varus stress test

Valgus stress test

Varus and valgus stress testing of the knee. Perform the test in full extension and 30° of flexion. *(Reproduced with permission from Smith BW, Green GA: Am Fam Physician 51:615, 1995.)*

in reduction of the posterior subluxed tibia if subluxation due to PCL injury is present.[7,8]

In addition to evaluating the PCL, posteromedial and posterolateral rotation require evaluation. One test that can evaluate both components is the "tibial rotation test," which compares the amount of increased internal (posteromedial) or external rotation (posterolateral) with the uninvolved side. Another test is the posterior drawer test with the foot in internal or external rotation. Still another test for posterolateral instability is the external recurvatum test (Fig. 8-9), which requires the patient to lie supine while one raises the extended legs by grabbing the toes.[10] An apparent bowlegged appearance due to hyperextension and external rotation of the tibia is a positive test.

Physical tests for evaluation of the menisci are of limited predictive value. Distinct joint line tenderness accompanying effusion and a history of mechanical symptoms, such as "locking or catching," are probably the most reliable indicators of a meniscal tear. If the patient can reproduce or demonstrate the motion that causes pain, that may provide valuable diagnostic information. Physical tests, such as the bounce test, McMurray's test (Fig. 8-10), and Apley's grind test (Fig. 8-11), can aid in making a diagnosis of meniscal injury. When performing varus and valgus stress testing, pain elicited on the contralateral, com-

Figure 8-5

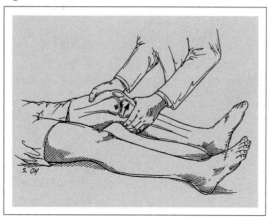

Lachman test. Place the tibia in neutral and flex the knee to 30°. Note the amount of anterior translation and the endpoint with examiner displacement. *(Reproduced with permission from Smith BW, Green GA: Am Fam Physician 51:615, 1995.)*

pressed side may suggest meniscal pathology. In addition, having the patient squat and duck walk may elicit the mechanical symptoms of a meniscal tear. Unfortunately, even if all these tests are negative, the possibility of a meniscal tear still exists.

Radiographic Evaluation

For patients with a nonacute injury, the role of radiography in the decision-making process depends largely on the physical examination and history. In the setting of acute trauma, radiographs should always be obtained to rule out fracture. At a minimum, anteriorposterior, lateral, notch, and sunrise or Merchant views are necessary (Merchant view is a standing sunrise view with the knee flexed 45°.) The presence of a fracture on x-ray suggests concomitant injury to adjacent soft tissue structures.[18] Stress radi-

Figure 8-6

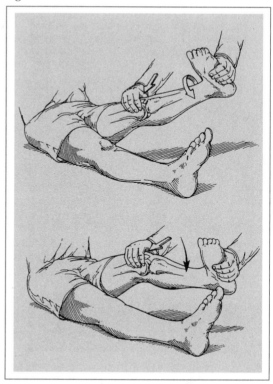

Pivot shift test. This test involves flexing the knee while the lower leg is internally rotated and a valgus stress is applied, resulting in subluxation of the tibia. The tibia can be relocated abruptly when the knee is extended. *(Reproduced with permission from Smith BW, Green GA: Am Fam Physician 51:615, 1995.)*

Figure 8-7

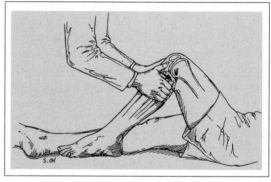

Posterior drawer test. *(Reproduced with permission from Smith BW, Green GA: Am Fam Physician 51:615, 1995.)*

Figure 8-8

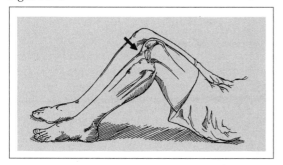

Sag test. Flex the knee to 90°. A posteriorly displaced tibia obscuring the tibial tuberosity is a positive test. *(Reproduced with permission from Smith BW, Green GA: Am Fam Physician 51:615, 1995.)*

ographs are rarely indicated, even in the pediatric population.

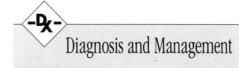

Diagnosis and Management

Following the complete history and physical examination, the decision-making process for determining the type of knee injury begins. Major soft tissue injuries that are essential for the clinician to recognize are patellar subluxation/ dislocation, meniscal injury, collateral ligament sprains, cruciate ligament sprains, and selected fractures. All of these injuries can lead to chronic knee problems. The remainder of the chapter discusses the diagnostic process and provides management options for these injuries.

Figure 8-9

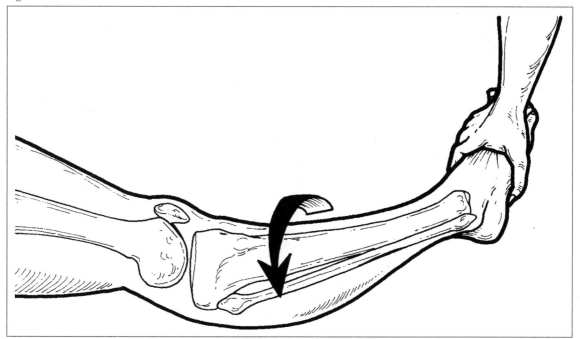

External recurvatum test. Grab the patient's toes and lift the feet off the table. If the patient's knee hyperextends laterally and the tibia externally rotates, the test is positive, giving a bow-legged appearance. *(Reproduced with permission from Hunter-Griffin LY: Athletic Training and Sports Medicine, 2nd ed. Park Ridge, IL: AAOS; 1991: 314.)*

Figure 8-10

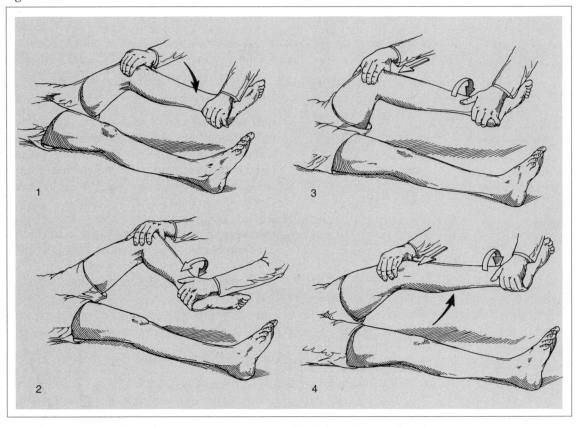

McMurray's test. (1) To evaluate the medial menicus, the knee is flexed 45° with the hip flexed slightly more. (2) While holding the foot in one hand, the medial joint is palpated with a finger and a valgus stress is applied. This action should open the medial compartment, and a torn meniscus may be displaced into the joint. (3) Next, a varus stress is applied with the knee flexed. (4) Finally, the knee is extended while still in varus. When the menicus relocates, a click may be heard, indicating a positive test. *(Reproduced with permission from Smith BW, Green GA: Am Fam Physician 51:615, 1995.)*

Patellar Injuries

Acute patellar injury usually requires differentiating patellar dislocation or subluxation from traumatic bursitis or fracture. Rarely, a quadriceps or patellar tendon rupture may be present. Other causes of anterior knee pain, such as patellar tendonitis, extensor mechanism dysfunction, and inflammation of a synovial plica, are usually insidious or chronic in presentation and are not pertinent in the setting of acute injury.

PATELLAR DISLOCATION/SUBLUXATION

The history and mechanism of injury can provide important clues to the nature of the injury. Traumatic bursitis is associated with direct trauma to the anterior patellar surface without rotatory force. The trauma may be sufficient to result in patellar contusion or fracture. In contrast, trauma from either side of the patella can result in a traumatic patellar dislocation or subluxation. A ripping or tearing sensation at the

Figure 8-11

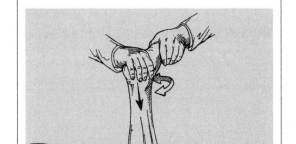

Apley's grind test. Place the patient in a prone position with the knee flexed to 90°. An axial load is placed on the heel and the lower leg is internally and externally rotated. Pain constitutes a positive test. Distracting the joint and repeating the rotation on the lower leg confirms the positive test if no pain is elicited. *(Reproduced with permission from Smith BW, Green GA: Am Fam Physician 51:615, 1995.)*

time of trauma to a semi-flexed knee is considered by some authorities to almost always be associated with patellar dislocation.[19]

Trauma is not necessary, however, for patellar subluxation or dislocation. Persons with inadequate, dynamic patellar stability are susceptible to nontraumatic patellar dislocation or subluxation.[20] According to Cash and Hughston, the typical mechanism for a nontraumatic patellar dislocation is a twisting injury with the femur internally rotating on a fixed foot.[21] This results in strong lateral forces created by the extensor mechanism with quadriceps contraction causing a lateral dislocation.[21] Garth et al. suggest that the knee should be in a flexed, valgus, and externally rotated position.[22] There are several predisposing conditions for nontraumatic patel-

lar subluxation or dislocation such as patella alta, increased lateral tilt, increased Q angle, genu valgum, long-standing Osgood-Schlatter disease, and abnormal patellar configuration.[14,23] Runow found a six times increased incidence of patellar dislocation in patients with articular hypermobility compared with age-matched controls.[24]

In both patellar subluxation and dislocation, the patient describes a sensation of instability and weakness and is reluctant to bear weight on the affected knee.[19,25,26] Swelling is often dependent on the degree of trauma and a large, painful or obstructive hemarthrosis may require aspiration. If aspiration is performed, the aspirate should be checked for fat globules, as these indicate that a fracture is present.

Physical examination findings of retinacular and facet tenderness along with patellar apprehension are typically found. Tenderness may be found over the lateral femoral condyle following reduction. Patellar dislocation can be associated with other injuries such as an ACL tear so a complete physical examination is warranted.

Many predisposing factors for re-injury may be found and checking for hypermobility in other joints is important for determining management options. The younger the patient is at the time of the initial injury, the greater the likelihood of recurrent subluxation and/or dislocation.[21]

Radiographs are essential for evaluating patellar injury. Predisposing conditions such as patella alta, patellar tilt, or an abnormal femoral sulcus can be detected.[27] But more importantly, studies indicate that 28 to 68 percent of patients with patellar dislocation have an associated osteochondral fracture.[21,26,28] Merchant and infra-patellar views with the knee in 45° of flexion, in addition to anteroposterior, notch, and lateral views, are optimal for identifying these fractures. Often, chondral lesions are not identified with plain radiographs. In the presence of a large effusion/hemearthrosis, chondral injury should be suspected even if the radiographs are negative, and an MRI should be obtained.

Treatment

Management of a patellar dislocation or subluxation varies. Options include closed reduction, immobilization and physical therapy, and acute surgical repair.[23] Many initial episodes of patellar dislocation or subluxation respond favorably to a program of bracing, physical therapy, and alteration of activities that aggravate the condition.[21,29]

Controversy exists regarding the degree of immobilization necessary when conservative therapy is used. In patients treated nonoperatively without immobilization, up to two-thirds continue to subluxate or dislocate and 50 percent have a fair or poor subjective outcome.[22,28] If nonoperative treatment is used, Cash and Hughston initially recommend the use of a knee immobilizer with aggressive physical therapy of quadriceps strengthening, straight leg raises, and progressive resistance exercises.[21] Every 2 weeks, the knee is evaluated and when the knee is stable and minimally tender, the immobilizer is discontinued with physical therapy continuing until the patient can return to play.[21] Garth et al. utilize a lateral buttressing knee sleeve along with aggressive physical therapy for 3 to 8 weeks.[22]

Rehabilitation consists of several phases that include soft tissue mobilization, patellar mobilization, and strengthening of appropriate muscle groups (e.g., vastus medialis, oblique, gluteus, and muscles of the foot and ankle). If after 6 months the patient is dissatisfied with the degree of recovery, surgery may be considered. Following rehabilitation, most patients begin a maintenance patellar stability program.

In most cases of patellar dislocation with an osteochondral fracture, surgery should be the initial treatment. In one study, over half of the patients with patellar dislocation and an accompanying fracture who were treated without surgery had a poor outcome.[23] Patients without articular hypermobility have been reported to have a much greater likelihood of chondral injury with patellar dislocation.[30] If the patient is predisposed to recurrent dislocation (e.g., has congenital patellar abnormalities or is performing at a high level of activity), the patient may be a candidate for early surgical intervention.[23,29]

Patellar Fracture

Patellar fractures may be transverse, longitudinal, stellate, or involve pole avulsions. Usually direct trauma is the mechanism of injury, but in some pole avulsions (e.g., the sleeve fracture seen in pre-teenagers, discussed in following sections) a jumping mechanism is at fault.[31] Distinguishing a fracture from a congenital bipartite patella can be achieved in most cases by comparison radiographs.

Nondisplaced (less than 2 mm) transverse or longitudinal patellar fractures require knee immobilization in extension for 3 to 6 weeks with physical therapy directed at maintaining strength. Progressive range-of-motion exercises can be added when pain-free on palpation. Stellate, displaced, and sleeve fractures require surgical intervention.

Sleeve fractures, in which a small sliver of bone may be attached to a large piece of articular cartilage, may be very difficult to appreciate on radiographs. Massive swelling is usually appreciated anteriorly, along with an inability to actively extend the knee.[32,33] There may be a palpable gap at the lower pole of the patella.[32,33] As noted, sleeve fractures require surgical repair.

Quadriceps Tendon Rupture

Quadriceps tendon rupture is rare in the young athlete. Eighty percent of injuries occur in persons over the age of 40. Basketball players are at greatest risk for injury.[34] Typically, the rupture site is one of preexisting tendonosis.[35,36] Treatment is early surgical repair.

The history is significant for feeling like one has been kicked or struck in the leg. Physical examination reveals a palpable defect and the patient usually cannot straight-leg raise. Radiographic signs of rupture are patella baja, no quad tendon shadow, suprapatellar mass, and suprapatella calcification.[36]

Patellar Tendon Rupture

This injury is rare, but typically occurs in athletes less than 40 years old. Athletes at risk are ones with preexisting tendonosis who play running/jumping sports.[34,36,37] Steroid injections in and around the tendon have been implicated with ruptures.[36]

Rupture typically occurs at the bone-tendon junction. History and physical examination are similar to the quadriceps rupture discussed previously. Lateral radiographs demonstrate patella alta. Surgical repair is required and the athlete typically returns to sport in 4 to 6 months.[37]

Meniscal Injury

A decision tree for the evaluation of meniscal injury is presented (Fig. 8-12). Meniscal injuries have always been a diagnostic challenge because there is no adequate clinical test available for diagnosis. In a study of more than 6,000 meniscal injuries (the ratio of men to women was 2.5:1.0), more than one-third of the injuries were associated with an anterior cruciate ligament tear.[38] In studies involving predominantly younger individuals, meniscal tears with a concomitant anterior cruciate ligament tear have been reported in as many as 92 percent of patients.[39] Sports most associated with meniscal injury are football, soccer, basketball, skiing, and baseball.[40]

Initially, meniscal injury may be difficult to discern if a large joint effusion hinders examination of the knee. Prudent management calls for reevaluation after a 1-week course of relative rest, icing, elevation, compression, and nonsteroidal anti-inflammatory medication. If the athlete is currently participating in sports or cannot delay training, an MRI is a reasonable next step to confirm the diagnosis without waiting for the swelling to subside.

A thorough history is essential to diagnosis considering the poor sensitivity of meniscal tests on physical examination. Mechanical symptoms such as locking or catching, are very suggestive of meniscal pathology. Joint line tenderness that does not extend over adjacent soft tissues is a predictive sign of meniscal pathology. When tenderness is combined with mechanical symptoms (such as locking or catching), inability to duck walk and a positive bounce, McMurray's or Apley's test, there is a strong likelihood that a meniscal tear is present. In this case, referral to an orthopedic surgeon is indicated for surgical evaluation. Although a peripheral meniscal tear, particularly in the lateral meniscus, may heal spontaneously or become asymptomatic, the majority of meniscal tears will require surgical intervention.[41]

With the availability of arthroscopy and magnetic resonance imaging (MRI), accuracy in the diagnosis of meniscal tears has increased to more than 90 percent.[42–44] MRI provides a noninvasive method for diagnosis and augments a thorough history and physical examination. However, the cost of an MRI can be as high as $1,500; it should be obtained only if the diagnosis is in doubt or if the results of the MRI will change the course of management.

MANAGEMENT

There is overwhelming evidence that the more meniscal tissue that can be preserved, the greater the degree of joint preservation and

Figure 8-12

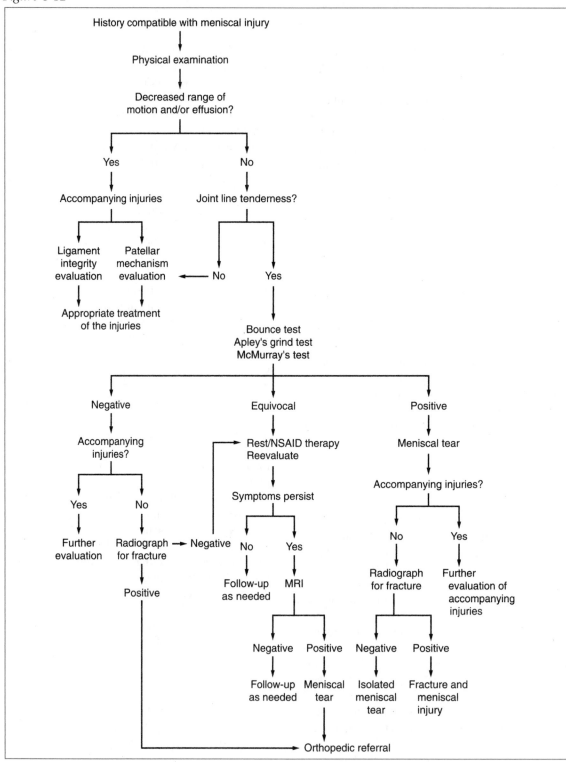

Decision algorithm for meniscal injury. *(Reproduced with permission from Smith BW, Green GA: Am Fam Physician 51:799, 1995.)*

Figure 8-13

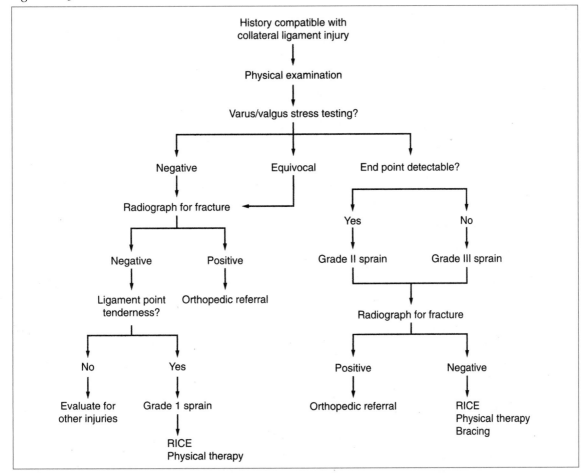

Decision algorithm for collateral ligament injury. *(Reproduced with permission from Smith BW, Green GA: Am Fam Physician 51:799, 1995.)*

future knee performance.[45] Meniscal repairs in the young athlete have been shown to have a higher success rate than in adults.[46] Treatment should be based on the type, location, and extent of the tear.[47] Currently, MRI is not accurate enough to determine the nature of meniscal tears.[44] Therefore, arthroscopy may be warranted to identify the type and extent of injury.

Aggressive rehabilitation after surgery reduces morbidity and allows the patient to return to daily activity sooner. However, how quickly the patient may return to activity is dependent upon which procedure is performed. Patients can bear weight in a day or two and can usually return to full activity within 2 to 4 weeks following arthroscopic meniscectomy. After meniscal repair, flexion is limited to less than 90° with partial weight for 4 to 6 weeks. Return to activity is prolonged, and it may be 4 to 6 months before participation in sports is possible.[41,48,49]

Collateral Ligament Injury

The layman's term "sprained knee" has come to mean a collateral ligament sprain. In a study of 160 knee injuries in athletes, 12 percent were collateral ligament tears; all but one occurred on the medial side.[50]

A diagnostic tree for the evaluation of collateral ligament injury is presented (Fig. 8-13). The history of a patient with a collateral ligament injury typically involves direct trauma to the contralateral side of the knee, usually in sports such as football or soccer, or excessive indirect force applied to the knee in a varus or valgus manner, such as often happens in wrestling. Pain and a sensation of tearing may have been noted by the patient at the time of injury. The amount of edema and ecchymosis depends on the severity of the injury, and a joint effusion may be noted if the capsular portion of the medial collateral ligament and/or the anterior and posterior cruciate ligaments are damaged.

Injuries to the medial collateral ligament usually occur at the proximal origin. Therefore, tenderness is usually localized along the distal femur and extends to the joint line. Minor sprains of the lateral collateral ligament may be missed because of the infrequency of this injury, the size of the ligament, and the inherent stability of the knee in a patient with a lateral collateral ligament injury. A careful history of the mechanism of injury will help determine whether a lateral collateral ligament sprain has occurred.

Ligament sprains are graded on a scale of I, II, and III, depending on the amount of ligament disruption. Comparison with the contralateral knee is essential because there are varying degrees of normal joint laxity. In the normal knee, collateral ligaments may permit up to 10 mm of joint opening when the knee is in 30° of flexion. A grade I sprain consists of microtears of the ligament, which corresponds to less than 5 mm of increased joint opening and no instability on clinical examination. A grade II sprain involves a partial macrotear of the ligament, as demonstrated by the presence of instability and significantly increased joint opening with an endpoint. A grade III sprain is a complete macrotear of the ligament with no end point distinguishable on examination.

MANAGEMENT

Initial treatment of isolated grade I and II sprains involves conservative measures such as rest, ice application, compression, and elevation, along with nonsteroidal anti-inflammatory medication, for the first 24 to 72 h. Prompt initiation of physical therapy should accompany initial treatment. In patients with a grade II sprain, bracing the knee for 4 to 6 weeks is recommended to protect against reinjury.

The treatment for a grade III collateral ligament sprain without accompanying injuries has changed. In the early 1980s, about one half of orthopedists surveyed favored surgical management.[51] A prospective study of nonoperative management of isolated grade III medial collateral ligament tears found no benefit from surgical management.[52] In a study of various operative and nonoperative management options involving canine knees, nonoperative management was superior to operative management and short-term immobilization.[53] Smith and Green recommend nonoperative, conservative management of isolated grade III collateral ligament sprains for 4 to 8 weeks, with emphasis on physical therapy and functional bracing during the rehabilitative period.[54]

Apparent collateral ligament injury in the child or adolescent may be confused with a growth plate injury. At greatest risk for growth plate injury is the mid to late adolescent whose physis is in the midst of an active growth period.[55] On the medial side, the femoral physis is almost always injured because the superficial MCL inserts on the tibial metaphysis. A proximal tibial physeal injury is usually associated with a high degree of trauma. Acute pain most prominently over the physis and immediate swelling are noted. Stress radiographs or MRI can be used for diagnosis. Comparison radiographs can be useful in distinguishing any widening of the physis of the affected knee with the unaffected knee.

For Salter-Harris grade I nondisplaced fractures, immobilization in a long-leg brace or cast in 15 to 20° of flexion for 4 to 6 weeks with accompanying physical therapy is recommended followed by range-of-motion and strengthening exercises before return to play.[56] Any Salter-Harris grade II (most common fracture) to V, or any displaced fracture, needs orthopedic referral for reduction and fixation. Close follow-up is recommended to check for displacement.

Cruciate Ligament Injury

ANTERIOR CRUCIATE LIGAMENT INJURY

NON-CONTACT INJURY Anterior cruciate ligament injury is one the most dreaded injuries for many athletes. Many of these injuries occur in a noncontact situation without warning, which is particularly devastating to the athlete psychologically. Until the 1980s, an ACL injury was seen as a career-ending injury for an athlete. Today, however, most athletes return to competition following reconstructive surgery, but the time loss from sport and the monetary cost of suffering an ACL injury are high.

Female athletes, particularly those playing soccer, gymnastics, and basketball, are at the highest risk for ACL injury.[57] The risk in women is two to eight times higher than male counterparts.[57] The likelihood of suffering an ACL injury at the World Cup/Olympic level for a female skier is nearly 100 percent over the course of a career.

Many factors have been postulated to explain the gender difference in noncontact ACL injuries. Intrinsic factors mentioned are joint laxity, hormonal influences (estrogen and progesterone), limb alignment, notch dimensions, and ligament size.[58] Extrinsic factors, including conditioning, skill, shoe, strength, muscle recruitment, and landing technique may also be involved.[58] A recent consensus symposium attempted to sort out the risk factors that had merit.[59] While no consensus was reached on many of these factors, neuromuscular activation factors were identified as an important reason for the differing ACL rates between men and women.[59]

The mechanism for ACL injury is commonly a change in direction and landing movement that occur simultaneously. Common force patterns are deceleration, valgus, external rotation or deceleration, internal rotation, or hyperextension of the knee.[60] Strong quadriceps activation during eccentric contraction is a major risk factor for ACL injury.[59]

Management. A thorough history and physical examination detect more than 90 percent of cases of cruciate ligament injury. A common presentation is the athlete who, while abruptly changing direction, feels or hears a pop and suddenly the knee gives way. Over the next 2 to 3 hours, the knee becomes swollen and difficult to bend.

A decision tree for the evaluation of cruciate ligament injury is presented (Fig. 8-14). About 75 percent of the time, a hemarthrosis following acute trauma is associated with anterior cruciate ligament injury.[61] There are excellent clinical tests, such as the Lachman and pivot shift, for the evaluation of an anterior cruciate tear. However, an initial equivocal examination warrants conservative management and reevaluation. Radiographs may demonstrate a lateral, tibial condylar avulsion fracture (lateral capsular sign or Segond fracture), which is highly suggestive of disruption of the anterior cruciate ligament (Fig. 8-15).[18]

CONTACT INJURY Whereas isolated ACL tears are common with a noncontact mechanism, traumatic contact ACL injuries are frequently associated with meniscal damage, MCL or LCL injury, and/or posterolateral corner injury. Careful physical examination, including vascular examination, is warranted. Up to two-thirds of traumatic ACL injuries are associated with a meniscal tear, usually of the posterior third, from compression as the tibia subluxates forward.[29,61] An MRI may be helpful in ruling out meniscal pathology because the rate of associated meniscal damage is high and the menisci are at increased risk for subsequent damage due to joint instability.[65] Structural damage to the anterior cruciate liga-

Figure 8-14

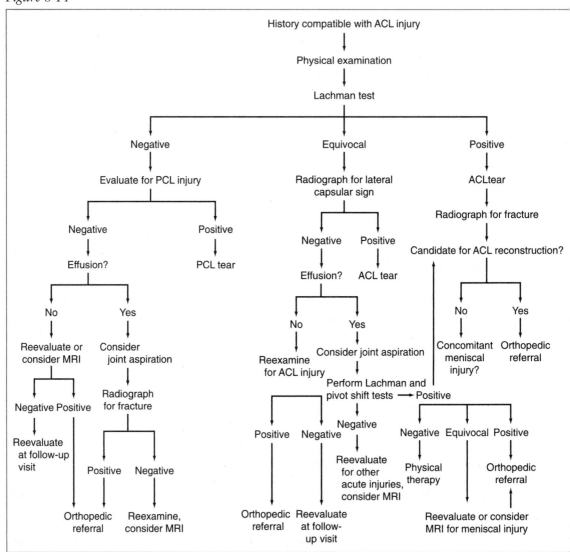

Decision algorithm for anterior cruciate ligament injury. *(Adapted from Smith BW, Green GA: Am Fam Physician 51:799, 1995.)*

ment that results in gross instability requires surgical repair.[64,66]

In determining when an anterior cruciate ligament requires reconstruction, the clinician faces three important concerns: (1) patient lifestyle factors, such as present and future activity levels; (2) patho-anatomical factors, such as associated structural damage; and (3) biomechanical factors, such as the degree of instability. Various options should be discussed with the patient. Athletic patients, especially those involved in sports that require "cutting" movements or jumping, should be offered the option of anterior cruciate ligament reconstruction. This approach

Figure 8-15

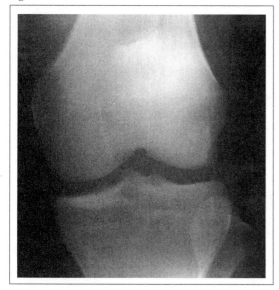

Lateral capsular sign. Anteroposterior radiograph demonstrating an avulsion injury of the mid-third of the lateral capsule indicative of an anterior cruciate ligament injury.

provides the greatest degree of knee stability for patients who wish to continue sports participation at their pre-injury level.

Sedentary individuals whose daily activities impose little chance for clinical instability may fare well with physical therapy and bracing. Also, if the patient is not committed to the 9- to 12-month period of rehabilitation required after surgery, surgery may be an unsuitable option. Bracing and rehabilitation alone may allow a select number of athletes to return to their athletic participation in an accelerated fashion.[62] However, the type of sport, the degree of post-injury instability and concomitant meniscal damage need to be factored into the decision. Patients who choose not to have surgery should be advised that less than one-half of people who do not undergo surgical repair are able to resume involvement in sports at their previous level, and up to three-fourths of patients have chronic activity-related symptoms.[63,64]

Post-ACL reconstruction rehabilitation has

evolved over the years and athletes are returning to sport 4 to 6 months following surgery. Early weight bearing and closed-chain kinetic exercises are the major components of an accelerated program.[67] However, many clinicians still advocate a 9- to 12-month rehab time frame to reduce graft stretching and reduce the failure potential.

ACL injury in the skeletally immature athlete is a controversial topic depending on the injury location and the type of management contemplated. Both tibial insertion avulsions and mid-substance tears can occur. The literature is less controversial with regard to avulsions. Any nondisplaced avulsion fracture may be treated in a long leg cast in 20° of flexion for 6 weeks, followed by gradual range-of-motion and strengthening exercise.[68]

Mid-substance tears are more controversial. Most surgeons try to plan surgery after skeletal maturity is reached since they do not want to damage the growth plate with surgery and have resultant growth arrest. However, rehabilitation and return to physical activity with a brace usually result in subsequent meniscal injury.[14] Therefore, the youngster must curtail his or her activities or undergo primary repair or early reconstruction. Primary repair has been attempted and is usually associated with a poor outcome.[68] Reconstruction techniques to avoid the growth plate such as extra-epiphyseal plate and trans-physeal approaches have had good success but have been attempted by few.[68]

At this time, most would recommend a non-operative plan for mid-substance ACL tears emphasizing rehabilitation and activity restriction until skeletal maturity develops and reconstruction can be performed with relative safety. The very young patient needs careful evaluation and early surgical consideration.

POSTERIOR CRUCIATE LIGAMENT INJURY

Injuries of the posterior cruciate ligament are relatively uncommon in athletes. Most posterior cruciate ligament tears in sports are the result of

Figure 8-16

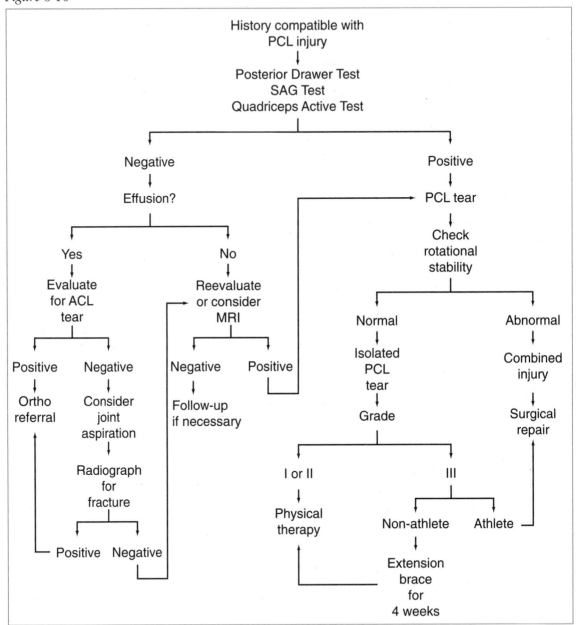

Decision algorithm for posterior cruciate injury.

a hyperflexion injury from a fall on a flexed knee. Other mechanisms of injury are hyperextension and pretibial trauma to a flexed knee (dashboard injury). Usually in the hyperflexion injury, only the anterolateral bundle of the PCL is injured and this injury may be overlooked given the inherent stability of the knee.

The primary complaints will be mild swelling, pain, and an inability to bear weight.[8] The posterior drawer test, sag test, and quadriceps active test complement a careful history and are usually sufficient to make a diagnosis (Fig. 8-16). With an isolated PCL injury, instability is rare. Evidence of instability or a complete PCL tear would suggest associated injury to the posterolateral or posteromedial capsule or the ACL. A complete tear (both bundles) requires more than 10 mm of posterior displacement and loss of medial stepoff.[7]

Radiographs, particularly the lateral view, are useful in ruling out a bony avulsion, either at the tibial insertion of the ligament or the femoral condyle.[8,70] Small tibial plateau fractures with a PCL injury suggest a combined ligament injury. Although MRI imaging is not routinely needed, it may have utility in more complex cases to guide treatment.

Displaced bony avulsions associated with PCL injury may require surgical fixation. Nondisplaced bony avulsions may be managed conservatively but require frequent follow-up during the immobilization period to evaluate the position of the fragment.[70]

An isolated, incomplete interstitial tear should be managed conservatively, even in the athlete. This involves protected weight-bearing, early range of motion, and quadriceps strengthening.[7,8,70] Return to sport takes 2 to 6 weeks, with no bracing normally required. The complete isolated tear can be managed conservatively but is less predictable. Two to four weeks of immobilization in a brace in full extension is usually required. Quadriceps strengthening, straight-leg raises, and partial weight-bearing come next. Following removal of the brace, range of motion and progressive weight-bearing can begin with progression to open and closed chain exercises and functional exercises such as biking and stair climbing. This rehabilitation usually takes 3 months before return to play is considered.[7,8] If the patient makes slow or poor progress, surgical reconstruction may be needed.

Surgical management is recommended for combined structure injury (i.e., the PCL and another structure) or symptomatic complete isolated PCL tears.[7,8] Aggressive rehabilitation follows with return to sport in 12 months.

Knee Dislocation

The knee can dislocate in a variety of directions. Anterior, posterior, and posterolateral dislocations are the most common.[71] Usually both the ACL and PCL are ruptured, but a complete dislocation can occur and leave either the ACL or PCL intact. The average number of concomitant injuries is: vascular, 30 percent; neurologic, 23 percent; and fractures, 10 percent.[71] The popliteal artery and peroneal nerve are most vulnerable.

Before the knee is reduced, lower extremity pulses should be evaluated and motor and sensory function should be documented. Reduction is performed by stabilizing the femur, applying traction to the tibia, and reversing the direction of dislocation.[71] Immediate immobilization and transport to a trauma center is warranted. Angiographic assessment of the popliteal artery is mandatory. Return to play following surgical reconstruction is unusual, but may be possible in selected instances.[72]

Tibial Fractures

TIBIAL PLATEAU FRACTURES

These are rare fractures but do occur in sports such as alpine skiing and cheerleading. They have an association with knee dislocation, ACL injury, and meniscal injury as well.

The usual mechanism of injury with skiing is a hyperextension, valgus displacement resulting in a compression fracture anterolaterally.[73] Falls from a height are another mechanism of injury. The lateral tibial plateau is more likely fractured than the medial side.

Clinically, a hemarthrosis is present. With varus/valgus stress, the compressed side is painful, in contrast to a collateral ligament injury in which abnormal laxity is also noted. Fat droplets are seen if the knee is aspirated.

Standard radiographs may not reveal the fracture. Therefore, either a lateral oblique radiograph or a CT scan should be obtained when there is clinical suspicion of a tibial plateau fracture.[73]

Cast bracing with early range of motion and delayed weight-bearing is used for nondisplaced fractures.[74] Depressed and displaced fractures require surgical treatment.

TIBIAL TUBEROSITY FRACTURES

These fractures occur in 12- to 16-year-olds who are performing a jumping maneuver. During this time, the tibial tubercle apophysis is closing from proximal to distal.[32,33,75] There is some controversy over whether preexisting Osgood-Schlatter's disease is a contributing factor. There are classification systems for these fractures on the basis of displacement and comminution.

Typically, the patient presents with severe pain, swelling, and tenderness at the tuberosity. Sometimes a bony prominence can be palpated, suggesting displacement. The patient usually cannot bear weight or extend the knee. Anterior compartment syndrome has been reported as a complication of this injury so a good neurovascular examination is indicated.[75] Lateral and oblique radiographs confirm the diagnosis.[75]

Minimal or nondisplaced fractures can be managed with immobilization in 0 to 15° of flexion for 4 to 6 weeks.[33] Displaced fractures require open reduction and internal fixation.[32]

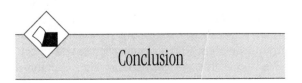

Conclusion

The physician should not only thoroughly understand the evaluation and treatment of the acutely injured knee, he or she should also be familiar with the patient's lifestyle and expectations regarding future performance ability.

Changing medical economics dictate that the primary care physician be able to efficiently evaluate the patient with an acute knee injury. If the patient is a candidate for surgery, a close working relationship between the primary care physician and the orthopedic surgeon is important so that a consistent and comprehensive treatment plan can be presented to the patient. Although medical technology continues to provide the clinician with expanding avenues for diagnosis, a thorough history and physical examination still form the foundation for diagnosis and management.

References

1. Pagnani MJ, Warren RF, Arnoczky SP, et al: Anatomy of the knee. In: Nicholas JA, Hershman EB (eds): *The Lower Extremity and Spine in Sports Medicine*, 2nd ed. St. Louis: Mosby; 1995;581.
2. Torzilli PA, Veltri DM: Biomechanical analysis of knee motion and stability. In: Nicholas JA, Hershman EB (eds): *The Lower Extremity and Spine in Sports Medicine*, 2nd ed. St. Louis: Mosby; 1995; 641.
3. Caldwell GL, Allen AA, Fu FH: Functional anatomy and biomechanics of the meniscus. *Oper Tech Sports Med* 2:152, 1994.
4. Renstrom P, Johnson RJ: Anatomy and biomechanics of the menisci. *Clin Sports Med* 9:523, 1990.
5. Levy I, Torzilli P, Warren R: The effect of medial meniscectomy on anterior-posterior motion. *J Bone Joint Surg* 64A:883, 1982.
6. Miller MD, Harner CD: Posterior cruciate ligament injuries: Current concepts in diagnosis and treatment. *Phys Sportsmed* 21:38, 1993.
7. Harner CD, Hoher J: Evaluation and treatment of posterior cruciate ligament injuries. *Am J Sports Med* 26:471, 1998.
8. Janousek AT, Jones DG, Clatworthy M, et al: Posterior cruciate ligament injuries of the knee joint. *Sports Med* 28:429, 1999.
9. St. Pierre P, Miller MD: Posterior cruciate ligament injuries. *Clin Sports Med* 18:199, 1999.

10. Swain RA, Wilson FD: Diagnosing posterolateral rotatory knee instability. *Phys Sportsmed* 21:95, 1993.

11. Hardaker WT, Whipple TL, Bassett FH: Diagnosis and treatment of the plica syndrome of the knee. *J Bone Joint Surg* 62:221, 1980.

12. Hoppenfeld S, Hutton R: *Physical Examination of the Spine and Extremities.* New York: Appleton-Century-Crofts, 1976.

13. Davidson K: Patellofemoral pain syndrome. *Am Fam Physician* 48:1254, 1994.

14. Henry JH: The patellofemoral joint. In: Nicholas JA, Hershman EB (eds): *The Lower Extremity and Spine in Sports Medicine*, 2nd ed. St. Louis: Mosby; 1995;935.

15. Katz JW, Fingeroth RJ: The diagnostic accuracy of ruptures of the anterior cruciate ligament comparing the Lachman test, the anterior drawer sign, and the pivot shift test in acute and chronic knee injuries. *Am J Sports Med* 14:88, 1986.

16. Lynch MA, Henning CE: Physical examination of the knee. In: Nicholas JA, Hershman EB (eds): *The Lower Extremity and Spine in Sports Medicine*, 2nd ed. St. Louis: Mosby; 1995;675.

17. Rubinstein RA, Shelbourne, KD, McCarroll JR, et al: The accuracy of the clinical examination in the setting of posterior cruciate ligament injuries. *Am J Sports Med* 22:550, 1994.

18. Woods GW, Stanley RF, Tullos HS: Lateral capsular sign: X-ray clue to a significant knee instability. *Am J Sports Med* 7:27, 1979.

19. Harvey J, Tanner S, Wotowey S: *Your Patient Fitness* 2:10, 1990.

20. Hughston JC: Patellar subluxation. A recent history. *Clin Sports Med* 8:153, 1989.

21. Cash JD, Hughston JC: Treatment of acute patellar dislocation. *Am J Sports Med* 16:244, 1988.

22. Garth WP, Pomphery M, Merrill K: Functional treatment of patellar dislocation in an athletic population. *Am J Sports Med* 24:785, 1996.

23. Hawkins RJ, Bell RH, Anisette G: Acute patellar dislocations: The natural history. *Am J Sports Med* 14:117, 1986.

24. Runow A: The dislocating patella: Etiology and prognosis in relation to generalized joint laxity and anatomy of the patellar articulation. *Acta Orthop Scand* 54 (Suppl): 201, 1983.

25. Henry JH: Conservative treatment of patel-lofemoral subluxation. *Clin Sports Med* 8:261, 1989.

26. Garrick JG: Knee problems in adolescents. *Pediatr Rev* 4:235, 1983.

27. Murray TF, Dupont J, Fulkerson JP: Axial and lateral radiographs in evaluating patellofemoral malalignment. *Am J Sports Med* 27:580, 1999.

28. Sallay PI, Poggi J, Speer KP, et al: Acute dislocation of the patella: A correlative pathoanatomical study. *Am J Sports Med* 24:52, 1996.

29. Zarins B, Adams M: Knee injuries in sports. *N Engl J Med* 318:950, 1988.

30. Stanitski CL: Articular hypermobility and chondral injury inpatients with acute patellar dislocation. *Am J Sports Med* 23:146, 1995.

31. Wu C, Huang S, Liu T: Sleeve fracture of the patella in children: A report of five cases. *Am J Sports Med* 19:525, 1991.

32. Smith AD, Tao SS: Knee injuries in young athletes. *Clin Sports Med* 14:629, 1995.

33. Pasque CB, McGinnis DW: Knee. In: Sullivan JA, Anderson SJ (eds): *Care of the Young Athlete.* Rosemont, IL: American Academy of Orthopaedic Surgeons, American Academy of Pediatrics; 2000;377.

34. Yost JG, Schmoll DW: Basketball injuries, In: Nicholas JA, Hershman EB (eds): *The Lower Extremity and Spine in Sports Medicine*, 2nd ed. St. Louis: Mosby; 1995;1411.

35. Connnell MD, Jokl P: The aging athlete. In: Nicholas JA, Hershman EB (eds): *The Lower Extremity and Spine in Sports Medicine*, 2nd ed. St. Louis: Mosby; 1995;167.

36. Kaylor, KL: Injuries to the patella and extensor mechanism, In: Levine AM (ed): *Orthopaedic Knowledge Update: Trauma.* Rosemont, IL: American Academy of Orthopaedic Surgeons; 1996;153.

37. Nichols CE: Patellar tendon injuries. *Clin Sports Med* 11:807, 1992.

38. Poehling GC, Ruch DS, Chabon SJ: The landscape of meniscal injuries. *Clin Sports Med* 9:539, 1990

39. Henning CE: Current status of meniscus salvage. *Clin Sports Med* 9:567, 1990.

40. Muellner T, Nikolic A, Vecsei V: Recommendations for the diagnosis of traumatic meniscal injuries in athletes. *Sports Med* 27:337, 1999.

41. DeHaven KE: Meniscus repair. *Am J Sports Med* 27:242, 1999.

42. Bessette GC: The meniscus. *Orthopedics* 15:35, 1992.

43. Pettrone FA: Meniscectomy: Arthrotomy versus arthroscopy. *Am J Sports Med* 10:355, 1982.

44. Matava MJ, Eck K, Totty W, et al: Magnetic resonance imaging as a tool to predict meniscal reparability. *Am J Sports Med* 27:436, 1999.

45. Mandelbaum BR, Finerman GA, Reicher MA, et al: Magnetic resonance imaging as a tool for evaluation of traumatic knee injuries. Anatomical and pathoanatomical correlations. *Am J Sports Med* 14:361, 1986.

46. Mintzer CM, Richmond JC, Taylor J: Meniscal repair in the young athlete. *Am J Sports Med* 26:630, 1998.

47. DeHaven KE: Decision-making factors in the treatment of meniscus lesions. *Clin Orthop* 252:49, 1990.

48. Vander Schilden JL: Improvements in rehabilitation of the postmeniscectomized or meniscal-repaired patient. *Clin Orthop* 252:73, 1990

49. Cooper DE, Arnoczky SP, Warren RF: Arthroscopic meniscal repair. *Clin Sports Med* 9:589, 1990.

50. Jensen JE, Conn RR, Hazelrigg G, Hewett JE: Systematic evaluation of acute knee injuries. *Clin Sports Med* 4:295, 1985.

51. Andrish JT: Ligamentous injuries of the knee. *Prim Care* 11:77, 1984.

52. Indelicato PA: Non-operative treatment of complete tears of the medial collateral ligament of the knee. *J Bone Joint Surg* 65:323, 1983.

53. Woo SL, Inoue M, McGurk-Burleson E, Gomez MA: Treatment of the medial collateral ligament injury. II: Structure and function of canine knees in response to differing treatment regimens. *Am J Sports Med* 15:22, 1987.

54. Smith BW, Green GA: Acute knee injuries: Part II. Diagnosis and management. *Am Fam Physician* 51:799, 1995.

55. Micheli L: Pediatric and adolescent sports medicine. In: Griffin LY (ed): *Orthopedic Knowledge Update: Sports Medicine*. Rosemont, IL: American Academy of Orthopaedic Surgeons; 1994;349.

56. Gray D: Femur fractures. In: Richards BS (ed): *Orthopedic Knowledge Update: Pediatrics*. Rosemont, IL: American Academy of Orthopaedic Surgeons; 1996;229.

57. Ireland ML, Gaudette M, Crook S: ACL injuries in the female athlete. *J Sport Rehab* 6:97, 1997.

58. Harmon KG, Ireland ML: Gender differences in noncontact anterior cruciate ligament injuries. *Clin Sports Med* 19:287, 2000.

59. Griffin LY: Non-contact ACL. *Consensus Symposium*. Hunt Valley, MD, June 10, 1999.

60. Zarins B, Fisk DN: Knee ligament injury. In: Nicholas JA, Hershman EB (eds): *The Lower Extremity and Spine in Sports Medicine*, 2nd ed. St. Louis: Mosby; 1995;825.

61. DeHaven, KE: Diagnosis of acute knee injuries with hemarthrosis. *Am J Sports Med* 8:9, 1980.

62. Shelton WR, Barrett GR, Dukes A: Early season anterior cruciate ligament tears. *Am J Sports Med* 25:656, 1997.

63. Buckley SL, Barrack RL, Alexander AH: The natural history of conservatively treated partial anterior cruciate ligament tears. *Am J Sports Med* 17:221, 1989.

64. Clancy WG Jr, Ray JM, Zoltan DJ: Acute tears of the anterior cruciate ligament. Surgical versus conservative treatment. *J Bone Joint Surg* 70:1483, 1988.

65. Finsterbush A, Frankl U, Matan Y, Mann G: Secondary damage to the knee after isolated injury of the anterior cruciate ligament. *Am J Sports Med* 18:475, 1990

66. Cross MJ, Harris J, Slater HK: Recent developments in the treatment and repair of anterior cruciate ligament injuries in the athlete. *Sports Med* 10:349, 1990

67. Schenck RC, Blaschak MJ, Lance ED, et al: A prospective outcome study of rehabilitation programs and anterior cruciate ligament reconstruction. *Arthroscopy* 13:285, 1997.

68. Fehnel DJ, Johnson R: Anterior cruciate injuries in the skeletally immature athlete: A review of treatment outcomes. *Sports Med* 29:51, 2000.

69. Graf BK, Lange RH, Fujisaki CK, et al: Anterior cruciate tears in the skeletally immature patients: Meniscal pathology at presentation and after attempted conservative treatment. *Arthroscopy* 8:229, 1992.

70. Kannus P, Bergfeld J, Jarvinen M, et al: Injuries to the posterior cruciate ligament of the knee. *Sports Med* 12:110, 1991.

71. Tornetta P: Knee dislocation. In: Levine AM (ed):

Orthopaedic Knowledge Update: Trauma. Rosemont, IL: American Academy of Orthopaedic Surgeons; 1996;145.

72. Bergfeld JA, Safran MR: Knee-ligaments. In: Safran MR, McKeag DB, Van Camp SP (eds): *Manual of Sports Medicine.* Philadelphia: Lippincott-Raven; 1998;431.

73. McConkey JP, Meeuwisse W: Tibial plateau fractures in alpine skiing. *Am J Sports Med* 16:159, 1988.

74. Steadman JR, Scheinberg RR: Skiing injuries. In: Nicholas JA, Hershman EB (eds): *The Lower Extremity and Spine in Sports Medicine*, 2nd ed. St. Louis: Mosby; 1995;1361.

75. Cohn SL, Sotta RP, Bergfeld, JA: Fractures about the knee in sports. *Clin Sports Med* 9:121, 1990.

John P. DiFiori

Chapter 9

Leg Pain

Introduction

Exercise-induced leg pain, defined as pain occurring in the lower extremity between the knee and ankle, is a common problem among competitive athletes involved in running and jumping sports. In addition, the majority of the most popular recreational sport and fitness activities place significant stress on the lower extremity. Thus, it is not surprising that leg injuries account for approximately 7 to 12 percent of injuries presenting to clinicians in the outpatient setting.[1,2] In some populations, the prevalence is much higher. A 1-year prospective study of track and field athletes found that 28 percent of all injuries were located in the leg, the most common site.[3] During military training, 26 to 36 percent of overuse injuries have been reported to occur in the leg.[4,5]

The causes of leg pain are extensive and varied (Table 9-1). Exercise-induced leg pain may be due to an acute injury (e.g., contusion, muscle strain) or develop from overuse. Referred pain sources, tumors, connective tissue disease, peripheral arterial disease, and deep venous thrombosis may also cause leg pain. The purpose of this chapter is to describe the diagnosis and treatment of the most common causes of leg pain in the athlete including medial tibial stress syndrome, stress fractures, exertional compartment syndromes, and acute strains of the gastrocnemius. Less common entrapment syndromes involving the popliteal artery and superficial peroneal nerve also are briefly discussed.

Anatomy

The leg is divided into anterior, posterior, and lateral compartments by the anterior and posterior intermuscular septa which emanate from

Table 9-1

Causes of Leg Pain in the Athlete

Frequently seen	Less frequent
Medial tibial stress syndrome	Exertional compartment syndromes
Stress fractures	Referred pain
Gastrocnemius strains	Acute (trauma-induced) compartment syndromes
Contusions	Popliteal artery entrapment syndrome
Muscle cramping	Superficial peroneal nerve entrapment
Delayed onset muscle soreness	Common peroneal nerve entrapment
Fractures	Common peroneal nerve contusion
	Effort-induced venous thrombosis
Other causes to keep in mind	
Deep venous thrombosis	
Tumors	
Peripheral vascular disease	
Connective tissue diseases (e.g., sarcoidosis, erythema nodosum)	
Bone diseases (e.g., rickets, hyperparathyroidism, Paget's disease)	

SOURCE: Adapted from Brukner P, Khan K: *Clin Sports Med*, Sydney: McGraw-Hill, 1993. p 407.

the crural fascia and attach to the fibula, and the interosseous membrane located between the tibia and fibula along most of their length (Fig. 9-1). The tibia is easily palpable along its entire length including its distal portion, the medial malleolus. The proximally located fibular head is also easily appreciated on examination, as is the common peroneal nerve just below it. Laterally, the fibula is covered by the peroneal muscles, making palpation difficult. The distal third and the distal end (the lateral malleolus) are readily discerned. The muscles, nerves, and vasculature of the leg are depicted in Fig. 9-1.

The posterior compartment includes superficial and deep layers. The superficial muscles in the posterior compartment are the gastrocnemius, soleus, and plantaris. The deep muscles are the popliteus, tibialis posterior, flexor digitorum longus, and flexor hallucis longus. The tibial nerve innervates all posterior compartment muscles. The major blood supply is provided by the posterior tibial artery, with the peroneal artery supplying the lateral portion.

The lateral compartment contains the peroneus longus and brevis muscles. They are innervated by the superficial peroneal nerve. The peroneal artery furnishes the blood supply.

The anterior compartment includes the tibialis anterior, extensor hallucis longus, and extensor digitorum longus muscles. The blood supply is contributed by the anterior tibial artery, with innervation from the deep peroneal nerve.

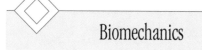

Biomechanics

The running gait cycle is composed of contact, stance, and swing phases. With initial ground contact three components of force are generated: a vertical force of 2 to 3 times body weight, a fore-aft component of 30 percent body weight, and a medial-lateral component of 10 percent body weight.[6] Dissipation of these forces occurs

in an extremely limited time, less than 200 msec.[7] Given such vertical forces, a 150 lb. runner with a stride length of 4.5 ft completing a 10K race would need to dissipate nearly 700 tons of energy over the course of the race.

A major site of the transmission of the ground reaction forces is the subtalar joint. As ground impact occurs, the foot is in a slightly supinated position and the tibia externally rotated. Eversion of the subtalar joint allows for pronation during the stance phase and internal tibial rotation on the talus follows. The peak forces do not occur with initial contact, but somewhat later during the stance phase. Pronation is followed by subtalar inversion and supination in preparation for toe-off. The foot remains supinated during the swing phase. This complex series of movements results in the transmission of forces proximally to the leg, knee, thigh, hip, and back. Variations in the timing or magnitude of these events (e.g., excessive or very rapid pronation), or factors that may hinder load-absorbing abilities (e.g., a rigid cavus foot), alter the distribution of forces throughout the lower extremity and may increase the risk for injury.

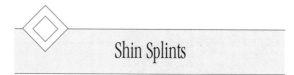

Shin Splints

Pain along the borders of the tibia that occurs with exercise has been described with a variety of terms. Perhaps the most commonly employed designation has been "shin splints." This is a nonspecific term defined in 1966 in the AMA *Standard Nomenclature of Athletic Injuries* as pain in the leg from repetitive running on hard surfaces involving forcible use of the foot dorsiflexors, excluding fractures and ischemic disorders.[8] Shin splints has been used to describe both acute and chronic injuries involving musculotendinous and bony structures. In the past, this diagnosis included injuries that would currently be recognized as stress fractures, fascial

Figure 9-1

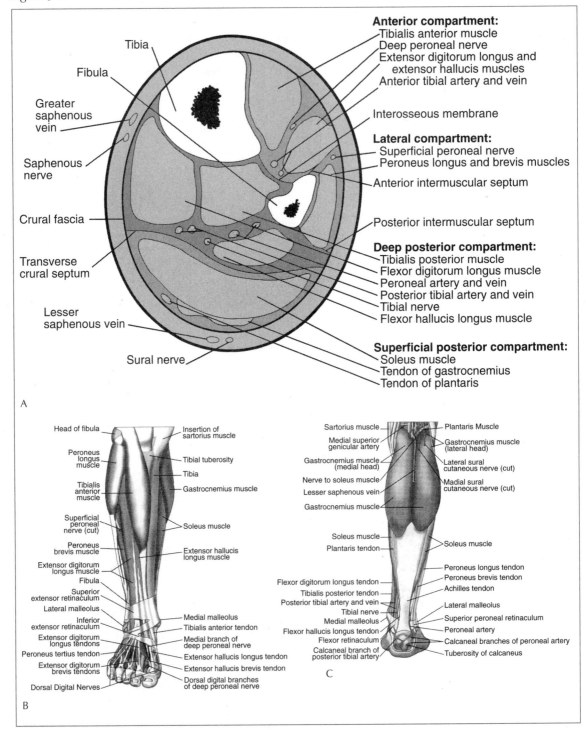

Anatomy of the leg. Cross section (**A**) of the leg showing the four compartments with their structures, and also an anterior (**B**) and posterior (**C**) view.

hernias, and exertional compartment syndromes.

More recently, in an effort to refine the definition, research and discussion has produced additional terms including the soleus syndrome and medial tibial stress syndrome.[9,10] At the same time, awareness of stress fractures and exertional compartment syndromes, and the ability to diagnose them has improved. Thus, it appears that the term "shin splints" has outlived its usefulness. It should be discarded and replaced with more specific, albeit at times still descriptive, diagnoses, such as those described as follows.

Medial Tibial Stress Syndrome

First proposed by Drez, medial tibial stress syndrome (MTSS) refers to exercise-induced pain of the posteromedial border of the distal two-thirds of the tibia.[10] It excludes pain due to a stress fracture, fascial hernia, or compartment syndrome, as well as causes of pain that are more laterally situated along the tibia, such as chronic anterior compartment syndromes. Because many of the reports describing leg injuries in athletes have used the less specific terminology, the true prevalence of MTSS is difficult to estimate. One recent study reported that shin pain not due to a stress fracture was responsible for about 10 percent of injuries among track and field athletes.[3]

Etiology

The etiology remains open to debate, but it appears to be due to a stress reaction involving the fascia, periosteum, or bone, or some combination of these structures at the posteromedial tibial border. The symptoms have often been attributed to a traction periostalgia, typically described to involve the tibialis posterior. More recently, the crural fascia, the flexor digitorum longus, and the soleus have been proposed as primary contributors.[9,11] One study utilizing magnetic resonance imaging in runners with medial tibial pain found periosteal edema at the attachment sites of all three muscles.[12]

History

Although the onset of pain may be acute, it more typically presents as an overuse injury, and is not uncommonly bilateral. The pain arises with the onset of exercise, but may become more tolerable as the exercise continues, allowing completion of the training session. Symptoms increase again after exercise, and eventually resolve with rest. As the injury progresses, pain is noted with routine activities, and begins to interfere with performance. Neurologic or vascular symptoms are inconsistent with the diagnosis.

Risk factors for overuse injuries should be reviewed in detail to determine why the injury developed (Table 9-2). Historical factors of particular interest include rate of training progression, running on hard training surfaces, prior level of conditioning, and recent changes in footwear (or the lack thereof). Even slight changes in training may result in injury, such as the use of spiked running shoes in place of training flats. Previous injuries and their treatment should be noted. An inadequately rehabilitated injury may serve as a weak link in force dissipation, resulting in further injuries. As in other overuse injuries, determining when the pain occurs in relation to the onset of activity helps to estimate the severity of the injury (Table 9-3).

Physical Examination

Tenderness to palpation along the posteromedial border of the tibia is the typical finding. This tenderness will be found a few cm proximal to the medial malleolus, extending proximally for several cm more. Slight swelling may also be seen. Resisted manual muscle testing in plantar flex-

Table 9-2

Factors Contributing to Overuse Injury

INTRINSIC FACTORS
Previous injury
Menstrual dysfunction
Growth-related factors in children
Muscle imbalance and inflexibility related to rapid growth
Increased susceptibility of growth cartilage to repetitive stress
Inadequate conditioning
Psychological factors
Poor flexibility
Muscle weakness or imbalance
Anatomic malalignment
Joint laxity

EXTRINSIC FACTORS
Training progression too rapid and/or inadequate rest
Inappropriate equipment and/or footwear
Incorrect sport technique
Peer and/or adult influences
Uneven or hard surfaces

SOURCE: Adapted with permission from DiFiori JP: Overuse injuries in children and adolescents. *Physician Sportsmed* 27:75, 1999.

ion, dorsiflexion, inversion, and eversion usually does not cause pain. Hopping on the affected leg may reproduce symptoms. Indirect percussion, however, is pain free. The neurologic and vascular portions of the examination are normal. Compared to control subjects, those with MTSS demonstrate an increased maximum pronation velocity and maximum pronation, varus alignment of the hindfoot and/or forefoot, and a standing foot angle of less than 140 degrees.[13,14] Observation of the patient standing and walking, or with videotaped gait analysis, may expose these characteristics. Shoes should be examined for signs of excessive wear and for their suitability for the activity.

Ancillary Tests

Routine radiographs of the leg are usually normal. Careful inspection, however, may reveal extensive thickening of posterior cortex of the tibia. A three-phase bone scan may demonstrate diffuse uptake along the posteromedial tibial border involving up to one third of the tibia, which is seen in the delayed phase of the scan only.[15] In contrast, tibial stress fractures exhibit findings in all three phases, with a more focal uptake pattern in the delayed phase. Magnetic resonance imaging (MRI) may display periosteal edema with or without associated mild to moderate bone marrow edema (Table 9-4).[12]

In some cases, differentiating MTSS from a tibial stress fracture can be difficult (Table 9-5).

Table 9-3

Clinical Assessment of Overuse Injury

SYMPTOM PATTERN	SEVERITY	REDUCTION OF LOADING TO INJURED SITE (%)
After activity only, or at onset, but not persisting	Low	≤ 25
During activity, late onset		25–50
During activity, early onset		50–75
Limits quality and/or quantity of training		≥ 75
Prevents training	High	Complete rest

SOURCE: Adapted with permission from DiFiori JP, Hosey R: Overuse injuries: diagnosis and treatment. *Clin Atlas Office Proced* 1:227, 1998.

Table 9-4

Magnetic Resonance Imaging Grading of Tibial Stress Injuries

| | | MRI FINDINGS | | |
GRADE	PERIOSTEAL EDEMA	MARROW EDEMA	FRACTURE LINE	CLINICAL CORRELATION
1	Mild to moderate on T2-weighted images	None	None	Stress reaction
2	Moderate to severe on T2-weighted images	Seen on T2-weighted images	None	Stress reaction
3	Moderate to severe on T2-weighted images	Seen on T1- and T2-weighted images	None	Stress fracture
4	Moderate to severe on T2-weighted images	Seen on T1- and T2-weighted images	Visible	Stress fracture

SOURCE: Modified with permission from Fredericson M, Bergman AG, Hoffman KL, et al: Tibial stress reaction in runners. Correlation of clinical symptoms and scintigraphy with a new magnetic resonance imaging grading system. *Am J Sports Med* 23:472, 1995.

Radiographs should be obtained in all such situations. If these are not helpful, either a three-phase bone scan or MRI should be obtained.

It may be even more challenging to rule out a deep posterior compartment syndrome. For patients in whom a stress fracture has been excluded, and who do not respond to a program of rest and rehabilitation, compartmental pressure measurements should be considered. Compartmental pressure studies in MTSS are normal.[10,16]

Treatment

For those with a typical history and diffuse tenderness of the posteromedial tibial border, treatment can be initiated without the need for imaging. The mainstay of the initial phase of treatment for MTSS is a reduction of impact loading to the leg to a level that will halt the overuse process. Complete rest may not be required (see Table 9-3). In some sports, only particular activities need to be curtailed. For example, in volleyball, blocking and spiking drills, which load the leg though repetitive jumping, should be reduced, but digging and passing may be continued if pain-free. Nonimpact activities such as cycling, swimming, or pool running should be used to maintain conditioning.

Ice massage can help in providing local pain relief. Other modalities such as iontophoresis and ultrasound have also been used, although their benefits have not been clearly demonstrated. Soft tissue therapy including digital pressure, transverse friction, and myofascial release applied to the soleus, flexor digitorum longus, and posterior tibialis can be helpful. A long pneumatic splint may be also used to alleviate symptoms that occur with daily activities.

Although nonsteroidal anti-inflammatory drugs (NSAIDs) are frequently used to treat MTSS, studies in which periosteal biopsies have been performed have not consistently shown an inflammatory reaction.[10,17,18] Thus, as in other overuse injuries, the use of NSAIDs remains somewhat controversial. Their main role may be as pain modifiers that enable controlled rehabilitation to proceed.

The rehabilitation program should focus on developing strength and flexibility of the entire lower extremity. Especially important are the

Table 9-5

Differentiating Medial Tibial Stress Syndrome (MTSS) from Tibial Stress Fractures

	MTSS	TIBIAL STRESS FRACTURE
SYMPTOMS		
Character	Bony, aching Often can continue activity with pain abating	Bony, aching Usually cannot continue without increasing pain
FINDINGS		
Pain location	Mid or distal third of posteromedial tibial border	Anywhere on tibia, including posteromedial border
Pain distribution	Several cm without distinct focal area	Distinct focal area, limited surrounding tenderness
Indirect percussion	Pain free	May be painful
Single leg hop	Usually painful	Usually painful
RADIOGRAPHS		
	Normal	May show periosteal reaction, fracture line
THREE-PHASE BONE SCAN		
	Diffuse uptake in delayed phase only	Focal uptake, all phases abnormal
MRI		
	Periosteal edema with or without mild to moderate marrow edema No discrete fracture line	Periosteal edema with extensive marrow edema May have discrete fracture

heel cord and dorsiflexors. Imbalances in strength and flexibility should be identified and corrected. Modification of malalignment with orthoses should be considered on an individual basis. Although malalignment has been associated with MTSS, prospective studies have yet to show a cause-and-effect relationship between malalignment and lower extremity overuse injury.[19,20] Thus, for those in whom an obvious cause for injury can be identified (such as the rapid introduction of plyometric training in a previously unfit individual) correction of malalignment may not be indicated. In other cases, over the counter or prescription orthoses may be beneficial.

Women should be advised to take 1,300 to 1,500 mg of elemental calcium per day. For those with a history of menstrual dysfunction, evaluation and management should be initiated (see Chap. 12.) In addition, those suspected of an eating disorder should receive appropriate consultation.

Return to Play

Return to impact-loading activities should occur on a gradual schedule, beginning with low-intensity training on softer surfaces. Training volume is slowly increased using symptoms and physical findings as a guide to the progression of activity. Intensity of training is increased as stable levels of volume are achieved. Although the return to unrestricted activity is quite variable, a 6-week time period is a reasonable estimate in most cases. The use of a long pneumatic splint in this phase of rehabilitation however, may allow an earlier return to activities.[21] As mentioned, many athletes will be able to continue to participate on a modified basis while undergoing treatment.

Prevention of Recurrence

It is important to review the factors that led to the injury with the athlete, coach, trainer, and parents (if the patient is a child or adolescent). Even a well-rehabilitated injury is no guarantee against a recurrence unless a specific plan is put in place directed at these issues. This plan should include a review of the training program, along with proper strength and flexibility training. The athlete should also ensure that footwear is appropriate, and replaced at regular intervals, to avoid excessive wear that may alter mechanics and load absorption.

Surgical Indications

Despite these measures, MTSS may occasionally prove resistant to conservative treatment efforts. In such instances, operative treatment, involving a posteromedial fasciotomy with release of the medial soleus fascial bridge, may be indicated.[9]

Stress Fractures

Prevalence

The tibia and fibula are among the most common sites for stress fractures. In studies using imaging techniques to diagnose stress fractures in athletes, the tibia was the site for 19 to 55 percent of these injuries, whereas the fibula accounted for up to 30 percent.[22] In the majority of these studies, the tibia and fibula were among the top three sites. The relative percentages vary depending on the activity performed. In track and field athletes, for example, stress fractures of the tibia and fibula are the predominant sites in middle and long distance runners.[3] In hurdlers, sprinters, jumpers, and multi-event athletes, however, tarsal and metatarsal stress fractures occur more frequently.

Etiology

Stress fractures occur as a result of the inability of bone to effectively remodel in response to repetitive loading. They represent one point in the spectrum of stress response in bone that also includes bone strain and stress reactions (e.g., MTSS). The etiology is likely multifactorial. Ground reaction forces, repeated muscle contractions across the bone, and muscle fatigue are each proposed as causes of this injury. One recent study suggests that strain rate, rather than strain magnitude, is responsible for stress fracture development.[23] The dynamic events that take place in bone due to repetitive loading and the risk factors for stress fractures are detailed in Chap. 20. This section addresses the specific clinical characteristics of tibial and fibular stress fractures.

Tibial Stress Fractures

LOCATION

Stress fractures of the tibia can occur at nearly any location. The posteromedial border of either the proximal or distal third of the shaft are the most common sites.[24] Stress fractures that arise in the proximal tibia (metaphysis) and the anterior midshaft are less frequent. Longitudinal stress fractures have also been reported.[25]

HISTORY

Patients with tibial stress fractures typically present with the gradual onset of leg pain localized to the tibia. Initially, the pain occurs only with exercise and is relieved by rest. With continued loading of the leg, the pain increases in severity, limiting the athlete's ability to complete training sessions. The pain is often described as aching in character. With progression of the injury, pain may occur with walking. Symptoms occasionally may be present at night. At this point, the symptoms may resolve after several days of rest, only to return when training is re-attempted.

A thorough search for risk factors for this overuse injury should be undertaken (see Table 9-2). Changes in training habits and/or equipment, particularly within the 3 to 6 weeks preceding the injury, should specifically be sought. Increases in running mileage or pace, new surfaces, worn or inappropriate footwear are typical examples. The patient's prior injury history, especially previous stress fractures, should be recorded. Changes in other facets of the athlete's training program (e.g., resistance training, plyometrics) should not be overlooked. New sport techniques should be reviewed in detail with the athlete, trainer, and coach. Menstrual history should be documented. A dietary history should estimate calcium intake. An assessment for signs of disordered eating should be also performed. Both menstrual dysfunction and disordered eating may be associated with osteopenia and increase the risk for stress fracture (see Chap. 12).

PHYSICAL EXAMINATION

Physical examination reveals well-localized tenderness to palpation over the tibia. At times the tenderness may span several cm, but within this area, there is usually a very sensitive focal point of pain. The painful site may be slightly swollen. In stress fractures that have been present for weeks or more, periosteal thickening may be palpable.

Hopping on one foot often reproduces symptoms. Indirect percussion—percussing at a distant point on the tibia or striking the heel—may also produce pain. Resisted manual muscle testing usually does not produce symptoms. Application of a vibrating tuning fork or ultrasound to the site in an attempt to reproduce symptoms has generally not been helpful.[26] The entire lower extremity should be evaluated for features of malalignment, which may affect load absorption. The presence of muscle imbalance, weakness, restricted range of motion, and poor flexibility should also be noted.

ANCILLARY TESTS

A history of exercise-related tibial pain accompanied by well-localized bony tenderness on examination, is very suggestive of a tibial stress fracture. In fact, such findings have been shown to correlate well with MRI results in athletes with tibial pain.[12] Imaging studies are useful, however, to exclude other causes of bony leg pain, such as tumors, and to confirm the diagnosis.

Radiographs are commonly ordered when stress fractures are suspected. Findings include a localized periosteal reaction, sclerosis, callus formation, or a lucent fracture line. Unfortunately, however, radiographs have a relatively low sensitivity for the diagnosis of stress fractures, particularly if the symptoms have been present for less than 2 to 3 weeks. Repeat radiographs may ultimately demonstrate the stress fracture, but it may be weeks or months before this occurs. In some cases radiographs will remain normal, and radionuclide or MR scanning will be needed to diagnose the fracture.

Three-phase radionuclide imaging is a highly sensitive and generally available method to diagnose stress fractures. All three phases of the study are abnormal in stress fractures. The delayed phase demonstrates a focal uptake pattern. Nearly all patients will have an abnormal scan within 3 days of symptom onset, although only rarely will a patient present this quickly. Although three-phase radionuclide scans are very sensitive, they can be nonspecific. For example, scans may show multiple abnormal areas that are not symptomatic. Thus, clinical correlation is important in such cases to develop a proper treatment plan.

MRI, as a technique for imaging stress fractures, is of comparable sensitivity to the three-phase bone scan. In addition, MRI depicts the surrounding soft tissues and provides greater specificity with respect to bony injury, and for these reasons, it is widely becoming the procedure of choice in evaluating suspected stress fractures. MR images in tibial stress injury are graded depending on the presence of periosteal edema, marrow edema, and a visible fracture line (see Table 9-4). A history of leg pain early after the onset of activity or with walking, and an examination with well-localized tibial tenderness, correlates with grade 3 or 4 findings on MRI.

TREATMENT

The cornerstone of treatment for tibial stress fractures is rest from impact activities. All activities that produce leg discomfort should be halted. For those patients in whom daily activities are painful (such as students who must negotiate treks across campus) a long pneumatic splint is helpful. If a splint is not available or not helpful, nonweight bearing or partial-weight bearing on crutches can be used until the pain has dissipated. Acetaminophen or NSAIDs may be used for pain relief.

Other forms of activity should be implemented to maintain fitness levels. Cycling, swimming, and pool running (especially in runners) are typical choices. Stair climbers and cross-country ski machines, however, may cause pain in the early stages of rehabilitation. Flexibility training for the entire lower extremity, along with progressive resistance exercises, should be performed throughout the rehabilitation process as long as they do not produce discomfort.

A gradual return to loading activities is begun once pain with daily activities and focal tenderness are resolved. It may take several weeks for this to occur. A recent study found that the median time to the beginning of light activities was 1 week for those using a pneumatic brace, compared to 3 weeks for those not using one.[27] Walking at a brisk pace on a soft surface (grass or synthetic track) is a reasonable starting point. On the following day, if the patient remains pain-free and is nontender on examination, the time spent walking may be increased. If at any point in the reintroduction of activities pain recurs, the progression is halted until the patient has been able to ambulate without pain for 2 to 3 days.

Although no firm guidelines exist, jogging is usually not introduced until the patient has been walking without symptoms for approximately 1 week. A useful test to determine when jogging may be resumed is the single leg hop. When this is pain free, jogging may resume on an every other day basis, beginning with 5 to 10 min per session. Small increases may be made each session as long as symptoms do not develop. Once the patient has been jogging on a daily basis for 1 week, periods of faster-paced running are introduced. Following this, functional activities are begun. Sprinting, cutting, and lastly, jumping are part of this phase. When the athlete is able to perform functional skills without pain, sport-specific training may be resumed.

RETURN TO PLAY

The use of a pneumatic brace significantly improves the time to return to unrestricted activity. Swenson et al reported that those using a brace had a median time to return of 21 days compared to 77 days for those not wearing a brace. Other authors have suggested a more aggressive approach in which athletes using a brace are permitted to continue their sport.[28] The basis for such treatment is that the additional support provided by the brace will allow bone remodeling to eventually overtake resorption, even in the face of continued loading. In the Swenson study, 11 of 13 athletes in various sports became pain-free within 1 month while continuing their sport with the addition of a brace. The brace is generally continued until the season is completed.

PREVENTION OF RECURRENCE

A return to play is an important goal to achieve; however, implementation of preventive measures should not be forgotten. A detailed plan should be put in place to address the factors that may have led to the stress fracture. Proper progression of training, the importance of regularly scheduled rest, and maintenance of strength and flexibility should be emphasized. Menstrual disturbances and disordered eating behavior should be carefully evaluated and treated, if such concerns are present. Calcium supplementation should be encouraged for all women.

Modification of malalignment should also be considered. In fact, a study of military recruits recently found that the use of custom orthoses decreased the incidence of stress fractures by more than 50 percent.[29]

SPECIAL SITUATIONS

ANTERIOR CORTEX STRESS FRACTURES   Stress fractures of the anterior cortex of the midshaft of the tibia are notorious for developing complications including delayed union, nonunion, and complete fracture. The cortical lucency sometimes seen on radiographs in these injuries has been referred to as the "dreaded black line." These stress fractures occur on the tension side of the tibia, and are most commonly reported in activities that require repeated jumping or bounding, such as basketball or ballet. Biopsies obtained from the stress fractures at this site have shown no evidence of remodeling, the absence of inflammatory cells, extensive ingrowth of fibrous tissue, and localized avascular bone necrosis.[30]

Given the difficulty in healing these injuries,

stress fractures occurring at this site should be referred to an orthopedic surgeon. Initial treatment of these injuries is usually a period of prolonged rest from impact loading with or without a cast or modified immobilization. Rettig et al. described successful conservative treatment in 7 of 8 basketball players with rest and/or pulsed electromagnetic fields. Average time to return to full activity was 8.7 months.[31] Monitoring of fracture healing should be done at regular intervals both clinically and with radiographs. If after 3 to 6 months there is no sign of clinical or radiographic healing, bone grafting with or without the use of an intramedullary rod can be considered.

LONGITUDINAL STRESS FRACTURES   The diagnosis of a longitudinal (vertically oriented) stress fracture of the tibia should be considered in patients presenting with poorly localized distal leg pain. This is a relatively rare stress fracture, with fewer than 50 cases reported in the literature.[32] Radiographs are often negative, but may show a longitudinal linear lucency, cortical thickening, or a periosteal reaction. Even though a bone scan is abnormal in these injuries, the appearance is variable and additional studies (either CT or MR) are usually needed to make the diagnosis. Management is similar to that for stress fractures of the proximal or distal tibia occurring at the posteromedial tibial border.

Fibular Stress Fractures

LOCATION

Stress fractures of the fibula most commonly occur in the distal shaft. Stress fractures of the proximal third are much less common, but have been reported.[33] Biomechanical studies have demonstrated that with the ankle in neutral position, the load distribution to the fibula is approximately 7 percent.[34] The load is increased with dorsiflexion and eversion, and decreased with plantar flexion and inversion. In addition, dorsiflexion produces torsional stresses that are dissipated at the proximal tibiofibular joint.[35]

HISTORY

Patients with fibular stress fractures present with lateral leg pain that is of gradual onset. In fact, because of the relatively small role the fibula plays in bearing weight, athletes typically will be able to "play through the pain" initially. Because of this, they may not seek care for several weeks after the onset of pain. As with tibial stress fractures, a complete history should be taken in an effort to identify factors that contributed to injury development.

PHYSICAL EXAMINATION

Physical examination should identify problems that may affect force dissipation including malalignment, muscle weakness or imbalance, and inflexibility. Palpation will reveal localized tenderness over the lateral aspect of the leg. This can be a bit more difficult to pinpoint than a tibial stress fracture due to the overlying musculature. However, applying a moderate amount of pressure will localize the injury to the fibula. Hopping on the injured leg will usually reproduce symptoms. Striking the heel, however, is not as helpful as it can be with tibial stress fractures.

ANCILLARY TESTS

Radiographs should be obtained, but many times are unrevealing. A three-phase bone scan or MRI can be ordered to secure the diagnosis if radiographs are negative (Fig. 9-2).

TREATMENT

Treatment for fibular stress fractures begins with a reduction in impact loading and the use of alternative conditioning activities. NSAIDs or acetaminophen may be used for pain relief. Once pain is controlled, a program of rehabilitation similar to that described for tibial stress fractures is begun. A long pneumatic splint is helpful to both assist in early pain reduction and to provide support during rehabilitation and return to activity.

Most patients will be able to proceed through the rehabilitation for fibular stress fractures in somewhat less time than for a tibial stress fracture. In fact, some cases may be successfully treated symptomatically with a long pneumatic splint without a significant reduction in training or competition. Measures to prevent future stress fractures should be taken as described previously.

SPECIAL SITUATIONS

PROXIMAL FIBULAR STRESS FRACTURES Stress fractures of the proximal one-third of the fibula are rare. They have been most frequently reported in military personnel involved in jumping activities.[36] Only nine cases have been described in athletes.[33] The etiology is unclear. It appears to involve loading of the fibula while the ankle is dorsiflexed (which produces external rotation at the proximal tibiofibular joint) and simultaneous eccentric activation of the plantar flexors.

Interestingly, these injuries appear to have two different clinical and radiographic presentations. In one type, the clinical history and imaging findings may be similar to those of more common distal stress fractures. Alternatively, they may occur acutely, and demonstrate a frank fracture on x-ray.

Because stress fractures at this site are so unusual, other causes of leg pain, such as tumors, should be carefully excluded. Once diagnosed, these injuries respond well to the typical treatment for stress fractures of the fibula.

Exertional Compartment Syndromes

Compartment syndromes occur when there is an increase in tissue pressure within a closed fascial space that causes a decrease in perfusion, compromising the function of the intracompartmen-

Figure 9-2

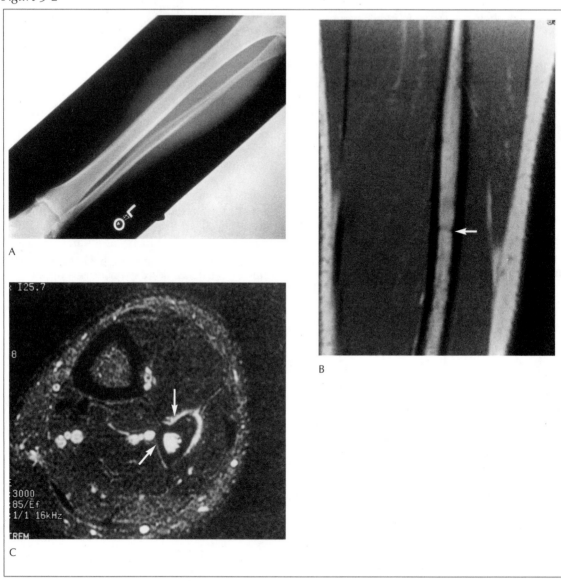

A 19-year-old collegiate softball player with a history of several weeks of left lateral leg pain when running. **(A)** Normal radiograph. **(B)** Sagittal MR image with visible fracture line. **(C)** Axial MR image demonstrating periosteal and marrow edema.

tal structures.[37] Acute compartment syndromes are recognized as true surgical emergencies. They are classically described to occur after significant trauma, such as limb fractures, but may develop after exertion in the absence of an obvious injury. Those due to acute injury are uncommon in athletes, but may occur in the leg secondary to tibial fractures and muscle ruptures. Acute exertional compartment syndromes—where severe unremitting pain develops after a bout of exercise—are also rare. More common in the athlete are chronic exertional compartment syndromes in which recurrent leg pain occurs with activity and resolves with rest. These latter two forms of compartment syndrome are rather unique to the athletic setting, and are discussed here.

Chronic Exertional Compartment Syndrome

The prevalence of chronic exertional compartment syndrome (CECS) of the leg is uncertain. In a highly selected series of 98 patients who were referred over a 5-year period because they were specifically thought to have CECS of the anterior compartment, only 26 were confirmed to have elevated compartment pressures by intramuscular pressure measurements.[38] Another study of over 2,400 patient visits to a sports medicine center reported that 3.5 percent of these patients were diagnosed as having true compartment syndromes.[1]

ETIOLOGY

CECS is known to involve an excessive increase in intracompartmental pressure during exercise.[37] Unlike the acute syndromes, however, CECS is reversible. Minutes to hours after exercise, the pressure returns to a normal level and symptoms resolve. The exact sequence of events is not well understood. In particular, the role of ischemia in this condition has been questioned.[39] It appears, however, that CECS entails an abnormal increase in intracompartmental volume, much of which is due to the increase in muscle volume that typically occurs with exercise. This may be coupled with an increase in extracellular fluid. The increased volume leads to increased pressures during muscle relaxation, inhibiting muscle perfusion. When this occurs, the metabolic demands of the intracompartmen-

tal tissues may be unmet, and compartment syndrome may result.

HISTORY

The most common sites for CECS are in the anterior and deep posterior compartments.[37] The patient typically describes the onset of leg pain over the affected compartment occurring only with exercise. The pain may be characterized as a cramping or aching pain, or a tightness. Transient neurologic symptoms (numbness or weakness) can also develop, but pain may be the only complaint. The symptoms continue to increase during exercise, often causing cessation of the activity. The pain gradually subsides once the activity is stopped. Occasionally, some or all of the symptoms may persist into the next day. The symptoms may be quite reproducible for a given level of effort, such as running a certain distance. Involvement of both legs is common, but each leg may not be affected simultaneously.

Familiarity with the structures contained within each compartment is helpful in establishing the diagnosis (see Fig. 9-1). Anterior leg pain (lateral to the border of the tibia) suggests an anterior compartment syndrome. Accompanying symptoms may include dorsiflexor weakness and paresthesias of the first web space of the foot. Pain or tightness deep within the leg is consistent with a deep posterior compartment syndrome. This may be associated with paresthesias of the instep.

PHYSICAL EXAMINATION

Without a preceding bout of provocative exercise, the physical examination is typically normal. In fact, symptoms of recurrent exercise-induced leg pain accompanied by a negative examination should prompt the physician to consider the diagnosis of CECS. Having the patient exercise to reproduce the symptoms may allow demonstration of palpable tightness or tenderness over the involved compartment. Pas-

Table 9-6

Criteria for the Diagnosis of Chronic Exertional Compartment Syndrome (CECS)*

	INTRAMUSCULAR PRESSURE (MM HG)
Pre-exercise	≥ 15
1 min post-exercise	≥ 30
5 min post-exercise	≥ 20

*One or more of the pressure criteria is considered diagnostic in the presence of clinical findings suggestive of CECS.

SOURCE: Reproduced with permission from Pedowitz RA, Hargens AR, Mubarak SJ, et al: Modified criteria for the objective diagnosis of chronic compartment syndrome of the leg. *Am J Sports Med* 18:35, 1990.

sive stretching may increase the symptoms. Pulses are normal.

ANCILLARY TESTS

Radiographs in patients with CECS are normal, but are helpful in excluding stress fractures or occult bone tumors. The diagnosis of CECS using bone scans and MRI has been reported; however, these imaging modalities are probably most useful in ruling out other causes of leg pain (e.g., stress fractures, MTSS, soft tissue and bony tumors).[39,40]

The standard of diagnosis remains the recording of intracompartmental pressures before, during, and after exercise. A variety of methods for measuring intracompartmental pressures have been described. Devices include the wick catheter, the slit catheter, and portable hand-held single needle systems. Elevated compartmental pressures, particularly after exercise, secure the diagnosis (Table 9-6).[41]

TREATMENT

Begin by assessing any extrinsic or intrinsic factors that may have contributed to the injury. Reduction in the level of exercise, flexibility

training, and deep soft tissue techniques often provide symptom relief. Despite these measures, symptoms commonly recur with the resumption of activity to the pretreatment level. In such cases, unless the patient accepts a level of activity that does not produce symptoms, referral for surgical intervention is necessary.

Surgical decompression of the involved compartment(s) is often successful, with success rates of approximately 90 percent for those with CECS of the anterior compartment.[37] The results of fasciotomy for patients with deep posterior compartment syndromes, however, are less favorable.[37] Insufficient fascial release or excessive postoperative scarring may result in a recurrence of symptoms.

Acute Exertional Compartment Syndrome

ETIOLOGY

Acute compartment syndromes occur as a result of prolonged, irreversible tissue pressure elevation within the fascial compartment.[42] If the elevated pressure is of sufficient magnitude or is maintained without treatment, nerve and muscle capillary perfusion is compromised, leading to muscle necrosis and/or permanent neurologic damage unless there is rapid decompression of the involved compartment.

HISTORY

AECS typically occurs following a high level of activity in a relatively unconditioned individual. Some cases of AECS have also been reported in patients with a prior history of recurrent leg pain consistent with CECS.[43] Severe pain over the involved compartment develops either during exercise or within several hours following the activity.

The presentation is similar to acute compartment syndromes that arise due to more common causes such as fractures, crush injuries, or acute muscle ruptures. The pain is not relieved by rest.

Table 9-7

Helpful Signs for Diagnosing Acute Exertional Compartment Syndrome

Pain out of proportion to the perceived severity of injury
Paresthesias in the distribution of the involved compartmental nerve
Palpable tension over the compartment
Increased pain with passive muscle stretching
Muscle weakness

Furthermore, the pain may continue to increase despite the cessation of limb movement. The skin may become shiny and warm.

PHYSICAL EXAMINATION

Signs that are helpful in making the diagnosis are shown in Table 9-7.[42]

Pulses are often present. The absence of pulses is indicative of severe ischemia and/or arterial injury.

ANCILLARY TESTS

The diagnosis of AECS is largely based on the clinical signs and symptoms described. Intracompartmental tissue pressure measurements can be useful to assist in making the diagnosis, but false positives and negatives do occur.[42] A number of pressure measurement cut-off levels ranging from 30 to 45 mm Hg have been proposed as indications for fasciotomy; however, it appears that the main factor in the development of muscle ischemia is the difference between the mean arterial and compartment pressures.[42] Those with arterial hypotension are particularly at risk for muscle damage. Thus, intracompartmental tissue pressure measurements should be interpreted in the context of the patient's systemic pressure.

TREATMENT

Patients suspected of having AECS should be referred to an orthopaedic surgeon at once. While this is being arranged, examinations of the leg should be repeated frequently to observe for progression of the injury. All splints, dressings, casts, or any other constrictive materials should be removed. Ice should not be used because it can interfere with the microcirculation. The leg should rest at the level of the heart to encourage arterial flow, but not impede venous drainage.

Fasciotomy is the definitive treatment for AECS. Mabee has proposed three criteria as absolute indications for fasciotomy for acute compartment syndromes.[42] First, for patients with clinical signs of an acute compartment syndrome from any cause, fasciotomy is indicated for those with (1) sensory loss, (2) motor loss, or (3) tissue pressure higher than 30 mm Hg. In addition, a second indication is more than 4 hours of interrupted arterial circulation to the extremity. Third, simply making the diagnosis of AECS is a relative indication in and of itself.

Early intervention is important in preventing sequelae including permanent neurologic and/or muscle damage, renal failure from myoglobinuria, arrhythmias, amputation, or death. In one series, fasciotomy performed within 12 h after the onset of an acute compartment syndrome resulted in normal extremity function in 68 percent of cases.[44] In those who had fasciotomy beyond 12 h, only 8 percent had normal function.

Acute Gastrocnemius Strain

Etiology

Strain injury of the medial head of the gastrocnemius at its myotendinous junction is a common cause of acute leg pain. The gastrocnemius muscle spans two joints with the medial and lateral heads inserting proximally in the supracondylar region of the femur. Distally, it combines with the soleus to form the Achilles tendon, which inserts onto the calcaneus. It is susceptible to injury when ankle dorsiflexion and knee extension occur simultaneously with muscle contraction.

Gastrocnemius muscle injury occurs when an athlete is in a position of knee flexion and ankle dorsiflexion and then suddenly extends the knee in combination with contraction of the gastrocnemius, such as leaping or sprinting from a crouched or "ready" position. In fact, the injury is also known as "tennis leg" because of its occurrence in middle-aged tennis players who incur the injury in this fashion. It may also happen in runners as the gastrocnemius contracts eccentrically to control the dorsiflexion produced by the ground forces that occur during the contact phase. Such loading is accentuated if the footstrike occurs on a curb or the edge of step. In either case, a previous strain injury, muscle soreness, tightness, or intermittent sharp pain (a "twinge") may be noted to precede the acute injury.

History

Patients report the sudden onset of posterior leg pain, and will often localize it medially. They may describe a sharp stabbing or tearing sensation, as if they were shot or kicked in the leg. The amount of pain is considerable, and patients are frequently unable to continue the activity. Later, as the acute pain dissipates, the athlete may describe the sensation as a painful knot at the site of injury.

Physical Examination

The medial head of the gastrocnemius will be tender to palpation at the myotendinous junction. Significant swelling and ecchymoses may be present. Due to the amount of swelling, it may be difficult to appreciate a defect in the muscle on initial examination. Pain is reproduced with passive ankle dorsiflexion with the knee extended. The patient may have difficulty performing a single leg heel raise.

In more severe injuries, even a double leg heel raise may be unachievable. Hopping on the injured leg produces pain in even the mildest of cases, but it should not be performed when the injury is obvious. In addition, patients will often note that when walking or attempting to run the pain is most prominent with footstrike, rather than during toe off. The severity of the injury is estimated by the amount of swelling, the presence or absence of a palpable defect in the muscle, and the ability to perform muscle functions.

Ancillary Tests

With a typical history and physical examination, imaging studies are generally not needed to establish the diagnosis. Although the clinical setting usually enables an accurate diagnosis to be made, it may be difficult to distinguish the injury from a deep venous thrombosis (DVT). A Doppler study may be used to confirm the diagnosis of a DVT. If this is not revealing, venography should be performed. It is important to make this distinction because the inadvertant use of anticoagulants in a patient with an acute gastrocnemius strain can result in an acute compartment syndrome due to bleeding.[45] Ultrasound and MRI may be used to confirm the diagnosis of an acute gastrocnemius strain when necessary.[46,47]

Complications

Serious complications of the injury include DVT and acute compartment syndrome. The extensive leg swelling that occurs can impede venous return, resulting in thrombophlebitis and DVT formation.[48] An acute compartment syndrome can develop as a direct complication of the muscle injury.[49] The symptoms and signs have been previously described in this chapter. If such a diagnosis is suspected, immediate surgical consultation should be obtained.

Treatment

Initial treatment for acute strains of the medial head of the gastrocnemius involves aggressive early management of pain and swelling. Frequent ice applications, the use of a compression wrap, NSAIDs, elevation, and a heel lift are helpful.

For many patients, ambulation is difficult after the injury. In these cases, crutches may be used for the first 24 to 48 h. During this time, gentle range-of-motion exercises (not stretching) that do not produce pain may be performed. This can be achieved by simply having the patient plantar flex and dorsiflex the ankle while the extremity is being supported on a table or bed. Initially, this should be attempted with a pillow or towel under the knee to provide slight flexion. The amount of extension can be increased if symptoms are not provoked. Progression to partial- and then full-weight bearing occurs during the first week.

As pain decreases and weight-bearing becomes tolerable, a gradual program of flexibility and strengthening is begun. It is important that these do not produce pain. Patients should begin with concentric training, such as a bilateral heel raise. This should be done in a pain-free range of motion, usually by starting on a flat surface. Over time, progression follows to performing this on a step with an increasing range of motion, followed by a unilateral heel raise, and finally, eccentrically loading the muscle by lowering the heel from the raised position. Weights can then be added for further progression. More dynamic loading may include sets of single leg hopping and the use of a recumbent sled to provide controlled plyometric training. Flexibility training and soft tissue techniques should be employed during this time as well. Icing after rehabilitation sessions is helpful to prevent swelling. Prolonged use of the heel lift (longer than 1 to 2 weeks) should be avoided to prevent loss of flexibility.

Return to Play

The return to training and competition is dependent on the restoration of pain-free range of motion, strength that is within 90 percent of the contralateral leg, and the ability to perform the functional skills required by the sport without producing pain. This may take as little as 2 weeks for mild strains, or 8 weeks or longer for severe injuries. Maintenance of a flexibility and resistance training program is essential to prevent re-injury.

Popliteal Artery Entrapment Syndrome

Entrapment of the popliteal artery causing claudication symptoms is an unusual cause of leg pain. The true incidence of this condition is not known. Eighty percent of cases have been diagnosed in men, 54 percent of whom are under the age of 30.[50] The syndrome has been reported to be bilateral in 33 percent, although both limbs may not be symptomatic. If left untreated, PAES can cause intimal damage leading to occlusive disease and its complications, including limb loss.

Etiology

Popliteal artery entrapment syndrome (PAES) occurs due to intermittent compression of the popliteal artery. The underlying cause has classically been described as anatomic in origin, but recently, several cases of "functional" PAES have been reported.[51,52] In the former type, PAES is a

Figure 9-3

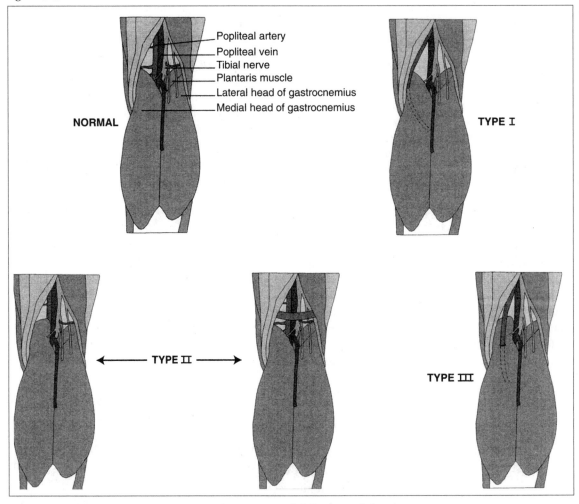

Classification of popliteal artery entrapment syndrome. Type I: the artery is medial to the gastrocnemius. Type II: abnormal muscular insertion. Type III: combination of I and II. *(Adapted with permission from Hoelting T, Schuermann G, Allenberg JR: Entrapment of the popliteal artery and its surgical management in a 20-year period. Br J Surg 84:338, 1997.)*

result of a variation in the anatomic relationship of the popliteal artery with the medial head of the gastrocnemius. There are many classification schemes used to describe the different forms of anatomic PAES. The Heidelberg classification, perhaps the simplest, separates PAES into three categories: type I: abnormal course of the popliteal artery in which it runs medial to the medial head of the gastrocnemius; type II: abnormal muscular insertion creating compression of the artery in its normal course; or type III: a combination of types I and II (Fig. 9-3).[53]

Originally described by Rignault, "functional" PAES occurs in the presence of an anatomically normal popliteal artery and gastrocnemius.[51] It has been reported in athletes as being due to muscular hypertrophy.[51,52] In these cases, plantar flexion causes deviation of the popliteal artery and nerve, resulting in compression laterally against the lateral condyle of the femur.

History

PAES should be suspected in young athletes who present with intermittent posterior leg pain or cramping with exercise. Paresthesias, coldness, and pallor of the foot may occur. Interestingly, the symptoms may develop with walking, but not running. Occasionally, symptom onset may be sudden due to acute occlusion of the artery. The symptoms may be unilateral, despite bilateral involvement. Rest usually results in symptom resolution.

Physical Examination

The physical examination may be normal. Although is important to assess pedal and posterior tibial pulses, intact pulses at rest do not exclude PAES. Resisted plantar flexion or passive dorsiflexion (which cause tension in the gastrocnemius, compressing the artery) may cause obliteration of the pulses, which is suggestive of the syndrome, although it can be observed in normal individuals. Palpation of a popliteal aneurysm or auscultation of a bruit should also alert one to the possibility of PAES. The examination should be performed on each leg because of the potential for bilateral entrapment.

Ancillary Tests

Doppler studies are usually normal in the absence of an occlusion. Duplex-scan examination along with pulsed Doppler of the popliteal fossa may reveal a deviation in the course of the artery or an abnormal spacing between the artery and vein, suggestive of an interposing structure.[50] It should be noted, however, that entrapment of the vein with the artery does occur. Entrapment may be provoked by dorsiflexion and/or plantar flexion during the study. The use of MRI with these provocation maneuvers has also been described.

The diagnostic study of choice is bilateral arteriography. A patent popliteal artery may be seen to deviate medially to the medial head of the gastrocnemius. Active plantar flexion and dorsiflexion should be performed during the study to demonstrate the entrapment. Stenosis, aneurysms, or occlusion may also be demonstrated. Studies should be performed in each leg to rule out bilateral involvement. Because compression of an anatomically normal popliteal artery may occur with provocation in asymptomatic individuals, it may be difficult to distinguish cases of "functional" PAES from a compartment syndrome. In such cases, intra-compartmental pressure measurements should be considered.

Treatment

The treatment for anatomic PAES and for symptomatic functional PAES is surgical. Release of the area of entrapment is the most common procedure.[50] For those with an anatomic form of PAES, this may be performed in combination with thromboendarterectomy and/or grafting procedures if necessary. Postoperative complications include graft occlusion, or in those in whom a graft is not initially performed, a future grafting procedure may be needed due to recurrent ischemia.[53] In a recent review of 19 patients with 23 limbs who underwent surgery for PAES, 16 of the 23 were free of complications at a mean follow-up period of 9.5 years.[53]

For those with a functional entrapment syndrome, surgical release of the soleus muscle from its tibial insertions, along with resection of its fascial band and the plantaris muscle has been described. In one series with a mean 20-month follow-up, 11 of 12 patients who underwent this procedure had good to excellent results, including a return to vigorous activity.[52]

Superficial Peroneal Nerve Entrapment

Entrapment of the superficial peroneal nerve is an infrequent cause of anterolateral leg pain. In a study of 480 patients with chronic leg pain, 3.5 percent were found to have this syndrome.[54]

Etiology

The superficial peroneal nerve arises from the common peroneal nerve at the fibular neck and runs distally in the lateral compartment of the leg. Entrapment typically occurs where the nerve pierces the deep fascia in the lower one-third of the leg, as it then divides into two subcutaneous sensory branches that supply the dorsum of the foot (Fig. 9-4). The tunnel in which the nerve travels at this site is normally of short length (less than 3 cm). In cases of entrapment, this tunnel may be found to be fibrotic or of excessive length. The syndrome may develop as a result of previous direct trauma to the leg, prior inversion ankle injuries (inversion and plantar flexion creates tension on the nerve at the point of exit from the deep fascia), fascial defects with muscle herniation, an abnormal course of the nerve, or as a complication of surgery for chronic anterior compartment syndrome. Interestingly, only 10 percent have a chronic lateral compartment syndrome.[54]

History

Patients complain of anterolateral leg pain that may be associated with pain and sensory loss of the dorsum of the foot. The symptoms may

occur only with exercise. In one study, the mean duration of symptoms was nearly 5 years before the diagnosis was made.[54]

Physical Examination

Styf described three provocation tests performed at rest and after exercise.[54] The first involves the application of pressure over the anterior intermuscular septum (approximately 8 to 10 cm above the lateral malleolus) during active ankle dorsiflexion. Passive plantar flexion and inversion of the ankle is the second maneuver. The third test adds pressure over the course of the nerve while this stretch is maintained. A clinical diagnosis can be made when the following criteria are met: (1) decreased sensation over the dorsum of the foot along with pain at rest or dur-

Figure 9-4

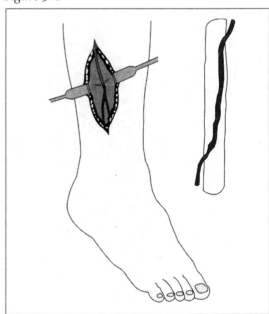

The course of the superficial peroneal nerve as it exits the deep fascia via the superficial peroneal tunnel. *(Adapted with permission from Lowdon IMR: Superficial peroneal nerve entrapment. A case report. J Bone Joint Surg 67(B):58, 1985.)*

ing an exercise test, and (2) at least the first two of the provocation tests are positive. The differential diagnosis includes chronic lateral compartment syndrome, referred pain, and lipomata.

Ancillary Tests

Radiographs of the leg are unremarkable and nerve conduction studies are also usually normal. Intracompartmental pressure measurements are generally normal too, but can be helpful to exclude those cases that are related to a chronic lateral compartment syndrome. A diagnostic injection of lidocaine at the painful site above the lateral malleolus has been described to relieve symptoms.[55] MRI has also been reported to assist in diagnosis by confirming the entrapment.[55]

Treatment

The treatment for this condition is surgical. Decompression is usually performed by complete opening of the superficial peroneal tunnel. In some cases the peroneal tunnel is absent, and treatment is then local fasciectomy. Complete fasciotomy is necessary when associated with a chronic lateral compartment syndrome. The results of surgical treatment are mixed. At a mean follow-up of 26 months, Styf reported 82 percent were satisfied with outcome of surgery, although 72 percent reported residual symptoms.[54] Nearly half had pain with walking, and only 4 of 17 were described to have returned to an unlimited level of activity.

References

1. Baquie P, Brukner P: Injuries presenting to an Australian sports medicine centre: A 12-month study. *Clin J Sport Med* 7:28, 1997.
2. Matheson GO, MacIntyre JG, Taunton JE, et al: Musculoskeletal injuries associated with physical activity in older adults. *Med Sci Sports Exerc* 21:379, 1989.
3. Bennell KL, Crossley, K: Musculoskeletal injuries in track and field: incidence, distribution and risk factors. *Aust J Sci Med Sports* 28:69, 1996.
4. Gordon NF, Hugo EP, Cilliers JF: The South African Defense Force physical training programme. Part III; Exertion-related injuries sustained at an SADF training centre. *S Afr Med* 69: 491, 1986.
5. Jordaan G, Schwellnus MP: The incidence of overuse injuries in military recruits during basic military training. *Military Med* 159:421, 1994.
6. Ounpuu, S: The biomechanics of walking and running. *Clin Sports Med* 13:843, 1994.
7. Cavanagh PR, LaFortune MA: Ground reaction forces in distance running. *J Biomechanics* 13:397, 1980.
8. Subcommittee on Classification of Injuries in Sports and Committee on the Medical Aspects of Sports. *Standard Nomenclature of Athletic Injuries*. Chicago: American Medical Association, 1966.
9. Michael RH, Holder LE: The soleus syndrome: A cause of medial tibial stress (shin splints). *Am J Sports Med* 13:87, 1985.
10. Mubarak SJ, Gould RN, Yu FL, et al: The medial tibial stress syndrome. *Am J Sports Med* 10:201, 1982.
11. Beck BR, Osternig LR: Medial tibial stress syndrome. The location of muscles in the leg in relation to symptoms. *J Bone Joint Surg* 76(A): 1057, 1994.
12. Fredericson M, Bergman AG, Hoffman KL, et al: Tibial stress reaction in runners. Correlation of clinical symptoms and scintigraphy with a new magnetic resonance imaging grading system. *Am J Sports Med* 23:472, 1995.
13. Messier SP, Pittala KA: Etiologic factors associated with selected running injuries. *Med Sci Sports Exerc* 20:501, 1988.
14. Sommer HM, Vallentyne SW: Effect of foot posture on the incidence of medial tibial stress syndrome. *Med Sci Sports Exerc* 27:800, 1995.
15. Deutsch AL, Coel MN, Mink JH: Imaging of stress injuries to bone: Radiography, scintigraphy, and MR imaging. *Clin Sports Med* 16:275, 1997.
16. Melberg P, Styf J: Posteromedial pain in the lower leg. *Am J Sports Med* 17:747, 1989.

17. Allen MJ, Barnes MR: Exercise pain in the lower leg: Chronic compartment syndrome and medial tibial syndrome. *J Bone Joint Surg, (Br)* 68:818, 1986.

18. Johnell O, Rausing A, Wendeberg B, et al: Morphological bone changes in shin splints. *Clin Orthop Related Res* 167:180, 1982.

19. Ilahi OA, Kohl III HW: Lower extremity morphology and alignment and risk of overuse injury. *Clin J Sports Med* 8:38, 1998.

20. Wen DY, Puffer JC, Schmalzried TP: Lower extremity alignment and risk of overuse injuries in runners. *Med Sci Sports Exerc* 29:1291, 1997.

21. Whitelaw GP, Wetzler MJ, Levy AS, et al: A pneumatic leg brace for the treatment of tibial stress fractures. *Clin Orthop Related Res* 270:301, 1991.

22. Bennell KL, Brukner PD: Epidemiology and site specificity of stress fractures. *Clin Sports Med* 16:179, 1997.

23. Fyrie DP, Milgrom C, Hoshaw SJ, et al: Effect of fatiguing exercise on longitudinal bone strain as related to stress fracture in humans. *Ann Biomed Engineer* 26:660, 1998.

24. Hulkko A, Orava S: Stress fractures in athletes. *Intl J Sports Med* 8:221, 1987.

25. Sherman CM, Brandser EA, Parman LM, et al: Longitudinal tibial stress fractures: A report of eight cases and review of the literature. *J Compute Assist Tomog* 22:265, 1998.

26. Boam WD, Miser WF, Yuill SC, et al: Comparison of ultrasound examination with bone scintiscan in the diagnosis of stress fractures. *J Am Board Fam Prac* 9:414, 1996.

27. Swenson EJ, DeHaven KE, Sebastianelli WJ, et al: The effect of a pneumatic leg brace on return to play in athletes with tibial stress fractures. *Am J Sports Med* 25:322, 1997.

28. Dickson TB, Kichline PD: Functional management of stress fractures in female athletes using a pneumatic leg brace. *Am J Sports Med* 15:86, 1987.

29. Finestone A, et al: A randomized prospective study of the effect of custom-made biomechanical shoe orthotics on the incidence of stress fractures in Israeli infantry recruits. Presented at the February 1997 Annual Meeting of the American Academy of Orthopaedic Surgeons, San Francisco, CA.

30. Rolf C, Ekenman I, Törnqvist H, et al: The anterior stress fracture of the tibia: An atrophic pseudoarthosis? *Scand J Med Sci Sports* 7:249, 1997.

31. Rettig AC, Shelbourne KD, McCarroll JR, et al: The natural history and treatment of delayed union stress fractures of the anterior cortex of the tibia. *Am J Sports Med* 16:250, 1988.

32. Shearman CM, Brandser EA, Parman CM, et al: Longitudinal tibial stress fractures: A report of eight cases and a review of the literature. *J Comput Assist Tomogr* 22:265, 1998.

33. DiFiori JP: Stress fracture of the proximal fibula in a young soccer player: A case report and a review of the literature. *Med Sci Sports Exerc* 31:925, 1999.

34. Goh JCH, Lee EH, Ang EJ, et al: Biomechanical study on the load-bearing characteristics of the fibula and the effects of fibular resection. *Clin Orthop Related Res* 279:223, 1992.

35. Ogden JA: The anatomy and function of the proximal tibiofibular joint. *Clin Orthop Related Res* 101:186, 1974.

36. Symeonides PP: High stress fractures of the fibula. *J Bone Joint Surg* 62(B):192, 1980.

37. Schepsis AA, Lynch G: Exertional compartment syndromes of the lower extremity. *Curr Opin Rheumatol* 8:143, 1996.

38. Styf J: Diagnosis of exercise-induced pain in the anterior aspect of the lower leg. *Am J Sports Med* 16:165, 1988.

39. Amendola A, Rorabeck CH, Vellett D, et al: The use of magnetic resonance imaging in exertional compartment syndromes *Am J Sports Med* 18:29, 1990.

40. Allen MJ, O'Dwyer FG, Barnes MR, et al: The value of 99Tcm-MDP bone scans in young patients with exercise-induced lower leg pain. *Nuc Med Comm* 16:88, 1995.

41. Pedowitz RA, Hargens AR, Mubarak SJ, et al: Modified criteria for the objective diagnosis of chronic compartment syndrome of the leg. *Am J Sports Med* 18:35, 1990.

42. Mabee JR: Compartment syndrome: A complication of acute extremity trauma *Emerg Med Rev* 12:651, 1994.

43. Goldfarb SJ, Kaeding CC: Bilateral acute-on-chronic exertional lateral compartment syndrome of the leg: A case report and review of the literature. *Clin J Sports Med* 7:59, 1997.

44. Sheridan GW, Matsen FA: Fasciotomy in the treat-

ment of the acute compartment syndrome. *J Bone Joint Surg (Am)* 58:112, 1976.

45. Anouchi YS, Parker RD, Seitz WH Jr: Posterior compartment syndrome of the calf resulting from misdiagnosis of a rupture of the medial head of the gastrocnemius. *J Trauma* 27:678, 1987.

46. Bianchi S, Martinoli C, Abdelwahab IF, et al: Sonographic evaluation of tears of the gastrocnemius medial head ("tennis leg"). *J Ultrasound Med* 17:157, 1998.

47. Gilbert TJ Jr., Bullis BR, Griffiths HJ: Tennis calf or tennis leg. *Orthopedics* 19:179, 182, 184, 1996.

48. Slawski DP: Deep venous thrombosis complicating rupture of the medial head of the gastrocnemius muscle. *J Orthop Trauma* 8:263, 1994.

49. Mohanna PN, Haddad FS: Acute compartment syndrome following non-contact football injury. *Br J Sports Med* 31:354, 1997.

50. Rosset E, Hartung O, Brunet C, et al: Popliteal artery entrapment syndrome: Anatomic and embryologic bases, diagnostic and therapeutic considerations following a series of 15 cases with a review of the literature. *Surg Radiol Anat* 17:161, 1995.

51. Rignault DP, Pailler JL, Lunel F: The "functional" popliteal entrapment syndrome. *Intl Angiog* 4:341, 1985.

52. Turnipseed WD, Pozniak M: Popliteal entrapment as a result of neurovascular compression by the soleus and plantaris muscles. *J Vasc Surg* 15:285, 1992.

53. Hoelting T, Schuermann G, Allenberg JR: Entrapment of the popliteal artery and its surgical management in a 20-year period. *Br J Surg* 84:338, 1997.

54. Styf J, Morberg P: The superficial peroneal tunnel syndrome: Results of treatment by decompression. *J Bone Joint Surg* 79(B):801, 1997.

55. Daghino W, Pasquali M, Faletti C: Superficial peroneal nerve entrapment in a young athlete: The diagnostic contribution of magnetic resonance imaging. *J Foot Ankle Surg* 36:170, 1997.

56. Lowdon IMR: Superficial peroneal nerve entrapment. A case report. *J Bone Joint Surg* 67(B):58, 1985.

57. DiFiori JP: Overuse injuries in children and adolescents. *Physician Sportsmed* 27:75, 1999.

58. DiFiori JP, Hosey R: Overuse injuries: Diagnosis and treatment. *Clin Atlas Office Proced* 1:227, 1998.

Edward J. Reisman

The Injured Ankle

Introduction

An injury to the ankle is one of the most common musculoskeletal problems encountered in the treatment of the athlete. Most of these injuries are simple sprains that can be adequately managed by the primary physician. However, many ankle injuries are treated too casually. More serious and potentially debilitating injuries can present as common sprains and will be missed if a careful evaluation and diagnosis are not made. Even if the injury is correctly diagnosed as a simple sprain, the common mistake of inadequate rehabilitation often leads to the expression "once a sprain, always a sprain."

This chapter provides a basic review of the anatomy of the ankle, mechanisms of injury, proper history, and physical tests and findings. A general overview of common ankle injuries emphasizes an accurate diagnosis and proper management. A special note points out those common injuries that will likely require a referral to an orthopedic surgeon for definitive treatment.

Anatomy

Bony Configuration

The anatomic characteristics of the ankle joint, including bony articulations and ligamentous and tendinous stabilizers, are important to the understanding of the types of injury that can occur in the athlete. Functionally, the ankle joint is a hinge joint allowing motion in one plane of dorsiflexion and plantar flexion. The ankle mortise is formed by the lateral malleolus of the fibula, the undersurface of the tibia, and the medial malleolus of the tibia. Inset into the mor-

tise is the body of the talus, which is wider anteriorly than it is posteriorly. Thus, when the foot is in mild dorsiflexion it is extremely stable, but as the ankle goes into plantar flexion the narrower posterior portion of the talus rotates into the mortise, resulting in some instability.

Note that extreme dorsiflexion causes the widest portion of the talus to force the fibula away from the tibia and can result in injury to the syndesmosis. Inversion and eversion movement actually takes place at the subtalar or calcaneotalar joint. Also, note that the lateral malleolus is longer than the medial malleolus, and combined with the strong deltoid ligament, results in lateral motion in the tarsus being more restricted than medial motion.

Ligamentous Stabilizers

The bony articulations are maintained by many ligamentous structures. The distal tibia and fibula are bound together by the anterior and posterior tibiofibular ligaments, which are really thickened expansions of the interosseous membrane. The syndesmosis between the tibia and fibula thus provides for the stability of the mortise joint. The ligaments, or joint capsule, are thin anteriorly and posteriorly to provide the most movement, but the collateral ligaments on each side are heavy and strong.

The medial collateral, or deltoid ligament, is the largest and strongest of the ankle ligaments (Fig. 10-1). It has a broad attachment to the medial malleolus and extends fanlike downward in many bands to support the medial ankle joint as well as stabilize the arch of the foot. It prevents abduction and eversion of the ankle and subtalar joint.

The lateral collateral ligament can be separated into three components—the anterior talofibular, calcaneofibular, and posterior talofibular ligament (Fig. 10-2). The anterior talofibular ligament runs parallel to the long axis of the foot, or perpendicular to the leg, and prevents anterior displacement of the talus within the

Figure 10-1

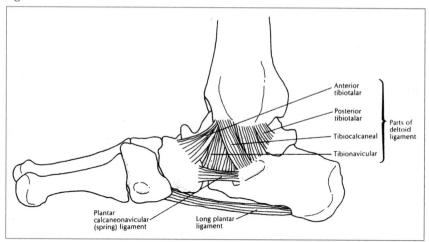

Medial view of the ligaments of the talocrural and proximal tarsal joints. *(Reproduced with permission from Hertling D, Kessler RM: Management of Common Musculoskeletal Disorders, 2nd ed. Philadelphia: J.B. Lippincott; 1990; 366.)*

mortise. It is the most commonly injured ankle ligament and is injured by inversion–plantar flexion movement. The calcaneofibular ligament runs vertically, deep to the peroneal tendons, and resists inversion. The posterior talofibular ligament is the smallest portion and is a weak restraint against posterior displacement of the talus.

Figure 10-2

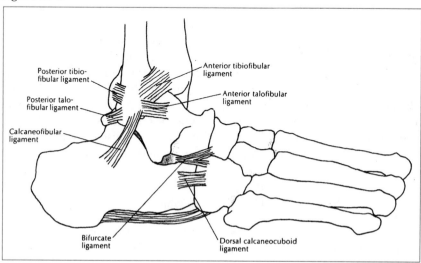

Lateral view of the ligaments of the right talocrural and proximal tarsal joints. *(Reproduced with permission from Hertling D, Kessler RM: Management of Common Musculoskeletal Disorders, 2nd ed. Philadelphia: J.B. Lippincott; 1990; 365.)*

Dynamic Stabilizers

The ankle is also dynamically supported by a number of tendons that arise from muscles of the lower leg. The peroneus brevis runs behind the lateral malleolus and inserts into the base of the fifth metatarsal. It is a powerful evertor of the ankle and foot and actively resists inversion. The peroneus longus runs with the brevis behind the lateral malleolus and at the cuboid, sharply changes direction, and runs across the bottom of the foot to insert on the head of the first metatarsal. Medially, the tendons of the posterior tibialis, flexor digitorum longus, and flexor hallucis longus, pass behind the medial malleolus and add their stability to the ankle joint. The posterior tibialis has its primary insertion on the navicular and functions to provide inversion and plantar flexion as well as to stabilize the arch of the foot. The anterior tibialis muscle crosses over the anterior ankle and inserts somewhat medially on the foot. It functions to dorsiflex and invert the foot. Posterior to the ankle is the powerful Achilles tendon, which provides plantar flexion.

Mechanisms of Injury

Functionally, the ankle is a hinge joint, allowing dorsal and plantar flexion; thus most injuries occur when the ankle is forced in a different direction or to extremes of its normal motion. The most common mechanism of injury to the ankle, accounting for 85% of all ankle sprains,[1] is an inversion injury combined with some element of plantar flexion and internal rotation. An eversion injury can also occur. It usually involves some component of dorsiflexion and external rotation. Less common, but still frequent and difficult to recognize, are hyperflexion or extreme dorsiflexion injuries.

Inversion

In an inversion injury the force typically consists of inversion, internal rotation, and plantar flexion. In other words, the foot is turned in and often pointed downward and the ankle and leg are forced to the outside. As the foot inverts in relation to the lower leg, strain is placed on the lateral collateral ligaments, first the anterior talofibular, then the calcaneofibular, and finally, the posterior talofibular ligament.

The ligaments will stretch slightly, then partially or completely tear depending on the severity of the force. Typically, the ligament will tear in the mid-substance, but occasionally it will avulse a small fragment off the tip of the lateral malleolus, or more rarely, especially in elderly, brittle bone, a larger portion of the lateral malleolus may break. If the inverting force continues, partially tearing the ligaments, then the ankle will open up on the lateral side and the talus is pushed against the medial malleolus.

Remembering the anatomy, the medial malleolus is short and stubby and only extends about halfway down the body of the talus. Thus, as the talus is pushed over, it often rotates over the tip of the medial malleolus opening up the lateral side of the ankle to more extensive tearing of the lateral collateral ligaments. If the inversion force is extreme, it can cause the medial malleolus to fracture. Typically, the fracture line extends vertically up the shaft of the tibia beginning at the lateral margin of the medial malleolus. If this type of fracture is seen with this mechanism of injury, one must presume the lateral ligaments are injured and torn.

Eversion

An eversion injury occurs when the foot is forced outward in relation to the lower leg. Initially, there is stretch and tearing of the medial deltoid ligament as the talus is pushed against the lateral malleolus. In eversion injuries, the anatomic difference between the two malleoli becomes significant. Whereas the medial malleolus is short, allowing the talus to rotate over its tip and add leverage to further opening up and tearing of the lateral ligaments, the lateral malleolus is at least as long as the height of the talus. Thus, eversion and external rotation produce direct outward pressure on the lateral malleolus. In addition, any component of dorsiflexion causes the wider, anterior portion of the talus to bring further outward pressure on the distal fibula, potentially resulting in fracture.

Several different types of injury can occur from the same eversion forces. The most common injury is a fracture of the distal fibula somewhere below the level of the ankle mortise. This can occur with only partial rupture of the deltoid ligament. The same eversion force can also cause the medial collateral ligaments to give way followed by the tibiofibular ligaments, and finally, the fibula to fracture anywhere along its length, although most commonly in the distal one-third. Given this eversion mechanism of injury, if a fibular fracture appears above the level of the ankle joint, it is likely that the tibiofibular ligament is torn and the stability of the ankle mortise has been lost. Note that most ankle injuries result in a lateral ligament sprain due to an inversion mechanism of injury, whereas most ankle fractures are to the lateral malleolus and due to an eversion injury.

Dorsiflexion

A dorsiflexion injury occurs when a hyperflexion force is applied to the ankle. As described previously, the anatomy of the talus shows it to be broad in the front and narrow behind. As the foot is brought into dorsiflexion, the wider anterior portion of the talus fits snugly between the two malleoli, held together by the strong tibiofibular ligament, creating a very stable joint. However, if excessive dorsiflexion occurs, the talus is forced against the malleoli, causing the

tibia and fibula to spring apart, partially tearing the tibiofibular ligaments. Once the force is resolved, the bones typically fall back together again and the injury initially does not seem so severe. This injury can occur in combination with rupture of the calf or Achilles tendon, or if there is enough eversion stress, fracture of the fibula as described in the previous paragraph.

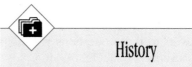

History

Mechanism of Injury

As is true for all injuries, obtaining a good history is the basis for performing a proper physical examination and ultimately reaching the correct diagnosis. First, determining the position of the ankle at the time of injury will lead to understanding the mechanism of injury. In other words, was the foot inverted, such as running on the basketball court and having the medial side of the foot step on the edge of another foot and then the leg roll over to the outside. Or, on the football field, the foot is planted on the ground, slightly turned out and then a hit to the lateral lower leg forces the ankle into more eversion. Perhaps the gymnast lands the vault slightly forward going into extreme dorsiflexion. Second, the activity at the time of injury, walking, running, jumping, or being hit by something else, will help to estimate the force behind the injury and understand the degree of damage. By understanding the mechanism and force of the injury, the areas most likely to be damaged can be carefully examined.

Symptoms

Next, try to determine the symptoms that were present immediately. A "pop" strongly suggests a torn ligament or fracture. The area of initial pain—medial or lateral ankle or radiating up the lower leg—can help pinpoint the injury. Did swelling occur immediately or not for several hours, and over what portion of the ankle. Similarly, did any ecchymosis or bruising occur; where was it located and when did it appear. Were they unable to stand and bear any weight or need assistance to walk with some partial weight on the injured ankle. Or, were they able to get up and walk, maybe even continue to play; did it feel stable or have a loose, unstable sensation. Answers to these questions will help to gauge the severity of the injury. It is also important to know of any initial treatment, such as ice, elevation, or compression, that would affect the amount of pain or swelling apparent in the injured ankle.

Past Injury

Other considerations to obtain in the history are any past injuries to either ankle, including information about the type of injury, length of disability, treatment, rehabilitation, and any subsequent problems or limitations that were experienced. If a few days or weeks have elapsed since the recent injury, then determine the type and area of pain, amount of swelling or bruising, and limitations of movement or activities, including any improvement, that have occurred over the time period since the injury.

Physical Examination

Inspection

The examination of the injured ankle is best done by developing a standardized approach and should always include a comparable examination of the opposite normal ankle. By beginning with careful observation and then proceeding to a slow and gentle examination of the injured ankle, the examiner can win the confidence of the apprehensive patient and obtain a better evaluation. Inspect for any deformity, swelling, or ecchymosis that may be present, and note the amount and location.

Palpation

Palpation should start in the area least likely to cause pain and should be directed to specific anatomic structures. Posteriorly, palpate the Achilles tendon and its insertion onto the calcaneous. On the medial side, palpate the broad expanse of the deltoid ligament and the entire medial malleolus, starting a few cms above the malleolus. Also feel along the course of the posterior tibialis tendon and its insertion onto the navicular. Anteriorly, palpate across the dome of the talus and anterior joint capsule fibers, including the anterior tibialis tendon. On the lateral side, palpate the anterior talofibular ligament and calcaneofibular ligament and posterior talofibular ligament, and lateral malleolus, and end with palpation of the peroneal tendon out to its insertion at the base of the fifth metatarsal. Any reports of pain in the lateral lower leg warrants palpation of the entire length of the fibula.

Neurovascular Assessment

A thorough examination should include a neurovascular assessment. Palpation of the dorsalis pedis and posterior tibialis pulses, assessment of capillary nail bed filling, feeling the temperature of the foot, and finally, assessing sensation.

Range of Motion

Range of motion, both active and passive, as well as abnormal motion with stress testing, should be evaluated. The amount of active, pain-free motion can be demonstrated by the patient and documented. Next, gentle passive motion can be attempted and any excessive inversion, eversion, plantar, or dorsiflexion movement noted.

Stress Testing

Specific stress testing includes the talar tilt, anterior drawer and squeeze tests. The talar tilt test (Fig. 10-3) is used to assess the integrity of the lateral or medial ligaments. The lower leg is stabilized with one hand and then the heel is

Figure 10-4

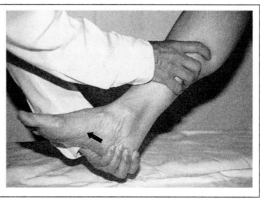

Anterior drawer test. Assesses stability of the anterior talofibular ligament. The test is performed by stabilizing the distal portion of the leg with one hand while the other hand attempts to move the talus anteriorly in the direction shown by the arrow. *(Reproduced with permission from Weiss, BD: 20 Common Problems in Primary Care. New York: McGraw-Hill; 1999, 342.)*

Figure 10-3

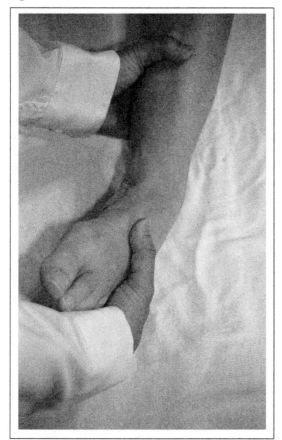

Talar tilt test. Integrity of the calcaneofibular ligament is assessed by stabilizing the distal leg with one hand while the other hand applies inversion stress to the ankle. *(Reproduced with permission from Weiss BD: 20 Common Problems in Primary Care. New York: McGraw-Hill; 1999, 342.)*

grasped with the other hand and either inverted (varus) or everted (valgus) and then compared to the other side.

The anterior drawer test is used to measure the laxity of the anterior talofibular ligament (Fig. 10-4). Again, the lower leg is stabilized with one hand, while the other hand cups the heel and displaces it forward or anteriorly. The amount of laxity is noted and compared to the other side.

The squeeze test assesses any injury to the tibiofibular ligaments. The examiner's hands are used to squeeze or compress the fibula against the tibia and any pain between the bones may indicate a syndesmosis injury.

Radiographic Evaluation

Ottawa Ankle Rules

The need for ankle radiographs is often debated. The use of the Ottawa Ankle Rules during the evaluation of ankle injuries can allow for the selective use of x-rays. In developing the Ottawa Rules, an initial prospective study evaluated 750 adult patients with ankle injuries with a goal of developing clinical "decision rules" to predict a fracture and allow for more selective use of x-rays.[2] The investigators conducted a follow-up study by applying these rules during the evaluation of 2,342 adult patients with ankle injuries presenting to two emergency centers. Using these criteria to determine which patients need x-rays decreased the use of radiography by 28 percent, and also saved emergency room time and cost without missing any fractures.[3]

The Ottawa Ankle Rules are simple. Ankle films are required if pain in the malleolar area is accompanied by bony tenderness at the posterior edge or tip of the lateral or medial malleolus, or the inability to bear weight (four steps) both immediately and in the emergency department. Radiographs of the foot are required if there is bony tenderness at the base of the fifth metatarsal or navicular. Note that these rules are valid only in individuals older than 18 years. In children, the growth plate is often weaker than the ligaments and thus more susceptible to injury. Fractures involving the growth plate are more common and require a greater use of x-rays in the evaluation of ankle injuries in children (see Chap. 18).

Standard and Stress Radiographs

If x-rays are obtained, they should preferably be done only after clinical evaluation. This would allow for proper application of the Ottawa Ankle Rules. In addition, it is possible that positioning by the x-ray technician to obtain the proper views may reduce deformities and make the true extent of injury less obvious.

Standard x-ray views of the ankle include anteroposterior, lateral, and mortise. Additional stress views can be obtained with inversion, eversion, or anterior drawer forces to help evaluate the amount of laxity in ligamentous injuries.

A mortise view is obtained while a varus or inversion stress is applied to the ankle. The angle of tilt between the talar dome and undersurface of the tibia is measured. There is a great deal of normal variation with a range from 0 to 27°. A tilt greater than 20°, or 10° greater than the uninjured side, strongly suggests a tear to the anterior talofibular and calcaneofibular ligaments.[4] When a valgus or eversion stress is applied, a tilt greater than 10° is considered a positive result for a tear of the deltoid ligament.[4] An anterior drawer stress radiograph is obtained on a lateral view by measurements of the amount of displacement of the talus with respect to the tibia. A displacement of 4 to 5 mm is probably normal, whereas greater than 8 mm suggests some disruption of the lateral ligaments.[4]

Additional Imaging

Arthography can be used to diagnose tears in the joint capsule and ligaments, but it does not quantitate the extent of the tear. Bone scanning can evaluate for stress fractures, osteochondral fractures, infection, and inflammatory reactions. Computerized tomography (CT) can localize osteochondritis dissecans, loose bodies, and subchondral cysts. Magnetic resonance imaging (MRI) shows the soft tissues of the ankle as well as osteochondral lesions such as osteochondritis dissecans and talar dome fractures. Tendons such as the Achilles, peroneals, and posterior tibialis are also well seen. The usefulness of routine MRI in the evaluation of ankle injuries is still being developed but can be very helpful in further evaluating the ankle in which more serious injury is suspected and in which initial x-rays are negative.

Ankle Injuries

In this section of the chapter, we discuss the lateral ankle sprains and their treatment along with many of the other common ankle sprains and injuries. Treatment of each of these sprains is briefly reviewed.

Acute Lateral Ligament Sprains

Ankle ligament sprains are typically lateral, medial (deltoid), or involve the syndesmosis. Lateral ankle sprains are by far the most common injury in sports, especially running and jumping sports such as basketball, soccer, cross-country running, and dance.[5] Injuries to the lateral ankle commonly occur at the moment of loading or weight-bearing with an added plantar flexion and inversion force. As the ankle rolls over, the anterior talofibular ligament first begins to stretch and tear, followed by the calcaneofibular and then the posterior talofibular ligaments. Most of the injuries are midsubstance tears to the ligament, but bony avulsion of the talus or fibula can occur.

Clinical presentation of a "typical" lateral ankle sprain usually involves the athlete describing how the injury occurred, feeling or hearing a popping or tearing sensation with pain, and a feeling of weakness or loss of support when trying to stand up or continue to play. Swelling can be localized or diffuse, immediate, or delayed several hours.

On examination, note the area of swelling or eccymosis, which suggests tearing or fracture of structures. The appearance of eccymosis can be delayed for several days. Careful fingertip examination, especially in fresh injuries, can often isolate the extent of injuries to the specific lateral ligaments—anterior talofibular, calcaneofibular, and posterior talofibular ligament. The anterior drawer test will cause discomfort and demonstrate laxity with tears to the anterior talofibular ligament. Laxity on the talar tilt test can indicate damage to the calcaneofibular ligament. Careful palpation and the use of the Ottawa Ankle rules can allow for selective use of radiographs for further evaluation if indicated.

A classification system for lateral ankle sprains can help describe the extent of injury and guide prognosis and treatment is described in detail later in this chapter (Table 10–1). A grade I or mild sprain will have minimal pain, swelling, and loss of function. Anatomically, the ligaments are intact with more of an overstretch resulting from the injury. Grade II sprains are due to a partial tear of the ligament which is still intact. Therefore, there is an increase in the amount of pain, swelling, and difficulty bearing weight functionally. Eccymosis from the tearing of the ligament fibers is typically present within a few days. A severe or grade III sprain is characterized by a complete tear of the lateral ankle ligaments and the corresponding loss of functional stability. There is even greater severity in presenting symptoms and physical signs.

Chronic Lateral Ankle Sprains

A subset of lateral ankle sprains to consider is the athlete with chronic symptoms. They will typically present with a mild acute sprain but a

Table 10-1

Grading Ankle Sprains

FINDINGS	GRADE I	GRADE II	GRADE III
Pain and Swelling	Mild	Moderate	Severe
Ecchymosis	None	Usually	Yes
Functional stability	Stable	Some laxity	Unstable
Ability to bear weight	Yes	Partially	Usually not
Ligament injury	Intact	Partial tear	Complete tear

history relating this as a recurring problem, or with a complaint of the ankle feeling "weak" or frequently "turning under" or "giving way." Pain, swelling, or eccymosis are often minor symptoms, but the physical examination will be remarkable for the amount of laxity found on anterior drawer and talar tilt testing, as well as weakness on muscle testing and loss of proprioceptive balance. Routine and stress views on radiography are often a useful part of the evaluation to help identify the instability and look for a frequently associated osteochondral lesion.

Management of Lateral Ankle Sprains

As a general rule, the treatment of grade I and II lateral ankle sprains is quite similar. The greatest difference is that grade II sprains, by definition, involve greater damage and loss of stability, and thus require more support to the ankle during treatment and longer time for healing. Grade III sprains often have associated injuries such as fractures, and these more serious injuries dictate treatment. For isolated grade III sprains, treatment is most often conservative with 1 to 3 weeks in a cast boot with limited mobilization and treatments, allowed only under the close supervision of a therapist or trainer. However, grade III sprains should be discussed with the orthopedist because surgery may be indicated based on the age of the athlete, level of athletic participation, and amount of instability.

INITIAL TREATMENT—RICE

The immediate management of ankle sprains involves implementation of the RICE protocol—Rest, Ice, Compression, and Elevation. The rapid, initial application of RICE will greatly minimize the amount of initial swelling, resulting in less time to resolve the swelling, and thus allow a quicker return to function for the ankle joint.

Rest implies taking the stress off the injured ankle. Continued play will delay healing and is more likely to lead to further, more serious

injury. Crutches are useful to allow ambulating while partial or nonweightbearing.

Ice will help control and minimize the initial pain and swelling. The immediate and frequent use of ice for 15 to 20 min every few hours during the initial 24 h following injury can result in a 50 percent decrease in the number of days required before full return to function.[4]

Compression will also aid in reducing the initial swelling. Methods of compression include wrapping with an elastic bandage, open taping, or a functional ankle brace.

Elevation means raising the ankle above the level of the heart. The ankle should be elevated as much as possible during the first 24 h. The addition of nonsteroidal anti-inflammatory medication can also reduce pain and swelling.

PHASES OF REHABILITATION

The general goal of ankle rehabilitation is for functional recovery and return to sport as quickly and safely as possible. An ankle rehabilitation program can be broken down into several phases (Table 10–2). The progression through each phase depends on the severity of the ankle injury. In an ideal situation, a qualified therapist or athletic trainer should monitor each step to accelerate the rehabilitation in a safe manner.[10]

The goals of phase 1 are to decrease pain and swelling and protect the ankle from further injury. The RICE protocol is the mainstay of treatment during this early acute phase. The injured ankle may be protected from further injury by taping, the use of a brace (such as an air stirrup) or a posterior splint, or casting, depending on the level of support needed. Weight-bearing is allowed as tolerated. Exercises are limited to pain-free range of motion while tracing the alphabet with the foot and large toe. Duration of this phase is a few days to weeks, mainly dependent on the amount of pain and swelling.

During phase 2, or subacute phase, the goals are to restore full mobility and strength and begin proprioceptive training. Ice bags or con-

Table 10-2

Ankle Rehabilitation

	ACUTE, PHASE I	SUBACUTE, PHASE II	RETURN TO ACTIVITY, PHASE III
Goals	Decrease pain and swelling, provide support	Improve ROM, strength, and balance	Normal ROM, strength, endurance, and balance
RICE	Frequently	As needed to control swelling	As needed after exercise
Weight-bearing activity	As tolerated	Full/walking	Full/running
Exercise	Limited ROM	Full ROM, alphabet Strength, elastic tubing Balance, BAPS	Closed kinetic chain Sport specific
Support	Tape, brace, or cast	Tape or brace	Tape or brace for injury prevention

ABBREVIATIONS: ROM, range of motion; BAPS, biomechanical ankle platform systems.

trast baths along with compression continues, as needed, to control any swelling. Weight-bearing has progressed to full weight-bearing with a close to normal walking gait. Exercises include range-of-motion, Achilles heel cord stretches, ankle resistance strength exercises with elastic tubing, and early balance exercises for proprioception. Progression through this phase will typically be 1 to 3 weeks dependent on the development of normal range of motion and initial strength.

Phase 3 goals are the preparation for return to full activity through a progression of functional exercises to fully restore flexibility, strength, power, endurance, and proprioceptive balance. Ice after exercise continues when needed to control any swelling. Support with taping or braces also continues to reduce chance of further injury. Rehabilitation advances to more closed kinetic chain exercises involving jogging and running patterns, jumping, and balance exercises.

CRUTCHES AND WEIGHT-BEARING

At the time of initial injury, crutches may be used. If it is too painful to fully bear weight, the use of crutches can allow someone to partially bear weight to tolerance while trying to walk with much of a normal gait. Crutches can also provide protection against full weight-bearing resulting in inversion or eversion, thereby preventing further injury. When tolerable, full weight-bearing is allowed as long as some support is provided.

TAPING, BRACE SUPPORT, AND CAST IMMOBILIZATION

There are various methods to protect and support the ankle from further damage. The traditional and most commonly used form of stabilization is adhesive ankle taping. Commercial stirrup type or lace-up braces help reduce inversion, but allow motion for plantar and dorsiflexion.

More rigid support can be obtained with a removable cast boot, which allows the trainer or therapist to still provide treatment. In some situations, applying a plaster or fiberglass cast for a short period of 1 to 3 weeks may allow someone the most protection and pain relief by not allowing any ankle movement, while still allowing weight-bearing. However, early mobilization, while protecting the ankle with a brace or taping, yields an earlier return to activity and sports.

A great variety of taping techniques are used, although they share many similar components. First, a tape adherent (e.g., benzoin) is placed on the skin. Underwrap may be used or the tape applied directly to the skin. Next, a number of layers of tape are applied in various sequences. Generally, a combination of anchors, stirrups (vertical), horseshoe strips (horizontal), heel locks, and figure of eights are used. Taping has the advantage of conforming to any ankle to provide a custom fit. The effectiveness of taping is due to improvement in ankle stability by reducing ankle motion while enhancing proprioception. However, taping loses its ability to restrict ankle motion within minutes into exercise. Another disadvantage is that daily taping is costly and requires trained personnel to apply.

Ankle braces include several different types. Elastic-type sleeves and lace-up ankle supports can add some variations with heel lock straps and plastic stays for more support. Stirrup type braces consist of medial and lateral plastic shells with air cells that are held together by straps on both sides of the ankle. Bracing also stabilizes the ankle by restricting ankle motion, but is able to provide support over a longer period of exercise time than taping. In addition, bracing, although initially more costly, is less expensive over time than daily taping.

It appears that both taping and bracing can stabilize the ankle joint and have a role in the treatment and rehabilitation of acute ankle injuries as well as prevention of recurrent injury. Their method of effectiveness may be slightly different with taping providing more proprioceptive stimulation and bracing longer-lasting mechanical support. There is ongoing debate about the superiority of ankle taping versus bracing as well as any effects on athletic performance. However, taping or bracing should never be used as a substitute for a complete strengthening and rehabilitation program.

REHABILITATION EXERCISES

The rehabilitation is frequently the most neglected part in the treatment and management of ankle sprains. Over time, the pain and swelling of an acute ankle sprain will resolve, but without exercise, the damaged ankle may forever remain weak and susceptible to further injury. This is due to the damage and loss of strength in the muscle–tendon unit from the initial injury and subsequent rest and support. The tearing of ankle ligament fibers results in a permanent loss of ankle stability and the need for even more strength about the ankle. An exercise program for the ankle is generally straightforward. The ankle only has four directions to strengthen—inversion, eversion, plantar, and dorsiflexion. There are various ways to provide resistance, but elastic tubing is the most common.

Another component in the rehabilitation program is restoring the sense of balance. Stretching and tearing of ankle ligament and musculotendinous fibers also damages stretch and proprioceptive receptors. Restoring this neuromuscular connection is critical for preventing future injury. These receptors are part of a reflex arc that allows for quick adjustments to maintain overall balance of the foot and ankle before it goes into an extreme position causing injury. There are many exercises designed to retrain this reflex mechanism. Just standing on one leg for 1 min, eventually doing so with eyes closed, will develop proprioception. Another method is the use of a BAPS (biomechanical ankle platform system) board under which half-spheres of various sizes can be attached to form a teeter-totter to practice balancing.

Throughout acute ankle injury treatment and rehabilitation, it is important to help the athlete remain active in ways that do not strain the injured ankle. Endurance conditioning can be maintained by cross-training, such as having a track athlete "run" in the water with a buoyancy vest. Strength training in the weight room can be continued for other parts of the body with minor modifications in some of the exercises. Some sport-specific skills may still be practiced if the ankle can be adequately protected and not placed under excessive strain, such as allowing a gymnast to work on the rings, but avoiding the dismount. Keeping the overall athlete active will minimize the loss of skills and conditioning and aid in returning to full sports as soon as the ankle injury has healed.

RETURN TO PLAY

The decision on returning to athletic activity is based on a number of factors, from functional ability, the particular sports demands placed on the injured ankle, the degree of protection or support that can be provided, and the risks of further injury. The ankle should be examined for absence of or minimal swelling, near normal range of motion, adequate strength on manual muscle testing, and demonstration of functional skills such as balance and sport-specific running or jumping drills. Decisions should also be made about continuing a certain level of ankle support through taping or bracing for a given period of time. Ideally, the early return to play should be monitored so that there is a gradual return to full activity. Adjustments can be made if the ankle shows signs of excessive load or stress with pain or swelling. The athlete should be encouraged to continue the ankle exercises indefinitely for injury prevention.

Atypical Ankle Sprains

Since lateral ankle sprains are such a common injury in the athlete, there is an understandable tendency to view all injuries around the ankle as an "ankle sprain." This is especially true when the athlete is unable to describe the exact mechanism of injury. Several points will suggest an injury other than, or in addition to, a simple lateral ankle sprain: (1) pain or swelling in the midfoot, (2) any deformity to the foot or ankle, (3) the inability to bear weight on the foot and ankle, or (4) the athlete' who continues to have excessive pain or swelling 3 to 4 weeks following the "sprain."

MEDIAL LIGAMENT SPRAINS

Medial ankle ligament sprains are often associated with concomitant injury to the lateral ligaments or fibula. Isolated medial (deltoid) ligament injuries do occur but constitute less than 10 percent of all ankle sprains.[5]

Athletes who suffer a deltoid ligament injury typically have a forced eversion injury, such as landing from a long jump with the foot abducted or landing on another player's foot. As the deltoid ligament stretches and tears, the talus is forced over against the fibula, leading to a syndesmosis sprain or fractures of the fibula. The clinical presentation, a "pop," pain, swelling and weakness, are often very similar to that of the lateral ankle sprain but the mechanism of injury, if known, will be a guide to evaluating medial injury.

On physical examination, carefully palpate for tenderness over the deltoid ligament and along the entire length of the fibula, including any deformity of the fibula. An eversion talar tilt and squeeze test can help identify injury to the deltoid or interosseous ligaments. Radiographs should be examined carefully for any widening of the mortise and may.need to include a complete view of the fibula.

Treatment of isolated grade I deltoid ligament sprains is similar to lateral ankle sprains, with the recognition that return to sports is generally more delayed (3 to 6 weeks) than a lateral sprain (1 to 3 weeks).[5] Grade II to III sprains are rare, however, and immobilization is longer (6 to 8 weeks), requiring a walking boot or cast to prevent any external rotation and allow tighter healing of the anterior deltoid fibers.

SYNDESMOSIS SPRAINS

Syndesmosis sprains are underdiagnosed and result in considerably more impairment than do lateral ankle sprains. Injuries to the interosseous structures (i.e., the syndesmosis) typically occur with eversion stress, as described previously, or with extreme dorsiflexion injuries, such as a gymnast landing a vault or dismount while leaning too far forward. Isolated syndesmosis injuries without fracture are difficult to recognize and require a careful history and physical examination. Again, the mechanism of injury, if it can be determined, is quite helpful, along with complaints of pain in the lower leg above the ankle. There may be increased pain and difficulty bearing weight.

The physical examination is remarkable for the lack of palpable bony tenderness in spite of the complaints of lower leg pain. The most provocative test is the squeeze test to indicate injury to the syndesmosis. Routine radiographs should be obtained if there is suspicion of syndesmosis injury and should be examined carefully for any widening of the mortise. Weight-bearing, stress, or comparison views to the opposite, uninjured ankle, may be needed to see any diastasis. If there is still any question, MR imaging can provide definitive diagnosis.

For an acute syndesmosis injury without widening of the mortise, treatment is typically a fracture boot for 3 to 4 weeks, followed by a stirrup brace for 6 weeks, and crutches initially with weight bearing as tolerated. Follow-up radiographs should be obtained at 2 weeks to confirm stability of the mortise. Return to sports is often delayed as long as 3 months. For a syndesmosis sprain with any widening of the mortise orthopedic consultation with probable operative stabilization is recommended.

Tendon Injury

There are 13 tendons crossing the ankle joint connecting muscles of the lower leg to bones in the feet. They are the dynamic stabilizers of the ankle and thus are subject to large loads. Tendons possess great mechanical strength but poor elasticity, and are most vulnerable to injury when a load is applied rapidly, obliquely, or during maximal eccentric contraction of the associated muscle. Examples of types of tendon injuries include inflammation, subluxation, and rupture. The most common tendons injured about the ankle include the peroneals, anterior and posterior tibialis, and Achilles tendon, and injuries of these tendons are discussed next.

PERONEAL TENDON SUBLUXATION

Injuries to the peroneal tendons are uncommon, but are easily misdiagnosed as a lateral ankle sprain. The peroneal tendons are strong evertors and weak plantar flexors of the foot and are the primary dynamic stabilizers of the lateral ankle joint. The peroneus longus and brevis are positioned posterior to the distal end of the fibula in the retrofibular sulcus. The sulcus is a shallow groove that just barely accommodates the peroneus brevis, with the longus lying just behind in a common synovial sheath. The whole complex is supported on the sides by the superior peroneal retinaculum, a thickened portion of the tendon sheath, forming a fibro-osseous tunnel. From the point of emergence at the end of the tunnel to its insertion at the base of the fifth metatarsal, the brevis tendon follows an anterior curve using the lateral cristae of the distal fibula as a fulcrum. When there is excessive forceful eversion of the foot, the brevis tendon slips in a lateral direction and forward, dragging the longus tendon with it in the common synovial sheath.

The subluxation or dislocation of the peroneal tendons can almost always be traced to a single traumatic event. The mechanism of injury involves a forceful, passive dorsiflexion with slight inversion movement with a violent reflex contraction of the peroneals, as can often be seen in skiing, soccer, figure skating, and basketball.[6] Note that this mechanism is different from the strong inversion force of a typical lateral ankle sprain and the athlete is often at a loss to explain exactly what happened.

Careful examination will reveal maximal tenderness and swelling along the posterior border of the distal fibula. Ligamentous examination, especially for pain and swelling over the anterior lateral ankle ligaments, or any laxity on stress testing, is absent. A hallmark finding on examination is extreme discomfort or apprehension during attempted eversion of the foot against resistance. Rarely do the tendons frankly dislocate with this office maneuver. In the chronic setting, the athlete often complains primarily of instability, giving way, or snapping, often with little discomfort. The physical examination is typically normal except for apprehension on eversion of the foot against resistance. Radiographs are often normal, although occasionally a fracture from the lateral ridge of the distal fibula indicates the avulsion of the superior peroneal retinaculum as the peroneal tendons dislocate.

Surgery is often recommended in the athlete with acute dislocation of the peroneal tendons when it is promptly diagnosed.[5] This is due to the high rate of recurrence seen in the athletically active population even with adequate conservative treatment, which involves the use of a nonweight-bearing short-leg cast for 4 weeks. In chronic injury to the peroneal tendons, conservative treatment has little to offer other than reduction of acute inflammation until the next subluxation occurs. Surgical treatment involves repair or reconstruction of the superior peroneal retinaculum, sometimes with the addition of a groove-deepening procedure. The postoperative management involves nonweight-bearing in a splint for 7 to 10 days, after which the athlete is placed in a walking brace for 4 to 6 weeks. Return to sports is typically 3–4 months.[5]

POSTERIOR TIBIALIS TENDON

The posterior tibialis tendon passes behind the medial maleolus to insert on the tarsal bones, primarily the navicular. The posterior tibialis

muscle and its tendonous insertion function to provide inversion and plantar flexion as well as to stabilize the arch of the foot. During the pronation phase, a great deal of stress is placed on the posterior tibialis tendon just posterior to the medial malleolus, which is an area of low vascularity. Sports that require quick changes in direction, such as basketball, soccer, football, and tennis, place increased stress on this tendon. Thus tendonitis from overuse stress is relatively common, but acute injury in the setting of an ankle sprain is rare. Rupture of the posterior tibialis tendon mainly occurs in the setting of chronic tendonitis, which weakens the tendon in an avascular zone posterior to the medial malleolus. Subluxation is not a problem as the tendon passes below the medial malleolus and underneath the strong deltoid ligament fibers.

ANTERIOR TIBIALIS TENDON

The anterior tibialis tendon runs down the anterior lower leg and passes medially to insert on the first cuneiform and metatarsal. Three overlying retinaculums hold the tendon close to the underlying bones. Due to its relatively straight course, minimal mechanical demands are placed on the anterior tibialis tendon. Tendonitis occurs in runners who train on hills or from direct irritation from ski or figure-skating boots. Rupture in association with an ankle sprain is rare; however, when it occurs, surgical repair is generally needed.

ACHILLES TENDON

Achilles tendonitis is a common injury, especially in sports involving running and jumping. The Achilles tendon is made up of fibers from the gastrocnemius and soleus muscles in the posterior lower leg and courses behind the ankle to insert on the calcaneous. Its function is to plantar flex the foot. Ankle injury involving extreme dorsiflexion can result in strain and partial to complete rupture of the Achilles tendon in addition to injury to the tibiofibular ligament.

Patients will usually complain of crepitus and pain with walking, particularly uphill. Physical examination will reveal tenderness along the distal aspect of the tendon and pain may be present at its insertion in the calcaneus. Tendon rupture should be ruled out with a Thompson test—the calf is squeezed and the foot should plantar flex if the tendon is intact.

Treatment of tendonitis consists of ice, NSAIDs, a heel lift, and gentle stretching of the heel cord. Ruptures should be referred for surgery.

Fractures

Several types of fractures can occur about the ankle and initially appear similar to a typical ankle sprain, but the treatment and prognosis can be quite different than for a sprain. Ankle fractures are much less common than ligamentous injury and are more likely to occur in nonathletes or young athletes with an immature skeleton. Primary ligamentous injuries may have associated subtle fractures that need to be accurately diagnosed and treated. Frank and occult ankle fractures are often an extension of ligamentous injuries, which must be recognized, respected, and included in the treatment plan for the fracture. Knowledge of the mechanism of injury can give clues to look for specific associated ligament and fracture injuries. The most important factors in the treatment of fractures about the ankle are maintenance of the integrity of the ankle mortise and weight-bearing surfaces of the tibia and talus.

FIBULA

Fractures of the fibula can occur at any level and may be due to any of several different mechanisms of injury previously described. In a typical inversion injury with tearing of the lateral ankle ligaments, a small avulsion fracture of the distal lateral malleolus may occur. As long as the fracture line is below the level of the ankle mortise or tibial plafond, the ankle joint is stable, and these fractures can often be treated conservatively similarly to an ankle sprain. In the young immature athlete, a fracture of the distal fibular epiphysis, usually a Salter–Harris type II fracture, might occur in lieu of a lateral ligament sprain with an inversion injury. With an eversion type of injury, as the deltoid ligament gives way, the talus pushes against the fibula and fractures can occur anywhere along the length of the fibula. Again, fractures below the level of the ankle mortise are relatively stable, and if there is no widening of the ankle mortise, they can be treated in a cast, initially nonweight-bearing, and followed closely for any change of position. Fracture of the fibula above the ankle mortise involves disruption of the deltoid and tibiofibular ligaments and is an unstable fracture often requiring open reduction and internal fixation. Beware of the Maisonneuve fracture of the proximal fibula, which occurs with a complete tear of the syndesmosis or tibiofibular ligament. Standard ankle radiographs will not show the proximal fibula fracture. This is an unstable fracture that must be recognized so that proper operative repair can be performed.

TIBIA

Several different fractures of the distal tibia can also occur with ankle sprains depending on the mechanism of injury. During the inversion injury of a typical lateral ankle sprain, as the lateral ligaments give way the talus is pushed over the tip of the medial malleolus to the point of fracture. Typically, the fracture line extends vertically up the shaft of the tibia beginning at the lateral margin of the medial malleolus. Recognizing this fracture line, the examiner must assume that the lateral ligaments are torn and the ankle mortise is no longer stable. An eversion injury can result in a bimalleolar fracture involving a lateral malleolar fracture and either a medial malleolar fracture or complete tear of the deltoid ligament. Again the integrity of the ankle mortise is not stable and if there is any displacement, particularly measured on the mortise radiograph, surgical open reduction and internal fixation is necessary. A bimalleolar fracture that involves the posterior lip of the tibial plafond, where there has been avulsion of the posterior tibiofibular ligament, is a trimalleolar fracture. This also requires surgical fixation. Extreme dorsiflexion injuries can cause fractures of the lateral or medial malleolus or both.

In the young athlete, an ankle sprain can damage the distal tibial physis in lieu of a ligament injury. These fractures require recognition and special consideration to avoid future growth disruption. The Tillaux fracture is an avulsion of the anterior lateral portion of the distal tibial epiphysis. Various Salter–Harris type I to V injuries can involve the distal tibial epiphysis due to different mechanisms of ankle injury (see Chap. 18).

Talus

Several occult fractures of the talus can initially appear similar to a typical ankle sprain. The lateral process of the talus is the wedge-shaped lateral portion of the talar body where it extends below the distal tip of the fibula. Fracture of this process is thought to result from inversion and dorsiflexion, which can result in a compressive force being delivered to the lateral talus.[5] The athlete may complain of significant pain with ambulating and significant ecchymosis can develop. Examination reveals minimal tenderness of the lateral ligaments, negative anterior drawer, and maximal tenderness somewhat below the distal tip of the fibula. Close attention to the AP or mortise radiographs will often reveal the fracture; if not, CT or bone scan may be necessary. Small undisplaced fractures are treated conservatively similar to a lateral ankle sprain. Chronic pain can develop from nonunion of the fragments and require surgical debridement. Large fragments may require internal fixation.

Posterior process fractures of the talus (os trigonum) rarely occur, but more commonly frequent extreme plantarflexion results in chronic impingement pain. A separate ossicle is found in 10 percent of the population and must be distinguished from a acute fracture. The athlete with a painful os trigonum will report posteriolateral or posteriomedial ankle pain without any complaints of instability. Conservative treatment with avoidance of extreme dorsiflexion is usually sufficient, although occasionally excision of the fragment is necessary.

Osteochondritis Dissecans

Osteochondral lesions of the talus include osteochondritis dissecans or osteochondral fractures involving the dome of the talus. These lesions are most common in the young athlete or young adult. The location of the lesions are either posteriomedial or anterolateral. These injuries are related to either acute trauma or repetitive microtrauma.[5]

Acute injury to the anterolateral dome of the talus can occur as the result of an inversion injury. If an inversion stress is applied while the foot is in dorsiflexion, the corner of the talus impinges on the inside of the fibula. As the talofibular ligaments tear and the talus tilts, the cartilage and a portion of the subchondral bone is peeled off the anterolateral corner of the talar dome. The force may be strong enough to dislodge an entire fragment or simply hinge it upward only to fall back into place.[7]

When the foot is in plantar flexion, such as a basketball player landing a jump on his or her toes with the foot slightly inverted, the applied force may damage the posteriomedial portion of the talus. Repetitive compressive microtrauma may lead to osteochondritis dissecans or an acute shear force may dislodge a flap of cartilage and subchondral bone.

The athlete with an osteochondral lesion is more likely to describe pain "inside" the ankle rather than laterally, and the painful symptoms will often persist longer than expected for a simple ankle sprain. Aching and stiffness are common complaints, especially when the problem is chronic.

Examination may reveal an ankle effusion and there may be palpable tenderness over the dome of the talus if the lesion is in an area that is accessible. Plain radiographs may not initially show the lesion and may have to be repeated later, though definitive diagnosis may require CT or an MRI to define the osteochondral lesion.[8]

Acute osteochondral fractures, if recognized early, are treated surgically through ankle arthroscopy in the highly active athlete, but if undisplaced, may respond to conservative treatment with early motion without weight-bearing for 6 to 8 weeks.[9] More commonly, osteochondral lesions are recognized in a more chronic setting of persistent ankle pain that has failed conservative treatment and are treated through arthroscopy.

CALCANEOUS

Another subtle fracture occurring with the typical lateral ankle sprain from plantar flexion and inversion is injury to the anterior process of the calcaneous. This is due to the avulsion of several ligament attachments to this process. Physical examination will reveal tenderness and swelling somewhat more inferior and anterior to the lateral malleolus than more typically seen in a lateral ankle sprain. The fracture is best seen on the lateral ankle or foot radiograph. Small fragments with little displacement are treated conservatively in a walking-cast boot. If chronic symptoms develop, then debridment of the fracture fragment usually relieves the pain. Large fragments with displacement require surgical treatment.

BASE OF THE FIFTH METATARSAL

A fracture at the base of the fifth metatarsal of the foot may occur with a lateral ankle sprain. The mechanism of injury is quite similar, involving a forceful inversion, which may avulse a fragment of bone from the tuberosity where the peroneus brevis has its attachment. However, sometimes the fracture occurs slightly more proximal at the metaphyseal diaphyseal junction approximately 1.5 cm from the base. This injury is typically referred to as a Jones fracture and has a different treatment and prognosis. Typically, the athlete describes landing a jump. The strong attachment of the peroneus brevis, plus the massive lateral ligament attachments tend to fix the base of the fifth metatarsal as the forefoot is sharply inverted and adducted, and a greater or lesser fragment may be pulled away. The prior history of aching in the lateral foot may indicate a prior stress reaction often leading to a Jones-type fracture. Pain and swelling with tenderness at the base of the fifth metatarsal will lead to radiographs demonstrating the fracture. Avulsion fractures at the base may be treated with a cast boot, early rehabilitation, and a return to sports with supportive taping based on symptoms, usually 4 to 6 weeks. Jones fractures, however, have a high incidences of nonunion. Vascular compromise and rigid stability of the base fragment with greater mobility of the shaft fragment contribute to poor healing. Treatment may be attempted with 4 to 6 weeks in a nonweight-bearing cast, followed by 2 to 4 more weeks weight-bearing in a fracture boot. Still, the incidence of nonunion is high with this treatment, especially if there is any evidence of prior stress reaction, and thus many prefer treatment in the highly active athlete with open reduction and internal fixation. This will allow reliable healing, early rehabilitation, and typically, return to sports in 6 to 8 weeks.

References

1. Wexler RK: The injured ankle. *Am Fam Physician* 57:474, 1998.
2. Stiell IG, Greenberg GH, McKnight RD, et al: A study to develop clinical decision rules for the use

of radiography in acute ankle injuries. *Ann Emerg Med* 21:384, 1992.

3. Stiell IG, McKnight RD, Greenberg GH, et al: Implementation of the Ottawa ankle rules. *JAMA* 271:827, 1994.

4. Rubin A: Ankle ligament sprains. In: Sallis RE, Massimino F (eds). *Essentials of Sports Medicine.* St. Louis: Mosby; 1996;450.

5. Clanton TO, Porter DA: Primary care of foot and ankle injuries in the athlete. *Clin Sports Med* 16:435, 1997.

6. Frey CC, Shereff MJ: Tendon injuries about the ankle in athletes. *Clin Sports Med* 7:103, 1988.

7. O'Donoghue DH: *Treatment of Injuries to Athletes,* 4th ed. Philadelphia: Saunders; 1984.

8. Manusov EG, Lillegard WA, Raspa RF: Evaluation of pediatric foot problems: Part II, the hindfoot and the ankle. *Am Fam Physician* 54:1012, 1996.

9. Stanish WD: Lower leg, foot, and ankle injuries in young athletes. *Clin Sports Med* 14(3):559, 1995.

10. Simons SM: Rehabilitation of ankle injuries. In Sallis RE, Massimino R (eds): *Essentials of Sports Medicine.* St. Louis: Mosby; 1996;458.

Foot Pain

Introduction

Foot pain is a common problem. Although highly adapted, the foot is prone to injury due to the tremendous amount of acute and repetitive stress it must endure, particularly during sport and exercise. Fortunately, with knowledge of basic foot anatomy and function, most foot problems can be confidently diagnosed and treated by the primary care physician.

The key to making the diagnosis in foot pain is simply the foot pain location. The most common areas of foot pain are shown in Fig. 11-1. Once accurately diagnosed, the athlete can be treated with specific and efficient measures that are usually available to the primary care provider. The need for referral is infrequent.

Basic Foot Anatomy

Bones and Soft Tissue

The bones and soft tissues that comprise the foot are illustrated in Figs. 11-2 through 11-4.

Arches

Three dynamic arches exist in the foot: (1) the medial longitudinal arch, (2) the lateral longitudinal arch, and (3) the transverse midfoot arch. These arches heighten and flatten pending foot position. This subsequently affects the foot's rigidity and flexibility respectively.

Foot Types

PES CAVUS

Pes cavas describes a foot with an inverted heel that creates a high, rigid arch. It is prone to over-supination and poor shock absorption. Stress is thus increased, not only in the foot, but up the kinetic chain to the back. This may predispose the lower extremity, pelvis, and back to stress-related injury.

PES PLANUS

Pes planus describes a foot with an everted heel that creates a flat, flexible arch. It is prone to over-pronation and lack of rigidity for propulsion. This may predispose the medial foot structures and those up the associated kinetic chain to injury.

Foot Function

HEEL AND FOREFOOT VARUS AND VALGUS

Heel varus alignment is simply heel inversion. Heel valgus is simply heel eversion. The forefoot may also have similar varus or valgus alignment. These alignments may predispose to biomechanical (functional) abnormality.

FOOT PRONATION

This is a three-dimensional movement that involves abduction, eversion, and dorsiflexion of the foot. When the foot pronates, its arches flatten and the foot becomes flexible. This allows the foot to accommodate the ground. Excessive foot pronation is the most commonly accused biomechanical abnormality contributing to, or causing, foot injuries.

FOOT SUPINATION

This is a three-dimensional movement that involves adduction, inversion, and plantar flexion of the foot. When the foot supinates it recreates its arch and becomes stiff. This allows the foot to act as a rigid lever for propulsion.

FOOT POSITION IN THE GAIT CYCLE

The foot goes through four phases during the gait cycle: heel strike/stance/toe off/swing. The

Figure 11-1

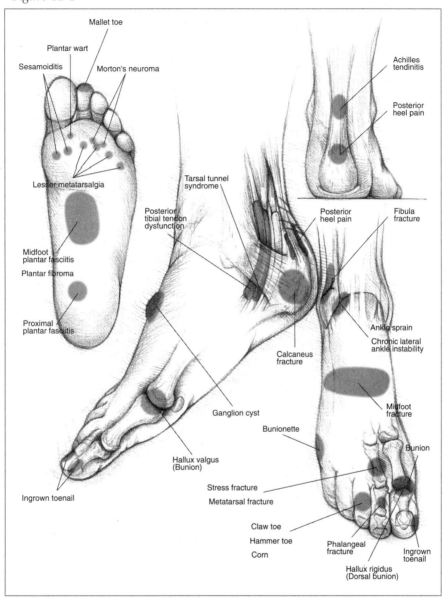

Pain diagram for foot and ankle. *(Reproduced with permission from Pfeffer GB, Clain MR, Frey C, et al: Foot and ankle. In: Snider RK (ed): Essentials of Musculoskeletal Care, 1st ed. Rosemont, IL: American Academy of Orthopedic Surgeons, 1997; 366.)*

Figure 11-2

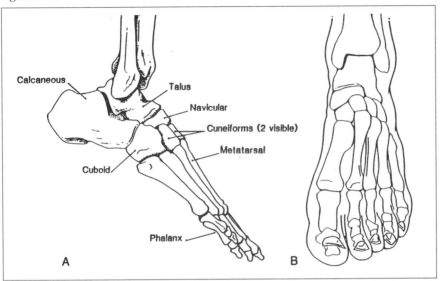

Calcaneous
Talus
Navicular
Cuneiforms (2 visible)
Metatarsal
Cuboid
Phalanx

A

B

(A) Normal bony lateral anatomy of the foot. **(B)** Normal bony dorsal anatomy of the foot. *(Reproduced with permission from Mellion MB, et al [eds]: The Team Physician Handbook. Philadelphia, PA: Hanley & Belfus, 1990.)*

Figure 11-3

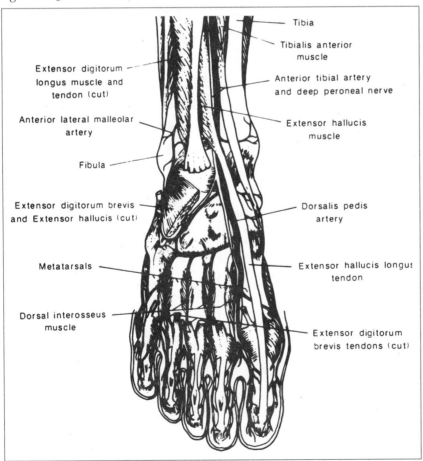

Extensor digitorum longus muscle and tendon (cut)

Anterior lateral malleolar artery

Fibula

Extensor digitorum brevis and Extensor hallucis (cut)

Metatarsals

Dorsal interosseus muscle

Tibia

Tibialis anterior muscle

Anterior tibial artery and deep peroneal nerve

Extensor hallucis muscle

Dorsalis pedis artery

Extensor hallucis longus tendon

Extensor digitorum brevis tendons (cut)

The anatomy of the dorsum of the foot. *(Reproduced with permission from Birrer RB [ed]: Sports Medicine for the Primary Care Physician, 2nd ed. Boca Raton, FL: CRC Press, 1994;562.)*

Figure 11-4

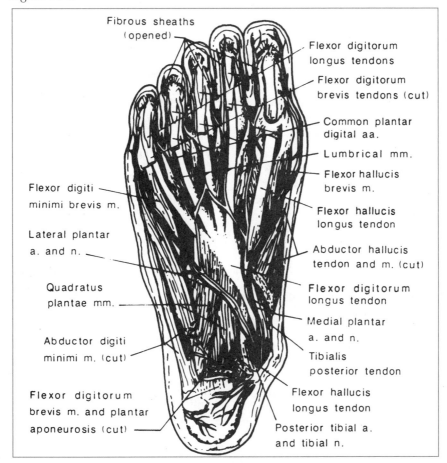

Fibrous sheaths
(opened)

Flexor digitorum
longus tendons

Flexor digitorum
brevis tendons (cut)

Common plantar
digital aa.

Lumbrical mm.

Flexor hallucis
brevis m.

Flexor hallucis
longus tendon

Abductor hallucis
tendon and m. (cut)

Flexor digitorum
longus tendon

Medial plantar
a. and n.

Tibialis
posterior tendon

Flexor hallucis
longus tendon

Posterior tibial a.
and tibial n.

Flexor digiti
minimi brevis m.

Lateral plantar
a. and n.

Quadratus
plantae mm.

Abductor digiti
minimi m. (cut)

Flexor digitorum
brevis m. and plantar
aponeurosis (cut)

Anatomy of the plantar surface of the foot. *(Reproduced with permission from Birrer RB [ed]: Sports Medicine for the Primary Care Physician, 2nd ed. Boca Raton, FL: CRC Press, 1994;563.)*

foot lands supinated in heel strike. It then pronates in the stance phase (which makes the foot more flexible to accommodate the ground) and finally, resupinates in toe off (which makes the foot more rigid for propulsion). *Remember, generally a pronated foot is flexible, and a supinated foot rigid.*

The Abnormal Gait

Several individual or grouped anthropometric abnormalities may lead to a biomechanically (dynamically) abnormal gait. The abnormal gait usually involves excessive foot pronation, or increased foot time in pronation.

However, the most common predisposing alignment abnormalities leading to excessive foot pronation are actual heel varus, forefoot varus, tibia vara, and tight heel cords. Abnormalities proximally may affect foot motion, such as femoral anteversion. In this case, the foot may simply be an innocent "victim" of pathology upstream (depending on your experience, utilizing a physical therapist may be of help in further evaluation of the kinetic chain).

It is important to remember, however, that static alignment abnormalities do not necessarily create dynamic, functional ones, and that dynamic gait abnormalities do not necessarily cause injury. Many people have "terrible biomechanics," yet are pain free. An individual's foot, leg, and gait can be highly adapted to its particular structure and movement. *Nevertheless, correcting the obvious biomechanical abnormality that logically ties with an injury is often useful, particularly in those with recalcitrant or recurrent injury.* Correcting these abnormalities may involve specific stretching, strengthening, cushioning, and/or mechanical support (i.e., orthotics) to correct the abnormality.

The Basic Foot Examination

As in any musculoskeletal examination, the basics include inspection, palpation, range of motion, and provocative tests. In the foot examination, it is especially important to carefully palpate to determine the point of maximal tenderness. This itself often gives the diagnosis. Additionally, when assessing foot structure and movement, the patient should be observed sitting, standing, and in gait. Finally, the entire kinetic chain from the foot to the back should be observed for obvious abnormalities that may

contribute to abnormal foot motion or stress. (For the examination details, see the specific injuries listed as follows.)

Hindfoot Pain

See Table 11-1.

Retrocalcaneal Bursitis

Retrocalcaneal bursitis occurs when either the superficial or deep retrocalcaneal bursa is inflamed. The most common culprit is direct irritation, usually from the shoe. There will be tenderness, swelling, and, perhaps, erythema just above the insertion site of the Achilles tendon on the calcaneous.

Treatment consists of (1) reducing the irritative focus, and (2) eliminating the inflammation. Changing shoes, utilizing a u-shaped cutout posterior heel pad surrounding the bursa, or even cutting out a portion of the shoe heel will reduce the irritation, as will Achilles tendon stretching. Ice and NSAIDs are the mainstay for reducing the inflammation.

Table 11-1

Hindfoot Injuries

Most Common	To Not Miss or to Refer
Retrocalcaneal bursitis	Calcaneal fracture, stress or acute
Posterior impingement syndrome	Talar fracture, stress or acute
Calcaneal stress fracture	Spondyloarthropathy
Sever's disease	Radiculopathy
Tarsal tunnel syndrome	
Plantar fasciitis	

At times, a cortisone injection of 10 to 20 mg of Depo-Medrol, or equivalent, is appropriate for recalcitrant bursitis. When giving this injection, however, make sure not to inject the Achilles tendon. Using a medial or lateral approach to the bursa reduces this risk.

Posterior Impingement Syndrome

Posterior impingement syndrome occurs when either an os-trigonum or posterior spur off the posterior talar process abuts the posterior tibial plateau on extremes of plantar flexion. This creates posterior heel pain deep to the Achilles tendon. On examination edema may be present along with tenderness in the posterior heel deep to the Achilles. Pain can often be produced with extreme active or passive foot plantar flexion. The diagnosis is confirmed radiographically with lateral ankle x-rays in plantar flexion showing the bony impingement.

Definitive treatment is often surgical resection of the offending bone. Reducing the associated edema with relative rest, ice, and NSAIDs and/or a cortisone injection may help relieve the pain. Some athletes are able to control their symptoms with activity modification. This, however, is not often compatible with continuing participation at the athlete's usual competitive level.

Calcaneal Stress Fracture

This is an important fracture to consider since treatment requires non-weightbearing, and progression to a completed fracture can lead to disastrous outcomes.[1] Suspect a possible calcaneal stress fracture in hindfoot pain when the point of maximal tenderness on examination is on the medial or lateral side of the calcaneus, or with side to side compression of the heel. Female long-distance runners who may be suffering from osteoporosis are obviously at higher risk. X-rays may show the stress fracture with a line of vertical sclerosis on the lateral calcaneal view.

If a stress fracture is not clearly seen, but still suspected, a bone scan or CT scan must be performed to rule it out.

Treatment, unlike most other stress fractures, involves non-weight-bearing on crutches for 6 weeks with slowly progressive activity thereafter as tolerated without pain. Heel cups or custom orthotics may be useful for shock absorption in selected athletes.

Sever's Disease

This is a condition seen in children. It involves irritation of the posterior calcaneal apophysis. The athlete will present with hindfoot pain and maximal tenderness on the medial or lateral calcaneus over the apophysis. X-rays are appropriate to rule out other bony lesions (see Chap. 17).

The mainstay of treatment is activity modification, Achilles tendon stretches, heel cups, and reassurance. Patients with this syndrome tend to do well and it will resolve. After becoming pain free, the athlete may slowly progress with activity as tolerated.

Tarsal Tunnel Syndrome

Tarsal tunnel syndrome results from irritation of the posterior tibial nerve as it curves around the posterior medial malleolus in the tarsal tunnel. Here, the tendons and nerve are covered by a fascial band and prone to injury, either by trauma such as an ankle sprain, or overuse in the pronated foot. Athletes with significant pes planus and subtalar pronation on examination, or excessive dynamic pronation with walking or running, produce increased tension in the tarsal tunnel and are at heightened risk of developing the syndrome.

Pain along with neurologic symptoms including numbness and tingling can occur around the medial malleolus with radiations along the distribution of the posterior tibial nerve up the leg or down into the medial arch, plantar foot, and toes. The most important finding on examination is a positive Tinel's sign on percussion over the tarsal tunnel (i.e., reproduction of neurologic symptoms). Edema may also exist in this area. Stretching the structures with the foot in extreme plantar flexion and eversion may reproduce the symptoms. If the examiner is unsure of the diagnosis, a nerve conduction study may show evidence of entrapment in the tarsal tunnel.

Treatment involves relative rest, NSAIDs, and/or a steroid injection to decrease the inflammation. Arch supports will help decrease the tension in the tarsal tunnel. Custom orthotics may be needed if significant underlying pronation abnormalities exist. Sometimes a short leg cast or walker boot is necessary to resolve the irritation and inflammation. If conservative measures are unsuccessful, surgical excision of the overlying fascial band is indicated.

Plantar Fasciitis

Plantar fasciitis is very common, and is caused by irritation and inflammation of the plantar fascia at its insertion site on the calcaneus. The plantar fascia is a strong fascial band that runs along the plantar foot from multiple attachment sites in the forefoot to its insertion on the medial process of the calcaneus. The fascial injury is secondary to relative overuse.

Athletes at risk are those involved in activities that require repetitive plantar flexion at the ankle and dorsiflexion of the forefoot, such as runners. This position stresses the plantar fascia. Other risk factors placing increased stress on the fascia include over-pronation, a flexible arch, tight heel cords, weak intrinsic arch musculature, being overweight, and wearing shoes with inadequate arch support.

The athlete with plantar fasciitis will complain of plantar heel pain with weight-bearing. This pain is characteristically greatest on rising from bed in the morning, or when active after resting for a period of time. On examination, maximal

tenderness is found over the plantar fascial insertion site on the calcaneus. This tenderness is often rather exquisite. Diffuse tenderness generally about the plantar heel is not uncommon and some edema may be noted. In addition, stretching the plantar fascia usually produces pain.

Radiographs may show a bony spur at the fascia's attachment site on the calcaneus. The spur develops as a result of the injury. It is not the cause, and rarely contributes to the pain unless very large.

Several levels of treatment may be used depending on the severity and chronicity of the injury. In general, the inflammation must be controlled, the possible anthropometric and biomechanical abnormalities addressed, and the tissue rehabilitated and strengthened. This is accomplished initially with relative rest, ice, NSAIDs, heel cups, Achilles and plantar fascial stretching, arch muscle strengthening (curling up a cloth with the toes), and, possibly, arch supports.

For those patients unresponsive to initial treatment, the next treatment option would include the addition of a posterior splint worn at night. The splint holds the foot in 90° or greater of dorsiflexion to put a prolonged stretch on the plantar fascia. Because the plantar fascia is fibrous tissue it is more difficult to stretch than muscle/tendon. A low-grade prolonged stretch, such as that provided by the posterior splint, is sometimes needed. The splint is easily constructed in the office with prefab material. Orthotics for arch support and motion control should be considered, particularly in those with pes planus and excessive pronation.

For those patients who do not respond favorably to the night splint, the addition of a short leg cast or walker boot to help diminish movement of the fascia may be useful. Use of a corticosteroid injection may be appropriate at this stage of treatment, or if extreme urgency exists in regard to the athlete's needs. Risks are involved with corticosteroid injection, and thus judicious use is warranted. The main risk with this injection is fat pad necrosis. This can result in chronic heel pain due to the loss of padding. Fortunately, if given correctly, this is a rare occurrence.

A common method to use when injecting the plantar fascia is a medial approach. The calcaneus is palpated distally to the point where it begins to curve up dorsally. This is approximately 2 cm from the plantar surface. The needle is inserted until it touches the calcaneus in this area, then is gently walked distally to the distal plantar surface. This is where the plantar fascia inserts. The needle is advanced a bit further and then the bolus of lidocaine and corticosteroid is injected (generally 4 mL lidocaine/1mL corticosteroid preparation). Make sure not to inject plantar to the plantar fascia.

For longstanding, recalcitrant cases, surgery may be necessary for a definitive cure.

Hindfoot Injuries to Not Miss or to Refer

Calcaneal Fracture

CALCANEAL STRESS FRACTURE

As mentioned previously, the point of maximal tenderness is generally on the medial or lateral calcaneus or with side to side compression of the heel. Treatment of a calcaneal stress fracture requires nonweight bearing for at least 6 weeks. Progression to a completed fracture can be disastrous. This fracture needs to be watched closely with serial radiographs to avoid this complication.

ACUTE CALCANEAL FRACTURE

This generally results from a high impact injury. Patients with this fracture are unable to bear weight. If radiographs are negative and the

fracture suspected, a CT or MRI should be obtained. Treatment is difficult and adverse outcomes, or complications, can be severe and disabling. Initial treatment by the primary care physician involves placing the patient in a posterior splint, elevation, and icing to give protection and reduce inflammation. Because many of these fractures require immediate surgical reduction and fixation to minimize complications, a completed stress fracture or acute calcaneal fracture should be referred immediately to an orthopedic surgeon after immobilization in a posterior splint has been accomplished.[1]

Talar Fracture

TALAR STRESS FRACTURE

This injury is infrequent. It usually involves the posterolateral talus. The patient complains of pain and swelling in the involved area accentuated by weight-bearing exercise.

Treatment differs from most other stress fractures in that it requires at least 6 to 8 weeks of cast immobilization, with non-weight-bearing during the initial 3 to 4 weeks. After bony healing is demonstrated and the cast removed, a semirigid arch support should be used during rehabilitation. Furthermore, these fractures are often associated with excessive pronation, which needs to be corrected before activity is resumed. As with calcaneal stress fractures, progression to a completed fracture can lead to serious complications and disability. Thus, this fracture also needs to be watched very closely. Unless experienced with this fracture, it is best referred or managed along with an orthopedist.[2]

ACUTE TALAR FRACTURE

This fracture generally results from a high-impact injury. The patient has difficulty bearing weight and tenderness with swelling over the anterior talocrural joint, talus, and talonavicular joint exists. Complications and outcomes from this fracture can be disastrous and should be managed in a similar way as calcaneal fractures, with immediate referral.[1]

Spondyloarthropathy

Be alert for a systemic disease in athletes with bilateral heel pain. Any of the seronegative spondyloarthropathies can cause heal pain, but the most common is Reiter's syndrome. Be certain to look for other manifestations of systemic disease, such as joint pain or swelling, back pain, or ocular symptoms when considering this possibility.

Radiculopathy

Numbness or tingling in the foot not reproducible locally on examination should lead to inquiry about a radiculopathy. It is not uncommon for initial radicular symptoms to present in the foot.

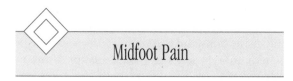

Midfoot Pain

See Table 11-2.

Posterior Tibial Tendonitis

The posterior tibial tendon courses around the posteroinferior medial malleolus in the tarsal tunnel and under the medial arch. It attaches at multiple places on the plantar arch including the navicular, cuneiforms, and second, third, and forth metatarsal bases. This tendon helps support the arch, and acts as an important foot plantar flexor and inverter. It is also important in the control of pronation, and therefore it is prone to being overstressed in the flat, pronated foot

Table 11-2

Midfoot Injuries

MOST COMMON	TO NOT MISS OR TO REFER
Posterior tibial tendonitis	Posterior tibial tendon tear
Navicular stress fracture	Navicular stress fracture
Mid tarsal sprain	Midfoot fracture/ dislocation
Plantar fascial strain	
Fifth metatarsal avulsion fracture	Tarsal coalition
	Jones fracture
Plantar fibroma	Köhler's disease
Ganglion cyst	Radiculopathy

and/or during repetitive dynamic over-pronation during gait.

With posterior tibial tendonitis the patient complains of pain along the course of the tendon. The posterior tibial nerve may also become irritated concomitantly with the tendon, creating neurologic symptoms, as in tarsal tunnel syndrome.

On examination, peritendinous swelling and crepitation may exist. Resisted inversion in the plantar-flexed foot stresses the tendon and can often reproduce the pain. Prior to treating posterior tibial tendonitis it is important to rule out a significant tendon tear. This is accomplished by observing the patient's heel appropriately invert on straight-leg toe raises. It should be compared to the opposite heel for symmetry. Fortunately, significant tears are rare and usually occur only in the older, middle-aged athlete.

Treatment is similar to that of tarsal tunnel syndrome with relative rest, ice, NSAIDs, and arch supports or orthotics. For resistant cases a walker boot or short leg cast may be necessary to eliminate the inflammation. After the inflammation and acute symptoms have resolved, rehabilitation may ensue. Resistance exercises with Therabrand (therapeutic elastic bands of varying resistance) are popular and easy to do any-where. Return to sport or exercise is gradual, and correction of abnormal biomechanics, if present, is essential.

Navicular Stress Fracture

Navicular stress fractures are a relatively com-mon stress fracture in athletes, and unfortu-nately, frequently overlooked. The navicular bone sits between the talus and the first, second, and third cuneiform bones articulating respec-tively with the first, second, and third meta-tarsals. It is in a sense the "cornerstone" of the foot arch, accepting and transmitting much of the foot's stress. Hence the navicular bone is prone to stress related injuries. Additionally, the navicular bone is notorious for poor healing after injury because of its tenuous blood supply, sim-ilar to the navicular (scaphoid) bone in the wrist.

A navicular stress fracture usually presents with a history of significant pain and maximal point tenderness over the bone on examination. Radiographs may demonstrate the fracture. This particular injury must be treated with non-weight-bearing, and potentially has serious con-sequences. If the examiner is clinically suspicious for a navicular stress fracture and x-rays are negative, a bone scan, CT, or MRI is required to detect or exclude it (see Chap. 20).

Treatment requires immobilization in a non-weight-bearing short leg cast for 6 weeks. If the navicular is still tender after 6 weeks, recasting and another 2 weeks of non-weight-bearing is necessary. Most clinicians use a semirigid arch support during the rehabilitation phase.[3]

The feet particularly at risk for navicular stress fractures are those with excessive pronation, poor dorsiflexion, and/or pes cavus. To prevent recurrent fracture, ensure appropriate heel cord stretching exercises are included in rehabilitation to allow adequate ankle dorsiflexion. And, if clinically indicated, prescribe the appropriate orthotics for arch support, motion control, and/or cushioning depending upon the situa-tion.

Midfoot Sprain

This injury occurs in high impact landing sports, such as gymnastics, or when the foot is in a fixed position and twisted, such as pulling away or falling when the foot is stepped on. On rare occasions, a midfoot sprain can potentially be a serious injury.

The athlete presents with the appropriate his-tory (high impact landing or twisting foot injury) and complains of midfoot pain. The midfoot has generalized tenderness on examination and the athlete usually has difficulty walking on his or her toes. Weight bearing anterior-posterior (AP) and lateral foot radiographs with comparison views of the opposite foot are needed to rule out midfoot subluxations or frank dislocations. If subluxation or dislocation is found, referral to an orthopedist is needed.

Most often, the radiographs are normal and the athlete can be treated conservatively with rel-ative rest, NSAIDs, and arch supports. Return to sport usually takes 2 to 3 weeks in mild to mod-erate sprains (the athlete should be able to walk on his or her toes, and perform appropriate sport-specific drills without pain before return). For severe midfoot sprains (the athlete with dif-ficulty bearing any weight, and significant swelling and tenderness on examination) non-weight-bearing for 3 to even 6 weeks may be necessary initially, followed by a walker boot or short leg walking cast for a couple of weeks.

In general, all displaced midtarsal dislocations need reduction and are prone to complications, often serious. The most common subluxation or dislocation is at the second metatarsal base. This is called a "LisFranc subluxation/dislocation." A weaker ligamentous link exists at this point between the base of the second metatarsal, first metatarsal, and the medial cuneiform. The weight-bearing radiographs will show an increased distance between the medial border of the second metatarsal base and the medial border of the middle cuneiform when compared to the opposite foot.[4]

Again, with any serious midfoot sprain make sure to obtain weight-bearing AP and lateral radiographs of the injured foot with comparison views of the noninjured foot to rule out gross midfoot instability.

Plantar Fascial Strain

A strain of the plantar fascia produces a plantar midfoot pain. This injury may occur from an acute event, or overuse. The foot with a dynamic (flexible) arch is at particular risk.

On examination tenderness is found over the plantar fascia. Sometimes a defect can be felt, indicating a partial tear. Stretching the plantar fascia will produce pain. As opposed to plantar fasciitis, where the primary pathology is at the plantar fascial insertion site on the calcaneus, a strain of the mid plantar fascia generally responds more quickly to treatment.

Treatment involves relative rest and inflammation control. Arch support may be helpful, and orthotics should be considered on return to sport to prevent re-injury. This condition usually resolves in 2 to 3 weeks.[5]

Fifth Metatarsal Base Fractures

Primarily two main categories of fracture occur at the base of the fifth metatarsal: (1) the avulsion fracture, and (2) the Jones fracture.

AVULSION FRACTURES

The peroneus brevis wraps around the lateral malleolus along with the peroneus longus and inserts at the base of the fifth metatarsal. An acute inversion ankle injury causes the peroneals to contract, resisting the inversion. This can cause an injury to the peroneal tendons themselves, but more commonly the bony attachment

of the peroneal brevis fails resulting in an avulsion fracture from the base of the fifth metatarsal (see Chap. 10).

The athlete complains of pain in the lateral foot. On examination exquisite tenderness exists at the base of the fifth metatarsal, and radiographs reveal the avulsed piece of bone. This fracture tends to heal well. Treatment is symptomatic. Often use of a walker boot or a stiff-soled shoe for a week or two is necessary secondary to the pain. Return to play requires pain-free walking and sport-specific drills. An ankle brace should be worn during strenuous activity over the next 6 to 8 weeks (this also is often necessary for the usually associated lateral ankle sprain).

JONES FRACTURE

A more serious fracture at the base of the fifth metatarsal is one through the diaphysis called a Jones fracture. This fracture tends to result either from an acute inversion ankle injury or repetitive stress. It is notoriously slow to heal and prone to non-union due to the tenuous blood supply in this part of the fifth metatarsal.

On examination the area will be quite tender and may be swollen or bruised. Radiographs will demonstrate a fracture through the diaphysis of the fifth metatarsal. Traditionally this fracture has been treated with a non-weight-bearing short leg cast for 6 to 8 weeks (some allow weight-bearing, particularly after 3 to 4). This fracture may, however, take from 3 to 4 months to completely heal, and non-union is common. Thus, in the active athlete, without the luxury of time, initial treatment with intramedullary screw fixation is now the treatment of choice. It allows for earlier return and overall improved outcome.[6]

Plantar Fibroma

Plantar fibromas are generally benign tumors of the plantar fascia that can vary in size up to 6 cm. They very rarely undergo malignant degeneration. They may be painful to the athlete, however, secondary to local irritation and mass effect.

On examination the nodule is firm, rubbery, and clearly attached to the planter fascia. Several discrete nodules may exist in any one patient. Plantar fibromas are best treated with shoe modification to accommodate the nodule. Surgical excision may be indicated if this is not possible, but is discouraged because they tend to recur. Elaborate work-up is usually unnecessary to exclude other etiologies of the foot mass such as a lipoma, neurofibroma, giant cell tumor of the tendon sheath, or malignant sarcoma.[7]

Ganglion Cyst

Ganglion cysts are small cystic tumors arising from synovial tissue surrounding a joint. They vary in size up to 3 cm and are filled with a straw-colored viscous fluid. Ganglion cysts most often occur on the dorsal or lateral midfoot, and are generally painless unless creating difficulties with shoe wear.

On examination the ganglion is usually soft and moveable. Aspiration with a large-gauge needle will yield the straw-colored viscous fluid. If symptomatic, the cyst should be aspirated, poking several holes in the cyst wall to hopefully prevent fluid from reaccumulating. If the cyst tends to recur, surgical excision is indicated. Again, as with plantar fibromas, elaborate work-up is generally not needed to confirm the diagnosis of a ganglion cyst and rule out others such as a lipoma, neurofibroma, giant cell tumor of the tendon sheath, or malignant sarcoma.[7]

Midfoot Injuries to Not Miss or to Refer

Midfoot pain can be problematic. There are several injuries in this area that should not be overlooked.

LisFranc or Other Midfoot Subluxation and Dislocation

As mentioned, a displacement or fracture of the second metatarsal base, or other midfoot bone, requires reduction and special attention. These injuries are prone to complications, some of which are serious. If not careful, these fractures and dislocations may be passed off as a midfoot sprain. Weight-bearing AP foot radiographs with comparison views of the opposite foot are essential in any significant midfoot sprain.

Tarsal Coalition

Fibrous and/or osseous bridges between certain tarsal bones may infrequently exist. The most common place is between the calcaneus and navicular bones. The second most common bridge is between the calcaneus and talus. Tarsal coalition should be suspected in the young athlete undergoing recurrent foot and ankle injuries, or unexplained recurrent midfoot pain with repetitive running or jumping.

On examination, the young patient may reveal a flat, rigid midfoot with decreased subtalar motion. Simple oblique foot radiographs may give the diagnosis. The "bridges," however, can be difficult to see on plain radiographs, particularly in the young, thus a CT scan or MRI may be necessary to visualize the coalition.

Tarsal coalition may be responsive to orthotic support. However, patients with tarsal coalition should be referred for considerations of surgical excision if the athlete sustains recurrent injury or suffers from pain resistant to conservative care.[8]

Köhler's Disease

Köhler's disease is an idiopathic avascular necrosis of the navicular. It is a disease of young children, especially between the ages of 2 and 8 years, and should be considered in any child with foot pain and maximal tenderness over the navicular.[8] Radiographs generally show increased density and narrowing of the bone typical of aseptic necrosis. If early, a bone scan or MRI may be needed to visualize the changes. Six weeks in a short leg walking cast may relieve the symptoms. If the examiner is uncomfortable with managing this condition, it should be referred.

Jones Fracture

As mentioned previously, a fracture through the diaphysis of the fifth metatarsal is prone to slow healing and non-union. Athletes should be considered for immediate intramedullary screw fixation for earlier return to play and improved overall outcome.

Displaced Midfoot Fractures

These fractures are fraught with complications. They also require reduction, and often, surgical fixation by an orthopedic surgeon.[9]

Radiculopathy

As mentioned, initial radicular symptoms may present in the foot. A radiculopathy should be considered whenever the neurologic symptoms are not reproducible on the foot examination. Further investigation of the back is then warranted.

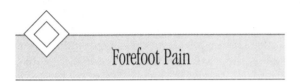

Forefoot Pain

See Table 11-3.

Metatarsal Stress Fracture

Metatarsal stress fractures are a common cause of forefoot pain. These injuries most often

Table 11-3
Forefoot Injuries

MOST COMMON	TO NOT MISS OR TO REFER
Metatarsal fracture, stress and acute	Displaced metatarsal fracture
Morton's neuroma	Multiple metatarsal fractures
Metatarsaligia	
First MTP joint sprain (turf toe)	First metatarsal fracture
Sesamoid dysfunction	First MTP joint fracture/dislocation
Hallux valgus	
Hallux rigidis	Freiberg's osteochondritis
	Radiculopathy

involve the second, third, or fourth distal metatarsal shafts. Particularly prone to stress fracture is the second metatarsal in an athlete with a "Morton's foot," which is an anatomic variant where the second toe extends beyond the first. Less likely are stress fractures of the proximal first and fifth metatarsals (see Chap. 20).

Patients complain of progressive pain with activity. On examination maximal point tenderness exists over the bone at the fracture site, not in the soft tissues. Edema is usually present. Radiographs will not show the fracture for 2 to 3 weeks after injury, and even then may still be negative. If radiographs are negative and/or the fracture is recent, a bone scan, MRI, or CT may be needed to confirm the diagnosis. The bone scan is less expensive and usually reveals the needed information.

Treatment involves 4 to 6 weeks of weight-bearing relative rest based on symptoms. A walker boot or stiff-soled shoe may be needed the first couple of weeks. Walking should be pain free before returning to activity. Return to sport is gradual, beginning 3 to 4 weeks after diagnosis by allowing progressive, protected pain-free activity. The athlete is most often able to return to sport in around 6 weeks.

The usual cause of metatarsal stress fractures is an error in training ("too much, too soon"). This should be addressed before returning to activity. Arch supports, particularly in the cavus foot, or semi-rigid orthotics with support and motion control may be appropriate in some, especially those with pes planus and excessive pronation.

Acute Metatarsal Fracture

Most acute metatarsal shaft fractures are non-displaced, or minimally displaced, and heal well. Usually a falling object is the culprit. The athlete presents in acute pain. On examination, there will be significant swelling and tenderness. Non-displaced fractures are treated symptomatically with a short leg cast or walker boot for the first 3 weeks, with repeat x-rays at that time to ensure that alignment is acceptable. Over the next 3 weeks, a stiff-soled shoe with good arch support can generally be used. Repeat x-rays at 6 weeks are recommended to ensure healing. Gradual return to sport may then ensue.

Multiple fractures, fractures with more than 4-mm displacement or 10° apical angulation, and first metatarsal fractures should be referred to an orthopedic surgeon. Reduction is often required with these fractures because a significantly higher incidence of complications (such as compartment syndromes with multiple fractures and dorsiflexed malunions creating chronic metatarsalgia) exist when compared to simple metatarsal fractures. First metatarsal fractures are high impact fractures and often require surgical management.[10]

Morton's Neuroma

This is a common condition involving irritation of the interdigital nerve between the metatarsal heads and beneath the overlying transverse ligament. Repetitive irritation creates scar tissue that organizes around the nerve and is called a "neu-

roma." This "neuroma," however, is not a true neuroma. Morton's neuromas most commonly occur between the second and third, or third and fourth, metatarsal heads. Shoe wear, particularly shoes with tight toe boxes, is thought to be a major culprit.

Symptoms of a Morton's neuroma may include localized plantar pain, the feeling of "walking on a marble," and numbness, tingling, and burning pain in the web space and/or associated toes. The symptoms are aggravated by shoe wear, particularly those with tighter toe boxes and higher heels. On examination tenderness exists in the web space between the metatarsal heads. A nodule may be palpable if the symptoms have been longstanding. Compression of the forefoot often reproduces the symptoms (a positive "squeeze test").

Treatment initially involves anti-inflammatory measures with ice and NSAIDs and a metatarsal pad placed in the shoe to spread out the metatarsal heads. If this fails, a corticosteroid injection is often helpful. Correction of overpronation, if it exists, should be accomplished with proper shoe wear or an orthotic (see section at end of chapter). If the symptoms are longstanding, a nodule is palpable on examination, and the above measures are unsuccessful, surgical excision should be considered.

Metatarsalgia

This is irritation of the metatarsal-phalangeal (MTP) joint. The second and third MTP joints are the most commonly involved. The etiology is repetitive trauma. Those with claw toes, pes cavus, and over-pronation are most susceptible. Improper shoe wear or worn-out shoes can also contribute.

The athlete complains of pain around the involved MTP joint aggravated by forefoot weight-bearing. On examination, the point of maximal tenderness is over the MTP joint, and pain may be created by passive flexion of the toe.

Treatment includes anti-inflammatory measures, such as ice and NSAIDs, along with appropriate metatarsal head padding to redistribute the load including arch support if inadequate and motion (pronation) control. All this can be included in an orthotic if necessary. In resistant cases, a corticosteroid injection, via a dorsal approach, is often very effective.

First Metatarsal-Phalangeal Joint Sprain (Turf Toe)

This is a common athletic injury, which typically occurs on hard surfaces when the athlete is wearing very flexible shoes. It involves a hyperextension injury to the first MTP joint, and has earned the popular name "turf toe" due to its dramatically increased incidence on "astroturf." As it turns out, the hard surface itself plays some role, but the predominant culprit is the type of shoe that tends to be worn on such surfaces.[11] Shoes with very flexible soles, especially in the forefoot, and which easily allow toe hyperextension, do not protect sufficiently against turf toe.

Turf toe is a forced excessive dorsiflexion event to the first MTP joint that injures the plantar capsuloligamentous complex, and the joint articular cartilage at times. In addition to improper shoes, predisposing factors include pes planus, hallux rigidis, and poor ankle flexibility. Severe joint injury is rare, yet possible. Sesamoid fractures may also be associated with the more severe injuries and should be assessed on examination.

The athlete with turf toe presents with varying degrees of first MTP joint pain and swelling. He or she can usually recall an acute event creating excessive toe dorsiflexion and pain. The severity of turf toe can be graded into three categories based on examination. Grade 1 has localized plantar joint tenderness, no or minimal swelling, and no ecchymosis. It represents a strain of the capsuloligamentous complex. Grade 2 presents with diffuse tenderness, moderate swelling, ecchymosis, and pain and decreased motion with active movement. It represents a partially torn capsuloligamentous complex. Grade 3 involves severe diffuse tenderness to palpation, greatest on the dorsal aspect, excessive swelling, considerable ecchymosis, and markedly restricted range of motion with significant pain. This represents a tear of the capsuloligamentous complex with compression injury to the articular surface. This injury may include a dorsal dislocation of the joint.[12]

Radiographs usually are normal in the patient with turf toe, although a planter avulsion fracture may be noted. With a compression fracture of the metatarsal head intra-articular loose bodies can be observed. A bone scan is helpful in selected severe sprains to detect significant impaction injury with possible articular cartilage damage and bony contusion. A bone scan may also help discern between a bipartite sesamoid and an acute sesamoid fracture that can occur concomitantly with more severe sprains.

Treatment depends on the severity of injury. Grade 1 injuries are treated with compression, frequent icing, NSAIDs, and taping to decrease toe dorsiflexion. The athlete may continue to participate in sports if the pain is minimal. Use of a rigid soled shoe or rigid forefoot insert is also helpful to allow continued participation and decrease the risk for recurrent injury.

Grade 2 injuries are treated as above; however, activity must be restricted until only minimal discomfort exists. This usually takes 1 to 2 weeks.

Grade 3 injuries are much more debilitating and may include a dorsal dislocation. If a dislocation has occurred and not spontaneously reduced, it should be relocated as soon as possible. The technique involves toe hyperextension with longitudinal traction and plantar-directed pressure with the other hand on the base of the proximal phalanx. Radiographs are necessary to rule out a fracture. Compression, ice, and immobilization follow the reduction. Articular cartilage injury probably occurs often with these injuries and may lead to long-term complications. If a dislocation did not occur, crutches are used with weight-bearing limited depending on the extent of pain. Walking may begin when it involves little discomfort. The toe should be taped, and progressive activity should proceed slowly. It is recommended that the shoe be fit with a rigid forefoot insole. Return to sport participation is generally between 4 to 8 weeks. Surgery is rarely indicated in the acute injury unless a significant fracture-dislocation has occurred. Surgery may also be considered in the athlete with chronic pain and decreased toe range of motion if it markedly interferes with his or her ability to perform.[11]

Sesamoid Dysfunction

The sesamoid bones of the first MTP joint play an important role in foot function. They are embedded in the flexor hallucis brevis tendon and articulate with the plantar facets on the first metatarsal head. The facets are concave and separated by an intersesamoidal ridge. Some make the analogy of this articulation with the patellofemoral articulation in the knee. The main function of this complex is to protect the flexor hallucis longus tendon and absorb most of the medial foot weight-bearing force. The sesamoid-first metatarsal complex may be affected by several conditions including an acute sesamoid fracture, sesamoid stress fracture, bipartite sesamoid strain, sesamoiditis, arthritis, and rarely osteonecrosis.[13]

SESAMOID FRACTURE

This may result from acute trauma or repetitive stress creating a stress fracture. The athlete complains of pain at the plantar aspect of the first MTP joint. In an acute fracture, the event can be recalled—usually a significant dorsiflexion event of the great toe (see also "Turf Toe"). Sesamoid stress fractures are most likely to occur in runners or dancers.

On examination, exquisite tenderness and swelling are noted over the involved sesamoid. Dorsiflexion of the great toe is usually painful. When such an injury is suspected, radiographs should be obtained that include AP, lateral, and axial views of the sesamoids. The medial sesamoid is the most often injured.

Fractures can be distinguished from bipartite sesamoid by their radiographic bone edges. Fractures have rough edges whereas the bipartite sesamoids have smooth, round edges. A bone scan will help to differentiate the two if unclear.

Sesamoid fractures have a fairly high incidence of non-union. Thus, most experts recommend these fractures be treated with nonweight bearing for 4 to 6 weeks followed by a stiff-soled shoe with sesamoid unloading padding. Gradual increase in activity and use of regular shoe wear may proceed if pain is minimal.

BIPARTITE SESAMOID STRAIN

Bipartite sesamoids exist in 25 to 30 percent of the population. On radiographs their edges are smooth and rounded. With repetitive trauma or an acute traumatic event, however, the joining ligament may be strained creating an intersesamoid strain. On examination tenderness exists over the involved sesamoid. Pain may occur at the sesamoid with forced great-toe dorsiflexion. Treatment is similar to that involved with sesamoiditis.

SESAMOIDITIS

This injury results from either repetitive trauma or an acute event that creates inflammation in the sesamoid-metatarsal articulation. It is a diagnosis of exclusion made after considering the possibility of sesamoid fractures and strain in a bipartite sesamoid, or osteonecrosis. The athlete complains of sesamoid area pain as described previously, and the examination is similar.

Treatment involves reducing the inflammation with ice and NSAIDs, relative rest, and a stiff-soled shoe. Taping the great toe to minimize dorsiflexion, along with use of a plantar footpad to unload the sesamoids, should also be considered. For resistant cases, a steroid injection into the sesamoidal-metatarsal joint may be helpful. Orthotics for motion control in those with over-pronation is also indicated.

SESAMOID OSTEONECROSIS

This presents as sesamoid pain, generally of long standing. The diagnosis is made by radiography showing fragmentation and mottling of the involved sesamoid. Conservative care as described above is indicated for early osteonecrosis. Extensive osteonecrosis usually requires surgical removal of the sesamoid.

Hallux Valgus

This is a common condition created by lateral (valgus) deviation of the great toe and medial (varus) deviation of the first metatarsal. This may lead to the development of a painful bony prominence on the medial head of the first metatarsal (a "bunion"). Genetics, shoe wear, and/or over-pronation seem to be involved in its development.[14] Most often, hallux valgus is asymptomatic; however, when painful, it can be very problematic.

The patient with symptomatic hallux valgus complains of pain and swelling in the area, usually aggravated by the shoe. The medial plantar sensory nerve may be irritated creating neurologic symptoms over the medial aspect of the great toe. On examination the alignment abnormality will be obvious along with a painful bony prominence of the medial first metatarsal head, sometimes with a hypertrophic bursa. Possible pes planus along with pronation during gait should be sought, and if found, these abnormalities should be corrected with an orthotic. Standing AP radiographs of the foot will show a hallux valgus angle of more than 15° and a first versus second intermetatarsal angle of greater than 9°. These radiographs can also assess for first MTP degenerative changes, lateral subluxation of the sesamoids, and the shape of the metatarsal head.

The treatment of symptomatic hallux valgus in an athlete is conservative. Surgery is only considered if the athlete's performance is significantly affected. Surgery usually results in stiffening of the joint and decreased functional ability, so it should be undertaken only with caution and with realistic expectations.[14] Conservative treatment involves proper shoe wear/modification, anti-inflammatories, and, possibly, orthotics. Shoes with a wide toe box should be selected. Stretching the shoe over the bunion may be all that is necessary to resolve the syndrome and should be considered early. Arch supports or orthotics to address over-pronation may be helpful in the selected athlete. If these measures fail and the athlete's resulting disability is unacceptable, surgery may be cautiously considered.

Hallux Rigidis

This condition is a degenerative arthritis of the first MTP joint, creating pain and stiffness, particularly on dorsiflexion. Similar to hallux valgus, it is a relatively common condition and tends to affect those greater than 30 years old. Not uncommonly, excessive pronation is involved placing greater stress on the first MTP joint.

The patient presents complaining of pain and stiffness of the joint. On examination, the joint may be tender and swollen. Toe alignment is proper; however, range of motion is limited and usually causes pain at the extremes, especially dorsiflexion. A dorsal exostosis may be visible as a dorsal nodule off the joint. Radiographs will show narrowing of the joint, often with spurs on the dorsal or lateral aspect.[15]

Treatment initially is conservative with anti-inflammatory measures including ice and NSAIDs, use of a stiffer soled shoe or stiff forefoot insert, and correction of excessive pronation, if it exists, with orthotics. If conservative measures fail, surgical spur excision and/or joint fusion may be needed to relieve the patient of painful symptoms.

Forefoot Injuries to Not Miss or to Refer

Displaced Metatarsal Fracture

As mentioned, significantly displaced metatarsal fractures may need reduction (those with more than 4-mm displacement or 10° of apical angulation) and are prone to developing complications. They are best referred.

Multiple Metatarsal Fractures

These also are prone to developing complications, as discussed, and are best referred if the examiner is not experienced in their care.

First Metatarsal Fracture

This generally results from a high-impact injury that may also have caused injury elsewhere. Fractures of the first metatarsal are prone to complications. Because the first ray is such an important weight-bearing structure, surgery is often considered for these fractures. If the clinician is not experienced with these fractures, they are best handled by an orthopedic surgeon.

First MTP Joint Fracture/Dislocation

A severe sprain of the first MTP joint (turf toe injury) may result in an articular fracture-dislocation. If noted on x-ray, fracture dislocations should be referred for surgical considerations and care.

Freiberg's Osteochondritis

Freiberg's disease is avascular necrosis of the metatarsal head, usually the second metatarsal. It occurs most often in adolescents. The patient complains of forefoot pain, especially on toe raising. Examination reveals maximal tenderness over the involved metatarsal head. Some swelling may also be noted. Radiographs may show flattening of the metatarsal head and growth plate fragmentation; however, these changes often lag behind the disease. Bone scan or MRI is the most sensitive. If diagnosed early, conservative measures will often be successful. These involve activity modification, padding to reduce pressure on the metatarsal head, and, perhaps, orthotics. Well-established cases, or resistant cases, may require surgical intervention.[16]

Radiculopathy

Again, neurologic symptoms in the foot are not uncommon. If not explained locally, the back should be investigated for evidence of a radiculopathy.

Recommending Shoes and the Orthotic Prescription

In general, there are three basic shoe types: (1) the cushioning shoe, (2) the stability shoe, and (3) the motion-control shoe. In general, there are also three basic foot types: (1) the rigid foot (the cavus foot), (2) the "normal" foot, and (3) the foot spending excessive time in pronation (often the flexible flat foot). The most accurate recommendations that can be made, with our knowledge thus far, are limited. The best a clinician can do is recommend: a cushioning shoe, which tends to have a more curved sole and be more flexible, for the rigid cavus foot; a stability shoe for the "normal" foot; and a motion-control shoe, which tends to have a straighter sole and be more stiff, thus providing better medial support, for the flat flexible foot or the foot with excessive time in pronation. Beyond this, further specifics are difficult to give. The remainder is usually trial and error.

The orthotic prescription is more complicated. The two main concepts to remember when considering orthotics are first, that a softer, "shock-absorbing" arch support is used for the rigid cavus foot, and second, that a heel counter for motion control with a semirigid arch support is used for the excessively pronating foot. The remaining specifics can be left to the orthotist. (As an aside, the softer arch support for cushioning the cavus foot may wear out too quickly for some, thus a semirigid cushioning design is better for certain athletes pending their weight and use).

References

1. Pfeffer GB, Clain MR, Frey C, et al: Foot and ankle. In: Snider RK (ed): *Essentials of Musculoskeletal Care*, 1st ed. Rosemont, IL: American Academy of Orthopedic Surgeons; 1997;427.
2. McBryde A: Stress fractures of the foot and ankle. In: DeLee JC, Drez D (eds): *Orthopedic Sports Medicine: Principles and Practice*, 1st ed. Philadelphia: WB Saunders; 1994;1975.
3. Brukner P, Khan K: *Clinical Sports Medicine*. Sydney: McGraw-Hill; 1993;468.
4. Renstrom PA, Kannus P: Injuries of the foot and ankle. In: DeLee JC, Drez D (eds): *Orthopedic Sports Medicine: Principles and Practice*, 1st ed. Philadelphia: WB Saunders; 1994;1753.
5. Brucker P, Khan K: *Clinical Sports Medicine*. Sydney: McGraw-Hill; 1993;470.
6. Connolly JF: *Fractures and Dislocations, Closed Management*, 1st ed. Philadelphia: WB Saunders; 1995;1029.
7. Pfeffer GB, Clain MR, Frey C, et al: Foot and ankle. In: Snider RK (ed): *Essentials of Musculoskeletal Care*, 1st ed. Rosemont, IL: American Academy of Orthopedic Surgeons; 1997;442.
8. Brucker P, Khan K: *Clinical Sports Medicine*. Sydney: McGraw-Hill; 1993;531.
9. Connolly JF: *Fractures and Dislocations, Closed Management*, 1st ed. Philadelphia: WB Saunders; 1995;1010.
10. Pfeffer GB, Clain MR, Frey C, et al: Foot and ankle. In: Snider RK (ed): *Essentials of Musculoskeletal Care*, 1st ed. Rosemont, IL: American Academy of Orthopedic Surgeons; 1997;429.
11. Michael JC: Conditions of the forefoot. In: DeLee JC, Drez D (eds): *Orthopedic Sports Medicine: Principles and Practice*, 1st ed. Philadelphia: WB Saunders; 1994;1859.
12. Clanton TO, Butler JE, Eggert A: Injuries to the metatarsophalangeal joints in athletes. *Foot and Ankle Manual* 7:162, 1986.
13. Michael JC: Conditions of the forefoot. In: DeLee JC, Drez D (eds): *Orthopedic Sports Medicine: Principles and Practice*, 1st ed. Philadelphia: WB Saunders; 1994;1866.
14. Michael JC: Conditions of the forefoot. In: DeLee JC, Drez D (eds): *Orthopedic Sports Medicine: Principles and Practice*, 1st ed. Philadelphia: WB Saunders; 1994;1842.
15. Pfeffer GB, Clain MR, Frey C, et al: Foot and ankle. In: Snider RK (ed): *Essentials of Musculoskeletal Care*, 1st ed. Rosemont, IL: American Academy of Orthopedic Surgeons; 1997;444.
16. Brucker P, Khan K: *Clinical Sports Medicine*. Sydney: McGraw-Hill; 1993;532.

Medical Problems

Kimberly A. Fulton
Aurelia Nattiv

Menstrual Dysfunction

Introduction

Menstrual cycle dysfunction manifests itself in a variety of ways and affects exercisers and nonexercisers alike. Although menstrual cycle irregularities can develop in any woman regardless of her activity level, the prevalence of menstrual dysfunction is greater among athletes than among the general population.[1,2] Retrospective survey data estimate the frequency of menstrual abnormalities, including luteal phase defects, anovulation, and delayed menarche, to be 2 to 51 percent in athletes compared with 2 to 5 percent in the general population.[2–4] The prevalence of amenorrhea, the most extreme form of menstrual dysfunction, is estimated to occur in as many as 10 to 20 percent of vigorously exercising women and as many as 40 to 50 percent of elite runners and professional ballet dancers.[1,2]

As the numbers of physically active women increase, it has become important to better understand the impact of exercise on the reproductive system. This chapter is intended to guide the clinician in the management and treatment of menstrual dysfunction and associated problems in the female athlete.

The Menstrual Cycle

Before discussing menstrual dysfunction, it is beneficial to briefly review the physiology of the menstrual cycle. The menstrual cycle is variable in length and is regulated by the hypothalamic-pituitary axis. The hypothalamus secretes gonadotropin-releasing hormone (GnRH) in a pulsatile fashion to stimulate pituitary production of follicle-stimulating hormone (FSH) and luteinizing hormone (LH). These gonadotropins are in turn responsible for the ovarian synthesis of both estrogen and progesterone. Each of these steroid hormones exerts different effects on the female reproductive system. Estrogen promotes the development of secondary sexual characteristics and can cause uterine growth, thickening of the vaginal mucosa, thinning of the cervical mucus, and development of the ductular system of the breasts. Progesterone is responsible for the secretory activity of the endometrial lining, decreased viscosity of the cervical mucus, and an increase in a woman's basal body temperature.

The menstrual cycle is divided into the follicular phase and the luteal phase (Fig. 12-1). The follicular phase begins with the onset of menses and culminates with the preovulatory surge of LH. The luteal phase begins with the LH surge and ends with the onset of menstruation. During the first several days of the follicular phase, FSH stimulates a cohort of ovarian follicles to mature and produce estrogen. Although many follicles are stimulated, only one becomes dominant. The rising levels of estrogen exert a positive feedback on the pituitary gland near the end of the follicular phase resulting in a relative increase in the production of LH compared to FSH. This LH surge triggers the mature follicle to rupture and release an egg, resulting in ovulation. The follicle involutes forming the corpus luteum, which secretes progesterone for the development and maintenance of the uterine lining.

The functional life of the corpus luteum is 14 ±2 days. If fertilization does not occur, the corpus luteum will degenerate and progesterone levels will decline. Without the presence of progesterone, the uterine lining sloughs and menstruation occurs. Low circulating steroid levels stimulate the hypothalamus and pituitary to produce GnRH, FSH, and LH. Higher levels of gonadotropins induce the next round of follicles to develop, and the ovarian cycle begins again. A normal menstrual cycle lasts 23 to 35 days. Because the functional life of the corpus luteum is relatively constant, variability in menstrual

Figure 12-1

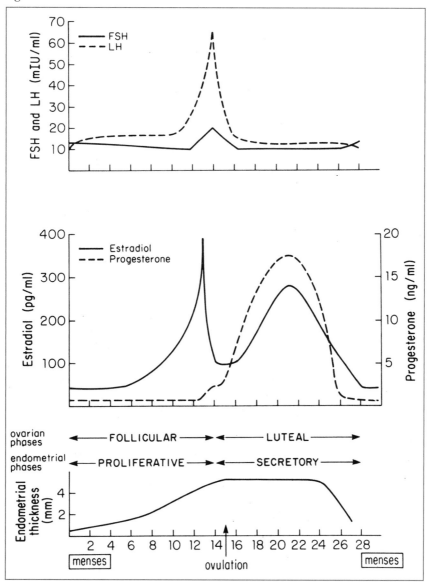

Hormonal events and phases of the normal menstrual cycle. *(Modified with permission from Shangold M: Menstruation and menstrual disorders. In: Shangold M, Mirkin G (eds): Women and Exercise: Physiology and Sports Medicine, 2nd ed. Philadelphia: F. A. Davis, 1994;155.)*

cycle length can be attributed to fluctuations in the follicular phase of the cycle.

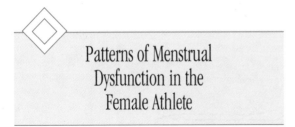

Patterns of Menstrual Dysfunction in the Female Athlete

The menstrual cycle involves a complex interaction between the reproductive and the neuroendocrine systems. Although menstrual dysfunction may have many etiologies, common patterns of menstrual irregularity in the female athlete include delayed menarche, luteal phase deficiency, oligomenorrhea, and amenorrhea.

Delayed Menarche

Delayed menarche, or primary amenorrhea, refers to the absence of menses by age 16 years. Numerous studies have demonstrated that menarche occurs later in athletes than in nonathletes,[5–8] although the actual prevalence in athletes is not known. Many have concluded that training for sport is the factor responsible for the delay in menarche. Allowing for the many factors that are known to have an influence on menarche, it is difficult to implicate training per se as the causative factor. The general consensus is that there is no conclusive evidence that participation in sports in and of itself delays sexual maturation.[9]

Luteal Phase Deficiency

Luteal phase deficiency is a shortened luteal phase length secondary to insufficient progesterone production. Some investigators hypothesize that this type of ovulatory disturbance may be an intermediate point in a progression toward amenorrhea.[10] Alternatively, other researchers postulate that it may be the end of successful acclimation to athletic training.[2,6,11] This disorder may be difficult to identify because the female athlete may often have a normal total cycle length despite the luteal phase dysfunction.

The first step in testing for luteal phase deficiency is to determine when ovulation occurs. A woman can monitor her basal body temperature or measure urinary LH mid cycle with an ovulation kit. A biphasic body temperature curve or a surge in urinary LH detected by the kit suggest ovulation has occurred. If the woman's next menses begins less than 10 days after the presumed ovulation, luteal phase inadequacy is probable. Assessment of serum progesterone levels during the mid-luteal phase can also be helpful, with a low progesterone level suggestive of luteal phase dysfunction. The gold standard for diagnosis of luteal phase deficiency is an endometrial biopsy, but most clinicians prefer to use less invasive techniques. Women with this menstrual pattern may suffer from infertility or recurrent spontaneous abortion, and require treatment when pregnancy is desired. The effect of luteal phase dysfunction on bone health is still controversial. The possibility of bone loss exists and should, therefore, be discussed with patients and appropriate preventive measures implemented.

Oligomenorrhea

Oligomenorrhea is characterized by cycles that are greater than 36 days in length and less than 90 days. These cycles may be associated with anovulation. Women with anovulation produce estrogen but lack a biphasic basal body temperature curve and have low levels of progesterone. These women often have menstrual bleeding that occurs at unpredictable intervals and it may be very heavy. Because these women have unopposed estrogen, there is a theoretical risk of endometrial hyperplasia and adenocarcinoma, although an increased risk in female athletes has not been identified.[4] Athletes with oligomenorrhea may also have periods of low estrogen and may experience significant bone loss and resultant osteoporosis if unidentified or untreated,[12] predisposing them to an increased risk for future fracture. A medical evaluation for athletes with oligomenorrhea is necessary and appropriate prevention and treatment are often indicated.

Amenorrhea

Secondary amenorrhea refers to the cessation of menses after menarche has occurred. There are no universally accepted definitions for secondary amenorrhea. Defining criteria have included the absence of menstruation for 3, 4, 6, or 12 months or less than three menstrual cycles per year.[2] In this chapter, secondary amenorrhea is defined as missing three or more consecutive periods in a year in women who have established menstrual cycles.

Hypothalamic amenorrhea is the most common cause of secondary amenorrhea in the female athlete (with the exception of pregnancy). There is evidence that secondary amenorrhea can have a significant negative impact on bone health, which is discussed in more detail later in this chapter.

Etiology of Amenorrhea

Cyclic menstrual bleeding requires the presence of an intact reproductive tract and a functioning neuroendocrine system. Abnormalities of the reproductive tract can be acquired or congenital. As outlined in Table 12-1, abnormalities in the reproductive anatomy or along the hypothalamic-pituitary-ovarian axis can result in menstrual dysfunction. Each of these etiologies must be considered in the female athlete with amenorrhea because the diagnosis of athletic amenor-

Table 12-1
Differential Diagnosis of Amenorrhea

Anatomic defects
  Labial agglutination
  Congenital defects of the vagina
    Imperforate hymen
    Transverse vaginal septae
  Müllerian defects
    Mayer–Rokitansky–Kuster–Hauser
      Syndrome
    Gonadal dysgenesis
    Testicular feminization syndrome
  Ashermann's syndrome
Ovarian failure
  Gonadal dysgenesis
    Turner phenotype 45,X
    Mosaicism 46,XX
    17- hydoxylase deficiency
    17,20 lyase deficiency
    Premature ovarian failure
Chronic anovulation with estrogen
  Polycystic ovarian disease (PCOD)
  Tumors
    Granulosa theca cell
    Brenner
    Cystic teratoma
    Mucus cystadenoma
    Krukenberg
Chronic anovulation in absence of estrogen
  and/or hypogonadotropic hypogonadism
  Athletic amenorrhea
  Kallmann's syndrome
  Stress
  Anorexia nervosa
  Pituitary tumors
    Prolactinoma
    Craniopharyngioma

rhea is made only after excluding more serious disease.

Amenorrhea may result from congenital defects of the vagina including imperforate hymen or transverse vaginal septae. These women will experience cyclic abdominal pain because menstrual bleeding occurs in the peritoneal cavity and accumulates behind the obstruction. These defects can be identified by examination of the external genitalia. Disorders of müllerian-derived structures involve the distal two-thirds of the vagina and the uterus. In müllerian agenesis, a woman will have only a short vaginal pouch and no cervix or uterus. A less severe müllerian defect is gonadal dysgenesis. Women with this syndrome have female secondary sexual characteristics, normal ovarian function, including cyclic ovulation, but have absence or severe hypoplasia of the vagina. A major diagnostic dilemma is distinguishing müllerian agenesis from complete testicular feminization. Although these persons have testes, they develop into phenotypic women with a blind vaginal pouch and an absent uterus. This condition is caused by a defect in the androgen receptor protein that causes profound resistance to the action of testosterone. A karyotype is the primary method for distinguishing between these two disorders: 46,XX for gonadal dysgenesis and 46,XY for testicular feminization.

Scarring of the cervix can occur from surgery or laser therapy and can create outflow obstruction similar to the vaginal disorders just described. In Asherman's syndrome, amenorrhea results from the development of intrauterine synechiae after destruction of the endometrium from postpartum hemorrhage, therapeutic abortion, or myomectomy.

Ovarian failure can be caused by gonadal dysgenesis. The germ cells or eggs are actually missing and the ovary appears like a fibrous streak under direct visualization. There are two karyotypes: 45,X Turner phenotype and the mosaic form 45,X/46,XX. Chronic anovulation can occur secondary to excess estrogen production or from the peripheral conversion of androgens to estrogen. Polycystic ovarian disease represents the latter type, and is characterized by infertility, hirsutism, obesity, and amenorrhea. Several tumors must be thought of when considering the differential diagnosis: granulosa-theca cell, Brenner, cystic teratoma, mucus cystadenoma, and Krukenberg.

Hypogonadotropic hypogonadism is chronic anovulation that occurs in the absence of estrogen. In Kallmann's syndrome, the affected women appear sexually infantile and eunochoid. They have a defect in the synthesis and release of LHRH. There are a variety of other etiologies including craniopharyngiomas and other hypothalamic tumors. Stress can cause hypogonadotropic hypogonadism as can anorexia and pituitary tumors like prolactinomas.

The ovaries must produce estrogen and progesterone in a sequential fashion. The production of these steroids requires oocytes. Cells in the pituitary need to be intact to produce FSH and LH. GnRH-producing cells may be absent or the pulse frequency deficient. Catecholamines and cortisol modulate GnRH-producing centers.[13] Problems in any of these areas may result in menstrual dysfunction.

Athletic Amenorrhea

Definition

Athletic amenorrhea (AA) is a subset of hypothalamic amenorrhea, and is the most common type of menstrual dysfunction in athletes. Pulsatile GnRH produced by the hypothalamus is deficient, absent, or inappropriately secreted. The resultant decline in the frequency of LH pulses from the pituitary gland causes ovarian suppression and resultant amenorrhea.[6] Without the monthly phasic elevations in gonadotropin and steroid hormone patterns in amenorrheic athletes, anovulation and no follicular or luteal phase development occurs.

Associated Factors and the Triad

When beginning an exercise training regimen, the body goes through changes in weight, body composition, hormone concentrations and secretion patterns, nutrient balance, as well as physical and psychological stress. Any or all of these factors may interact and be associated with the development of athletic amenorrhea. An increase in training intensity and high running mileage have also been found to contribute to AA. Additional risk factors include younger age, previous history of menstrual irregularity, low body weight, nulliparity, genetic factors, and disordered eating.

The drive to be thin and achieve a certain preconceived percent body fat or weight for appearance and performance is believed to underlie the development of the female athlete triad. The female athlete triad refers to the interrelationship and often coexistence of disordered eating, amenorrhea, and osteoporosis.[14,15] The true prevalence of the triad in the female athlete is unknown. Although all athletes are at risk, those at the highest risk appear to be those who compete in appearance or endurance sports, including gymnasts, figure skaters, ballet dancers, and distance runners.

It is important to recognize the association of disordered eating with the possible development of amenorrhea and resultant bone loss. Disordered eating refers to a spectrum of eating behaviors ranging from the restriction of certain food groups to frank anorexia and bulimia nervosa. These disordered eating patterns include: occasional fasting, restricting food intake, self-induced vomiting, using laxatives, diet pills and/or diuretics, and over-exercising to lose weight. The majority of female athletes with disordered eating fail to meet the criteria for anorexia or bulimia nervosa as defined by the *American Psychiatric Diagnostic and Statistical Manual* (DSM) IV. The diagnostic category of Eating Disorder Not Otherwise Specified acknowledges the existence of a variety of eating disturbances including individuals who binge-eat infrequently. More research is needed in methods of early recognition, prevalence, comorbidity, and recommended treatment for individuals along the disordered eating continuum. Because these disorders often involve denial, guilt, and secrecy, it is important for the health care professional to screen all athletes with menstrual dysfunction for disordered eating, as well as those with a history of stress fractures.

Pathophysiology

The energy availability hypothesis provides the most widely accepted mechanism to date that explains the suppression of reproductive function in amenorrheic athletes.[16] Energy availability is defined as the difference between dietary intake and exercise energy expenditure. Loucks demonstrated that strenuous training in and of itself may not be a sufficient stimulus to disrupt the reproductive hormone secretion unless accompanied by dietary restriction.[16] Rather, insufficient availability of energy is the critical factor. There may exist a specific threshold whereby further negative energy balance signals the inhibition of hypothalamic GnRH neuronal activity.[17] Loucks and colleagues demonstrated that LH pulsatility depends on carbohydrate availability and that the supply of glucose may be less compromised by exercise than by dietary restriction or by a combination of dietary restriction and exercise.[16] Exercise, therefore, appears to contribute to menstrual dysfunction only when the energy expended is not adequately replenished. Tomten also suggests a combination of high mileage and increased level of nutritional conflict gives reason to suggest that menstrual dysfunction is associated with a negative energy balance, and that the cessation of menses is part of a metabolic adjustment to prevent loss of body weight.[8]

Laughlin and Yen have shown that the hormone product leptin may play a role in the reproductive status of female athletes.[18] A diurnal pattern of 24-h leptin levels was present in normal cycling athletes and controls but was absent in amenorrheic athletes. This finding provides additional evidence supporting the interrelationship between energy and diet in the reproductive system.

Although no causal link between exercise per se and menstrual disorders has been established, a prospective study by Bullen presents the strongest evidence to indicate that amenorrhea in athletes may be related to exercise itself.[19] The investigators imposed a strenuous training program on a group of conditioned women with regular menstrual function. Within the first month, the LH surge, follicular and luteal development, and ovulation were suppressed in a large proportion of subjects. During a second month of training, the proportion of women displaying these reproductive abnormalities increased. Although exercise did induce menstrual irregularities, it is unclear whether this was from the stress of training or reduction in energy availability caused by the profound increase in energy expenditure.

Body composition was previously thought to impact menstrual cycle function. The notion is derived from clinical observation that severe weight loss through anorexia nervosa or other forms of starvation is inevitably associated with secondary amenorrhea. Sanborn et al[20] analyzed long-distance runners and found that body fat percentages were equal between amenorrheic and regularly cycling athletes who were matched by weight, height, age, menarcheal age, weekly training mileage, and maximum oxygen uptake. Tomten showed that the most important indicator of menstrual dysfunction was a reported feeling of conflict in association with food.[8] Not all competitive runners became amenorrheic, suggesting that there are individual variations in the resiliency of the reproductive system.

Loucks and Heath demonstrated that there is

an induction of a low-T3 syndrome in exercising women that occurs at a threshold of low energy availability and that was independent of the level of exercise.[21] She demonstrated altered LH pulse frequencies during both the day and night in athletes given a restricted diet. The LH pattern resembled that shown in amenorrheic athletes: LH pulse frequency was reduced during the day and the amplitude was increased during sleep. Williams and colleagues have demonstrated similar findings.[17]

Consequences of Athletic Amenorrhea

Until the early 1980s, it was felt that exercise-associated amenorrhea was temporary and reversible and posed no risk to the affected female athlete. Historic studies demonstrated that when women stopped training, their menses resumed and they had normal fertility.[11] However, with more research, the scientific community now understands that the hypoestrogenic state does have long-term consequences. Women with hypoestrogenic amenorrhea lack the beneficial effects of estrogen on calcium metabolism and bone, urogenital epithelial maturation, and lipid metabolism.

Effects on Bone

The majority of bone mineral density (bmd) is genetically determined but environmental variables including hormone status, nutrition, and mechanical factors can play a significant role. Bone resorption begins after the attainment of peak bone mass at approximately age 25 to 30 years at a rate of 0.3 to 0.5 percent per year. Bone loss in women is accelerated after menopause at a rate of 1 to 2 percent per year, and can be as high as 3 to 5 percent per year after menopause in the presence of hypoestrogenemia. Similar losses of bmd can occur in premenopausal hypoestrogenic women[23,24] and weight-bearing exercise alone will usually not prevent this loss.[4,25,26]

Although weight-bearing exercise is beneficial in promoting bmd when dietary calcium and estrogen are adequate, it may not be a sufficient stimulus in the presence of hypoestrogenic amenorrhea. In addition, many hypoestrogenic athletes consume inadequate dietary calcium. The combination of poor nutrition during adolescence and low estrogen may result in lack of bone accretion during critical years of skeletal consolidation.[14,22] Of additional concern is evidence that bone loss in the amenorrheic athlete may be irreversible, even with return of menses or use of oral contraceptive pills (OCP).[14,24]

The concern for athletes with low bmd secondary to hypoestrogenemia revolves around the risk for fractures during their competitive years and the risk for osteoporotic fractures later in life. Studies report a higher incidence of injuries and stress fractures among athletes with menstrual dysfunction as compared to eumenorrheic athletes.[8,26–29] There is evidence that delayed menarche may be associated with scoliosis and stress fractures in dancers[29] as well as stress fractures in female runners.[27]

It is important to recognize that it appears to be the sum total of estrogen exposure over a women's lifetime that in part determines her risk for bone loss and the development of osteoporosis. The decrease in bmd noted in the amenorrheic athlete is often generalized bone loss, demonstrated in the lumbar spine as well as at multiple skeletal sites.[26] However, not all athletes with amenorrhea have low bmd. Although prior menstrual history has been demonstrated to be the best predictor of current bone mineral density,[12,26] skeletal status depends on a number of other factors as well, including nutritional status, genetic factors, and mechanical loading factors.[14,30] For example, there are some sports

where the high mechanical loads involved at certain skeletal sites may outweigh the negative effects of estrogen on bone, such as has been noted in the female gymnast.[30]

The skeletal effects of amenorrhea depend on the length and severity of the irregularity and nutrition, skeletal loading, and genetics.[14] Body weight and months of amenorrhea have been predictive of bone mineral density of amenorrheic and eumenorrheic athletes, suggesting that the treatment for athletic amenorrhea involves changes, which should include proper nutrition and weight gain, resulting in resumption of normal menses.[26]

Effects on Urogenital Epithelium

Estrogen promotes maturation of the urogenital epithelium and maintains a thick vaginal epithelium that is resistant to many disorders. Estrogen deficiency leads to thinning of the vaginal epithelium and increased susceptibility to atrophic urethritis and vaginitis. These may be reversible with estrogen treatment. Development of urogenital atrophy can take years to develop and is not commonly reported in the athletic woman.

However, urinary stress incontinence has been reported in the female athlete. The role of estrogen deficiency in this disorder is not entirely certain. A review of this problem can be found elsewhere and is not covered in this chapter.[31]

Effects on Lipid Metabolism

Increased risk of cardiovascular disease occurs in the postmenopausal hypoestrogenic woman. The benefits of strenuous exercise on apolipoprotein levels can be reversed by exercise-induced amenorrhea and decreased estradiol levels.[4] The adverse effects of estrogen deficiency on low-density lipoprotein cholesterol levels, however, may be offset by aerobic training. High density lipoproteins (HDL) are increased with exercise and may be cardioprotective. It is unlikely that the younger hypoestrogenic amenorrheic athlete is at increased risk for cardiac disease, but more research is needed in this area.

Clinical Evaluation

Athletic amenorrhea is a diagnosis of exclusion. All female athletes with menstrual dysfunction should be thoroughly evaluated for other causes of amenorrhea, including pregnancy. If the athlete is age 14 and prepubertal, or 16 and premenarchal, she should be further evaluated for primary amenorrhea. If the athlete is post-menarchal, but has had cessation of menses for 3 months or more, she should undergo further evaluation for secondary amenorrhea. Those athletes with oligomenorrhea and other types of menstrual irregularities should also be evaluated. The preparticipation physical examination presents an excellent opportunity to screen and prevent potential problems associated with menstrual dysfunction in the athlete. An approach to the evaluation of secondary amenorrhea in the athlete is illustrated in Table 12-2.

A review of pubertal milestones is important, particularly for the athlete with primary amenorrhea. Congenital defects and chromosomal abnormalities need to be considered in the athlete with primary amenorrhea. Lack of pubertal development may occur with hypothalamic dysfunction, pituitary abnormalities, and gonadal failure/dysgenesis. If secondary sexual characteristics are present but menstrual bleeding has not occurred, the absence of the reproductive organs needs to be considered. Foremost in the differential diagnosis is androgen-insensitivity syndrome and congenital absence of the uterus. Other anatomic defects should be considered such as labial fusion, congenital defects of the

Table 12-2

Suggested Evaluation of Secondary Amenorrhea

History
   Athletic training
   Nutrition
   Menstrual
   Injury
Complete physical examination
   Pelvic examination if indicated (over age
      18 years and/or sexually active)
Laboratory tests*
   Urine pregnancy test
   TSH
   FSH
   Prolactin
   Consider estradiol (E_2) and/or provera
      challenge
   LH, DHEA-S, and testosterone if the physical
      findings are consistent with androgen
      excess
   E_2 and LH if the patient has disordered
      eating or anorexia nervosa
Bone density assessment
   Consider obtaining a DEXA in women with
    a prolonged history of oligomenorrhea
    and/or greater than 6–12 months of
    amenorrhea, especially in women with
    low weight, disordered eating, or other
    risk factors

*If the patient has athletic amenorrhea, expect low levels of FSH, LH, E_2 and the absence of withdrawal bleeding with the provera challenge.

vagina (imperforate hymen, transverse vaginal septae), and müllerian defects (müllerian agenesis/Mayer-Rokitansky-Kuster-Hauser syndrome, gonadal dysgenesis, testicular feminization syndrome).

History

When taking a history, the clinician should obtain a detailed menstrual history, including age of menarche and the frequency of cycles. An emphasis on the overall cycle pattern since menarche is important because menstrual history has been found to be a significant predictor for current bone mineral density in the lumbar spine, hip, femoral mid-shaft, and whole body.[12,16]

A family history should include a history of delayed puberty, age of menarche, menstrual irregularities, congenital anomalies, as well as endocrinopathies, including thyroid disease, and osteoporosis. A sexual history including contraception methods and previous pregnancies should also be obtained, as well as a history of uterine curettage for pregnancy loss/termination as this can increase the risk of scarring resulting in Ashermann's syndrome.

It is important to obtain a dietary history because poor nutritional habits and low energy balance can be predisposing factors to the development of menstrual dysfunction. Explore whether the athlete has restrictive eating habits or avoids certain food groups. Inquire about bingeing or purging behaviors including laxative use. Assess for weight fluctuations over the past year. Abrupt changes in body composition or weight may contribute to menstrual dysfunction. Exercise training history should be obtained, including the type, frequency, and duration of exercise as well as the number of years of training and intensity level. Obtaining a history of stress fractures is important. A history of femoral neck or sacral fractures are especially concerning and suggest low bone mineral density.

Assessing for symptoms of ovulation is also important. Ovulation is suggested by changes in cervical mucus at mid cycle and common premenstrual symptoms like mittleschmertz, cramps, and breast tenderness. A history of hirsutism, acne, striae, or other signs of androgen excess would suggest polycystic ovarian syndrome. Vasomotor symptoms and hot flashes suggest ovarian failure. Inquire about visual changes and headaches, which may be a sign of a pituitary or hypothalamic mass. A history of galactorrhea is suggestive of a pituitary adenoma.

An important part of the history involves taking note of medications such as OCPs or other methods of contraception. Of note is that use of Depo-Provera has been recently shown to have a negative effect on bone, primarily due to low estrogen levels. Additional medications to inquire about include anabolic steroids and thyroid supplements, among others. Use of radiation or chemotherapy may also be associated with amenorrhea.

Physical Examination

It is important to perform a complete physical examination to assess for underlying problems that may contribute to menstrual dysfunction. Obtain the patient's height, weight, blood pressure, and pulse. Assess the athlete's general appearance and keep in mind the stigmata of chromosomal disorders such as Turner's syndrome and androgen-insensitivity syndrome. Evaluate the skin for acne and male-pattern hair development, which would signify androgen excess from polycystic ovarian syndrome or exogenous steroid use. Abnormal pigmentation or striae would suggest Cushing's disease. Palpate the thyroid for enlargement or nodularity. Evaluate breast and pubic hair development by Tanner staging. Assess for galactorrhea in the breast examination, which would suggest excess prolactin.

The American College of Obstetrics and Gynecology and the American Academy of Pediatrics recommend screening all sexually active women and all women over 18 years with annual Pap smears and pelvic examinations.[32–34] Some investigators have questioned the rationale for this strategy and purport screening is necessary only in women over the age of 20 years.[35] If a pelvic examination is not performed, an examination of the external genitalia will help exclude some anatomic abnormalities. For example, the presence of a vaginal septum or imperforate hymen may help elucidate the cause of primary amenorrhea. For those obtaining a pelvic examination, the vaginal mucosa should be assessed. The presence of moderate to abundant cervical mucus suggests that estrogen is produced. Alternatively, if it is dry and thin, it suggests either estrogen deficits or atrophic vaginitis. Check the size and presence of the uterus and ovaries and intact vagina to assure normal anatomy.

Laboratory Studies

The symptoms and laboratory profile of AA resemble other types of hypothalamic amenorrhea. LH and FSH are normal or low. Estradiol is low and there is often an absence of withdrawal bleeding after a progestin challenge. Prolactin and androgen (testosterone, DHEA-S) levels are normal, as is thyroid-stimulating hormone. Both daytime and nocturnal cortisol may be slightly elevated in both amenorrheic and eumenorrheic runners.[36]

Initial laboratory analysis of the athlete with menstrual dysfunction should include a pregnancy test, TSH, FSH, prolactin, and consideration of an estradiol level. Indirect testing of estrogen levels is performed by giving a progesterone challenge with medroxyprogesterone acetate 10 mg a day for 7 to 10 days. Failure to produce vaginal bleeding within 10 days suggests a hypoestrogenic state, an obstructed outflow tract, or pregnancy. If the history and physical examination suggest androgen excess or polycystic ovarian disease, LH, free testosterone, and DHEA-S should be obtained.[4,10] A woman who is less than 30 years old and has either an elevated FSH or absence of her uterus should have a karyotype analysis. An elevated prolactin should be followed up with pituitary imaging, usually with an MRI. The clinician should be aware that prolactin levels might be falsely elevated if obtained early in the morning, after a breast examination, or in close relation to a high protein meal.

Bone density assessment should be considered in individuals with hypothalamic hypoestrogenic amenorrhea for greater than 6 to 12 months or a prolonged history of oligomenorrhea, disordered eating, and/or stress fractures. Dual x-ray absorptiometry (DEXA) represents the state of the art measurement tool for assessment of bmd. However, there is no consensus regarding guidelines for bone density assessment for children, adolescents, or young adults. There are technical limitations to assessing bone mineral density in the growing child given that not all DEXA equipment includes the appropriate age-matched reference range for girls less than 18 years of age. Radiographic bone age determination is an alternative when pubertal development and menarche are delayed.

Those "at risk" individuals hesitant to undergo treatment or implement preventive strategies may be more likely to be compliant with treatment programs with the objective finding of a low bone density. If specific treatments are to be instituted, a baseline bmd may be helpful to monitor effectiveness of the treatment.

Treatment

Physically active girls and women should be educated about proper nutrition, safe training practices, and the warning signs and risks of the triad.[14,15] All individuals working with active girls and women should promote athletic training that is medically and psychologically sound.[14] An approach to the use of nonpharmacologic and pharmacologic treatments in the management of athletes with menstrual dysfunction is presented in Table 12-3 and discussed below.

Nonpharmacologic Treatment Options

ENERGY BALANCE

In the female athlete with luteal phase dysfunction, oligomenorrhea, and amenorrhea, a trial of nonpharmacologic therapy including

Table 12-3

Treatment of Hypoestrogenic Oligomenorrhea and Amenorrhea in Athletes

Oligomenorrhea or amenorrhea without osteopenia (or if bone status unknown and lower risk of osteopenia)
  Nonpharmacologic treatment for 3–6 months
    Decrease physical activity and/or increase caloric intake with goal of obtaining positive energy balance
    Increase weight if needed (within 10 percent of ideal weight range)
    Screen and treat for disordered eating if present
    Obtain 1,200–1,500 mg/d of calcium
  Consider pharmacologic trial if no results after 3–6 months of nonpharmacologic treatment
    Oral contraceptive pills (preferable) or estrogen replacement therapy
  Re-evaluate frequently
Oligomenorrhea or amenorrhea present for less than 6 months and osteopenia
  Nonpharmacologic trial for 3 months
    Decrease physical activity and/or increase caloric intake with goal of obtaining a positive energy balance
    Increase weight if needed
    Screen and treat for disordered eating if present
    Obtain 1,200–1,500 mg/d of calcium
    Consider adding resistive weights or adding impact activity while maintaining a positive energy balance
  Pharmacologic trial if no spontaneous menses with nonpharmacologic treatment
    Oral contraceptive pills (preferable) or estrogen replacement therapy
    Consider nasal calcitonin if significantly osteopenic
  Re-evaluate frequently
  Repeat DEXA in 1 year
Oligomenorrhea or amenorrhea present for greater than 6 months and osteopenia/osteoporosis
  Pharmacologic and nonpharmacologic therapy simultaneously as in oligomenorrhea or amenorrhea present for less than 6 months and osteopenia
  Consider nasal calcitonin
  Re-evaluate frequently
  Repeat DEXA 1 year

dietary intervention and possible adjustments in training should be implemented with the goal of restoring a state of positive energy balance. Nonpharmacologic therapy is reasonable and focuses on what is believed to be the underlying mechanism involved in AA.

Dueck reported the effect of a 15-week diet and intervention program on energy balance, hormonal profiles, body composition, and menstrual function of an amenorrheic endurance athlete.[37] With the reduction of training by only 1 day per week and the addition of a sport nutrition beverage containing 360 kcal/day, the athlete experienced a transition from a negative to a positive energy balance. Her body fat and LH increased while her cortisol decreased. Kopp-Woodroffe reported the effect of a 20-week program with 1 day off a week and the same sport nutrition beverage.[38] Athletes changed to positive energy balance, gained weight (1 kg), and resumed menses.

Treatment needs to be individualized to the athlete. If she is significantly underweight (20 percent ideal weight) efforts to gain weight may help resume menses and preserve bmd. In the presence of significant osteopenia or osteoporosis and evidence of ongoing bone loss, a pharmacologic approach will likely be needed in addition to the nonpharmacologic treatments.

NUTRITION AND WEIGHT

The adolescent diet is often lacking in adequate calcium intake. Adequate calcium is needed to maintain proper bone health. The physically active woman needs to supplement the diet with 1,200 to 1,500 mg of calcium a day.[33] It is recommended to obtain 400 IU of vitamin D a day to assist in the absorption of calcium and maintenance of bone health. In addition, maintenance of a normal weight range is important, as low body weight is predictor for bone loss in the young athlete with AA.

EXERCISE

The optimal exercise program for bone health has yet to be determined. In the presence of amenorrhea, the goal should be to restore a positive energy balance with improved nutrition and possible decreased training intensity in the effort resume normal menses.[4,11,37] What is known is that regular weight-bearing exercise above and beyond the individual's usual activities is beneficial to bone. The magnitude of the load (higher impact) seems to be a better osteogenic stimulus than the frequency of the load. Resistive exercises with weights are also recommended 2 to 3 days per week for optimal bone health. Recent analysis from Witzke and Snow have demonstrated that lean body mass and leg power best predicted bone mineral content and bmd of the whole body, lumbar spine, femoral shaft, and

hip in adolescent girls.[39] This study suggests the important role for muscle mass development during growth to maximize peak bmd.

Pharmacologic Therapy

ORAL CONTRACEPTIVE PILLS/ESTROGEN REPLACEMENT THERAPY

Normal reproductive function is important to prevent the effects of estrogen deprivation on bone. For athletes with low estrogen levels, estrogen replacement therapy will usually result in resumption of menses. Longitudinal studies on the effect of estrogen replacement on bone health, however, are lacking. Keen and Drinkwater[24] found that bmd of former oligomenorrheic and amenorrheic athletes remained low despite several years of OCP use or resumption of normal menses. The American Academy of Pediatrics recommends that women with primary amenorrhea should not start estrogen therapy before 16 years of age due to concern for premature closure of the growth plates. If contraception is desired, OCPs can lessen blood loss and dysmenorrhea. Many young women have concerns regarding the side effects of such therapy. Weight changes, acne, nausea, effects on performance, and mood alterations are common concerns although many of the newer OCPs have fewer adverse effects.

Conflicting data exist regarding whether or not there is a protective effect of OCP use on stress fracture development in the female athlete. Most of the studies assessing the effect of OCP use on stress fractures have been in runners and have been cross-sectional or retrospective. A prospective cohort study in track and field athletes by Bennell and colleagues[27] showed no evidence of stress fracture reduction in those using OCP. Other investigators have demonstrated a protective effect.[28]

Insufficient studies exist showing postmenopausal doses of premarin and provera lead to gains of bmd or prevention of fractures in young women with menstrual dysfunction. Cumming's[40] retrospective study demonstrated an increase in bone mineral density in the lumbar spine and femoral neck in amenorrheic women runners ages 24 to 34 followed for 24 to 30 months on hormone replacement therapy. In contrast, Warren[41] showed no changes in bmd of the spine, foot, and radius in women with hypothalamic amenorrhea randomized to hormone replacement therapy with premarin 0.625 mg daily and medroxyprogesterone acetate 10 mg a day for 10 days each month for 2 years when compared to placebo. The subjects were then randomized in a crossover protocol into treatment versus no treatment for 1 year. No differences were noted in bmd of the amenorrheic athletes who received placebo or hormone replacement except in those with weight gain.

Most of the discussions of bone loss have implicated low estrogen levels. Other investigators have postulated that in some young athletic women with ovulatory disturbances and spinal bone loss, decreased progesterone but not estrogen production was found.[42] In her intervention study, Prior demonstrated that cyclic medroxyprogesterone treatment for 1 year was found to increase lumbar bmd in young (21 to 45 year old) premenopausal women with a history of amenorrhea or ovulatory disturbances and low progesterone.[43] However, the trial had insignificant power and did not evaluate any potential for decreased fracture risk.

In the oligomenorrheic athlete with hormone levels in the normal range, including FSH and estradiol and a positive progesterone challenge test, periodic withdrawal with medroxyprogesterone acetate (10 mg/d for the last 14 days in the cycle) should serve to prevent endometrial hyperplasia. The frequency of withdrawal needed is debatable. One can withdraw the athlete once a month or up to once every 3 months. Physician and athlete preference, guided by the athlete's symptoms, may be used as a guide for the frequency of progesterone.

There are some studies that have evaluated the effects of depot medroxyprogesterone acetate (Depo-Provera) on bone metabolism. The initial work indicates this form of progesterone may have a negative impact on bone metabolism particularly in the younger women, and should not be recommended in the amenorrheic athlete, especially in the presence of osteopenia.

OTHER MEDICATIONS

Because many AA are reluctant to take hormones, other pharmaceutical agents may be indicated, especially in the presence of osteopenia or osteoporosis. Insufficient prospective data exist, however, that consistently demonstrate an increase in bmd from any pharmacologic treatment in the female athlete with hypoestrogenic amenorrhea or oligomenorrhea and osteopenia.

Drinkwater and colleagues found that nasal calcitonin (miacalcin) use for 2 years in young amenorrheic athletes with osteopenia resulted in significant bone gain in the lumbar spine and proximal femur.[44] Miacalcin is approved for the treatment of postmenopausal osteoporosis. It has been found to be safe and has a relatively short half-life. More research is certainly needed in the use of this medication in the amenorrheic athlete with osteopenia before recommending it for widespread use.

The bisphosphonates, including Alendronate, are approved for the treatment of postmenopausal osteoporosis but have not been fully studied in the growing child or in women of childbearing age. The long half-life of Alendronate and other bisphosphonates is concerning, especially in the latter group. In addition, the mechanisms involved in bone loss and formation in children and young adults with hypothalamic hypoestrogenic amenorrhea and disordered eating may be different from those involved with postmenopausal women.

The selective estrogen receptor modulators (SERMs), such as raloxifene, have been approved for the prevention and treatment of postmenopausal osteoporosis. These medications, however, should not be used in the premenopausal woman at this time because there are insufficient data on safety in this age group. A recent study of another SERM, tamoxifen, showed bone loss in the lumbar spine and hip in premenopausal women but a gain in bone in postmenopausal women.[45]

Conclusion

Determining the role that exercise may play in the etiology of adolescent development and menstrual disturbances is critical to our understanding of how to promote and protect the health of women. The cardiorespiratory and other physiologic benefits of regular physical exercise are well established, but an accumulating body of evidence indicates that several types of reproductive system disorders occur disproportionately in exercising females. There are clinical consequences to states of chronic hypoestrogenism. Maximizing peak bone mass and preventing bone loss are important goals in the pediatric, adolescent, and young adult age groups. Ensuring adequate calcium nutrition and vitamin D intake, encouraging exercise, and maintaining hormonal balance are important preventive measures for optimizing skeletal integrity and preventing the risk of future fractures.

Correcting energy deficits in the athlete with menstrual dysfunction is an important prevention and treatment strategy. The goal is for the athlete to resume menstrual periods through establishment of a positive energy balance. Athletes with low weight and disordered eating are also predisposed to significant bone loss. Prevention and treatment of AA and osteopenia in these high-risk groups is imperative.

There is controversy regarding the long-term effects of hormonal treatment on bone density in hypothalamic hypoestrogenic female athlete or in the female athlete with established osteoporosis. More research is needed to determine additional risk factors that may be contributing to bone loss in young athletic women, in addition to elucidating other risk factors for stress injury. There is a need for outcome studies to assess treatment options for athletes with menstrual dysfunction and osteopenia, leading to increases in bmd and skeletal integrity as well as treatments leading to a reduction in stress injury in the female athlete.

References

1. DeSouza MJ, Metzger, DA: Reproductive function in amenorrheic athletes and anorexic patients: A review. *Med Sci Sports Exerc* 2 3:995, 1991.
2. Loucks AB, Horvath SM: Athletic amenorrhea: A review. *Med Sci Sports Exerc* 17:56, 1985.
3. Highet R: Athletic amenorrhoea: An update on etiology, complications, and management. *Sports Med* 7:82, 1989.
4. Shangold M, Rebar RW, Wentz, AC, et al: Evaluation and management of menstrual dysfunction in athletes. *JAMA* 2 63:1665, 1990.
5. Claessens AL, Malina RM, Lefevre J, et al: Growth and menarcheal status of elite female gymnasts. *Med Sci Sports Exerc* 24:755, 1992.
6. Loucks AB, Vaitukaitis J, Cameron JL, et al: The reproductive system and exercise in women. *Med Sci Sports Exerc* 24:S288, 1992.
7. Malina RM: Menarche in athletes: a synthesis and hypothesis. *Ann Human Biol* 10:1, 1983.
8. Tomten SE: Prevalence of menstrual dysfunction in Norwegian long-distance runners participating in the Oslo Marathon games. *Scand J Med Sci Sports* 6:164, 1996.
9. Malina RM: Physical growth and biological maturation of young athletes. *Exerc Sport Sci Rev* 22:389, 1994.
10. Shangold M: Menstruation. In: Shangold M, Mirkin G (eds): *Women and Exercise*. Philadelphia: 1988; 129[C1].
11. Otis CL: Exercise-associated amenorrhea. *Clin Sports Med* 11:351, 1992.

12. Drinkwater BL, Bruemmer B, Chestnut III CH: Menstrual history as a determinant of current bone density in young athletes. *JAMA* 263:545, 1990.

13. Laughlin GA, Yen SS: Nutritional and endocrine-metabolic aberrations in amenorrheic athletes. *J Clin Endocrinol Metab* 81:4301, 1996.

14. American College of Sports Medicine. Position stand on the female athlete triad. *Med Sci Sports Exerc* 29:i, 1997.

15. Nattiv A, Agostini R, Drinkwater B, et al: The female athlete triad: The interrelatedness of disordered eating, amenorrhea and osteoporosis. *Clin Sports Med* 13:405, 1994.

16. Loucks AB, Verdun M, Heath EM: Low energy availability, not stress of exercise, alters LH pulsatility in exercising women. *J Applied Physiol* 84:37, 1998.

17. Williams NI, Young JC, McArthur JW, et al: Strenuous exercise with caloric restriction: Effect on luteinizing hormone secretion. *Med Sci Sports Exerc* 27:1390, 1995.

18. Laughlin GA, Yen SS: Hypoleptinemia in women athletes: Absence of a diurnal rhythm with amenorrhea. *J Clin Endocrinol Metab* 82:318, 1997.

19. Bullen BA, Skrinar GS, Beitins IZ, et al: Induction of menstrual disorders by strenuous exercise in untrained women. *New Engl J Med* 312:1349, 1985.

20. Sanborn CF, Albrecht BH, Wagner WW: Athletic amenorrhea: Lack of association with body fat. *Med Sci Sports Exerc* 19:207, 1987.

21. Loucks AB, Heath EM: Induction of low-T3 syndrome in exercising women occurs at a threshold of energy availability. *Am J Physiol* 266:R817, 1994.

22. Slemenda CW, Reister TK, Hui SL, et al: Influences on skeletal mineralization in children and adolescents: Evidence for varying effects of sexual maturation and physical activity. *J Pediatr* 125:201, 1994.

23. Drinkwater BL, Nilson K, Chestnut III CH, et al: Bone mineral density content of amenorrheic and eumenorrheic athletes. *N Engl J Med* 311:277, 1984.

24. Keen AD, Drinkwater BL: Irreversible bone loss in former amenorrheic athletes. *Osteoporosis Intl* 7:311, 1997.

25. Petterson U, Stalnacke BM, Ahlenius GM, et al: Lowbone mass density at multiple skeletal sites, including the appendicular skeleton in amenorrheic runners. *Calcified Tissue Intl* 64:117, 1999.

26. Rencken ML, Chestnut CH, Drinkwater BL: Bone density at multiple skeletal sites in amenorrheic athletes. *JAMA* 276:238, 1996.

27. Bennell KL, Malcolm SA, Thomas SA, et al: Risk factors for stress fractures in track and field athletes. *Am J Sports Med* 24:810, 1996.

28. Myburgh KH, Hutchins J, Fataar AB, et al: Low bone density is an etiologic factor for stress fractures in athletes. *Ann Intern Med* 113:754, 1990.

29. Warren MP, Brooks-Gunn J, Hamilton LH, et al: Scoliosis and fractures in young ballet dancers. *New Engl J Med* 314:1348, 1986.

30. Robinson TL, Snow-Harter C, Taafe, DR, et al: Gymnasts exhibit higher bone mass than runners despite similar prevalence of amenorrhea and oligomenorrhea. *J Bone Min Res* 10:26, 1995.

31. Nygaard IE, Thompson FL, Svengalis SL, et al: Urinary incontinence in elite nulliparous athletes. *Obstet Gynecol* 84:183, 1994.

32. Committee on Professional Standards. *Guidelines for Women's Health Care*. Washington, DC: American College of Obstetricians and Gynecologists, 1995.

33. Committee on Sports Medicine, American Academy of Pediatrics: Amenorrhea in adolescent athletes. *Pediatrics* 84:394, 1989.

34. Green M (ed): *Bright Futures: Guidelines for Health Supervision of Infants, Children, and Adolescents*. Arlington, VA: National Center for Education in Maternal and Child Health, 1994.

35. Schachter J, Shafer M, Young M, et al: Routine pelvic examinations in asymptomatic young women. *New Engl J Med* 335:1847, 1996.

36. Marshall LA: Clinical evaluation of amenorrhea in active and athletic women. *Clin Sports Med* 13:371, 1994.

37. Dueck CA, Matt KS, Manore MM, et al: Treatment of athletic amenorrhea with a diet and training intervention program. *Intl J Sport Nutr* 6:24, 1996.

38. Kopp-Woodroffe SA, Manore MM, Dueck CA, et al: Energy and nutrient status of amenorrheic athletes participating in a diet and exercise training intervention program. *J Sport Nutr* 9:70, 1999.

39. Witzke KA, Snow C: Lean body mass and leg power best predict bone mineral density in adolescent girls. *Med Sci Sports Exerc* 31:1558, 1999.

40. Cumming DC: Exercise-associated amenorrhea,

low bone density, and estrogen replacement therapy. *Arch Intern Med* 156:2193, 1996.

41. Warren MP, Fox RP, DeRogatis AJ, et al: Osteopenia in hypothalamic amenorrhea: A 3 year longitudinal study (abstract). Proc Endocrine Soc, 1994.

42. Prior JC, Vigna YM, Schecter MT, et al: Spinal bone loss and ovulatory disturbances. *New Engl J Med* 323:1221, 1990.

43. Prior JC, Vigna YM, Barr SI, et al: Cyclic progesterone treatment increases bone density: A controlled trial in active women with menstrual cycle disturbances. *Am J Med* 96:521, 1994.

44. Drinkwater BL, Healy NL, Rencken ML, et al: Effectiveness of nasal calcitonin in preventing bone loss in young amenorrheic women [Abstract #592]. *J Bone Min Res* 8(Suppl 1):S264, 1993.

45. Powles TJ, Hickish T, Kanis JA, et al: Effect of tamoxifen on bone mineral density measured by dual energy x-ray absorptiometry in healthy premenopausal women. *J Clin Oncol* 14:78, 1996.

Andrew W. Nichols

Chapter

13

Exercise-Induced Bronchospasm

Historical Perspective and Definition

"If from running, gymnastics, or any other work breathing becomes difficult, it is called asthma." Aretaeus of Capadocia, 2nd century AD.[1]

The association between asthma, bronchospasm, and exercise has been recognized for centuries. In 1946, Herxheimer documented that pulmonary spirometry measurements decline after exercise in patients with exercise-induced bronchospasm (EIB).[1]

The diagnosis can be confirmed by demonstrating a reduction in pulmonary function tests (FEV_1 or PEFR) of 20 percent or greater when comparing postexercise values to pre-exercise baseline readings.

Even though exercise may provoke bronchospasm, many young asthmatics benefit greatly from regular exercise programs. Nearly all individuals with EIB may participate in athletic activities by selecting appropriate sports, using techniques to reduce the asthmogenicity of exercise, and by taking EIB-inhibiting medications. A 1989 American Academy of Pediatrics Policy Statement asserted that: "Asthmatic children should be encouraged, not discouraged, from participating in all athletic endeavors . . . they should pursue their athletic goals with the knowledge that various anti-asthma drugs may be taken without being considered doping."[2]

Incidence and Epidemiology

EIB affects 80 to 90 percent of individuals with chronic asthma, and 40 percent of those with allergic rhinitis but no history of asthma. Only 3 to 4 percent of individuals who have neither asthma nor allergic rhinitis have EIB. A strong association between positive skin prick test atopy and EIB is reported in elite runners.[3] Substantial rates of unrecognized EIB—highly associated with previous wheezing, childhood asthma, residence in a poverty area, and African-American versus European-American ethnicity—have been reported among urban varsity athletes.[4]

The prevalence of EIB in the general population is estimated to be 7.5 to 15 percent. Table 13-1 shows the incidence of EIB among various athletic population groups. The higher than expected rates of EIB reported for several athletic groups—such as figure skaters—suggests that some types of exercise may actually predispose to EIB via repeated exposures to airborne allergens and cold air.

Clinical Characteristics

Characteristics of an Exercise-Induced Bronchospasm Attack

EIB is characterized by bronchospasm that occurs within 6 to 12 min of beginning exercise

Table 13-1

Incidence of Exercise-Induced Bronchospasm among Various Athletic Population Groups

POPULATION GROUP	INCIDENCE (%)
Elite figure skaters	30–35[5, 6]
Distance runners exposed to cold	25[7]
High school/college football players	12–23[8–10]
USA Olympic team members 1984/1996	11.2/10.4[11, 12]
Australian Olympic team members 1976/1980	9.7/8.5[13]
General population	7.5–15

and becomes maximal 5 to 15 min after completing exercise (Fig. 13-1). Bronchospasm typically resolves spontaneously over 30 to 90 mins, with children improving faster than adults.[5] The intensity of exercise must be relatively high (more than 85 percent of the maximum heart rate) to provoke an attack of EIB. Although status asthmaticus is rare, EIB-induced deaths have been reported in the medical literature. In particular, highly publicized EIB deaths affected a collegiate basketball player at North Carolina Central University in 1992 and the 1994 first-round draft pick of the major league baseball Colorado Rockies.

Signs and Symptoms

The clinical manifestations of EIB often vary significantly. The most common signs and symptoms are wheezing, dyspnea, and chest tightness induced by vigorous exercise. Among the more subtle signs of EIB are cough, chest congestion, feeling "out of shape," a lack of energy, inconsistent or erratic athletic performance, frequent "colds," better tolerance of short as compared to long duration exercise sessions, and more frequent occurrence of symptoms during running sports than swimming activities.

Refractory Period

Many individuals with EIB experience a "refractory period," which lasts for up to 90 min after exercise, during which repeated exercise exposures induce relatively milder or no bronchospastic responses. Athletes can take advantage of this refractory period by performing an adequate warm-up an hour or so before the competition so as to eliminate or blunt the subsequent bronchospastic effect during competition.

Late-Phase Response

Thirty percent of individuals with EIB experience a delayed "late phase" bronchospastic

Figure 13-1

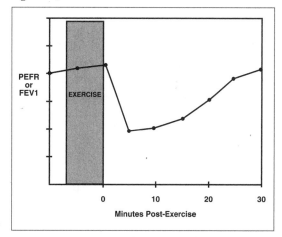

PEFR
or
FEV1

EXERCISE

0   10   20   30
Minutes Post-Exercise

Transient post-exercise reduction in peak expiratory flow rate (PEFR) or 1-sec forced expiratory volume (FEV₁), which affects individuals with EIB.

response (LPR), which occurs 4 to 8 hrs after the initial EIB episode. Notably, this LPR occurs in the absence of an immediately preceding exercise bout (Fig. 13-2). The LPR occurs more commonly in children than adults, and appears to involve primarily the smaller airway structures.

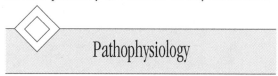

Pathophysiology

Mechanism of Disease-Hypotheses

Although no single theory explains the pathophysiology of EIB in all patients, four separate hypotheses—airway cooling, osmolarity, mediator, and rebound rewarming—appear to contribute to EIB. Certain environmental conditions such as cold, dry, or polluted air predispose to EIB. Atopy also plays a prominent role in the pathogenesis of EIB in susceptible individuals.

AIRWAY COOLING HYPOTHESIS

The airway-cooling hypothesis proposes that airway cooling (via increased respiratory water

Figure 13-2

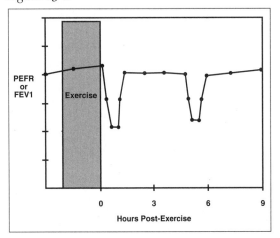

Demonstrates an initial reduction in FEV_1/PEFR, which occurs immediately after the completion of vigorous exercise and a delayed late-phase bronchospastic response (LPR), which may occur 4 to 8 hr after the original episode. Both episodes resolve spontaneously.

and heat loss) stimulates bronchial tree receptors that produce cough and bronchospasm through vagal nerve activity. The magnitude of airway cooling is defined by the respiratory heat exchange equation (RHE):

$$RHE = VE[HC(T_i - T_e) + HV(W_i - W_e)]$$

VE = minute ventilation
HC = specific heat density of air (constant)
$(T_i - T_e)$ = the temperature difference between inspired and expired air
HV = the latent heat of water vaporization (constant)
$(W_i - W_e)$ = the water content difference between inspired and expired air.

Regardless of the temperature and water content of inspired air, expired air typically becomes fully humidified and warmed to body temperature. Conditions that maximize RHE and thus provoke EIB include intensive exercise, cold air, and dry air. The finding that EIB occurs more commonly in cold, dry air and less frequently in

warm, humid conditions supports the airway-cooling hypothesis. Clinical features of EIB that are not logically explained by the airway cooling hypothesis, however, include the late phase bronchospastic response, and the fact that bronchospasm can persist for up to an hour after the airways have rewarmed following exercise in cold, dry conditions.

OSMOLARITY HYPOTHESIS

The osmolarity hypothesis suggests that increased respiratory heat exchange causes evaporative water loss from the airways, thereby producing hyperosmolarity of the airway-lining fluids, which consequently provokes bronchospasm. Evidence in favor of the osmolarity hypothesis is that EIB episodes can be prevented by breathing nebulized normal saline during exercise and provoked by inhaling hypertonic saline during exercise.

MEDIATOR HYPOTHESIS

The mediator hypothesis proposes that increased minute ventilation during exercise irritates the airways resulting in mast cell and basophil degranulation with the release of inflammatory mediators such as histamine, neutrophil chemotactic factor of anaphylaxis (NCFA), leukotrienes, and other substances that induce bronchospasm.

Individuals with EIB have been shown to develop increased circulating levels of inflammatory mediators after exercise in cold, dry environmental conditions, whereas subjects without EIB do not exhibit such increases. The transient depletion of inflammatory mediator stores is one plausible explanation for the occurrence of the refractory period in which subsequent exercise sessions closely spaced together result in lesser degrees of bronchospasm. The therapeutic efficacy of the mast cell stabilizers and leukotriene antagonists also indicate the importance of mediators in the pathogenesis of EIB. Younger children recover from EIB more rapidly than older children, a finding that may be due to age-related changes in mediator production or release.[5]

REBOUND REWARMING HYPOTHESIS

The rebound rewarming hypothesis suggests that airway "rewarming" after exercise—rather than the airway "cooling" during exercise—produces bronchial edema and subsequent bronchospasm. This theory may account for the peak in bronchospasm that occurs post-exercise in EIB.

Predisposing Factors

Numerous extrinsic factors may increase an individual's susceptibility to EIB, including exposure to cold air, dry air, dusty air, allergen-polluted air, smoke-filled air, automobile exhaust pollution, and the smog components ozone, sulfur dioxide, and nitrogen dioxide. Respiratory viral infections and previous neonatal meconium aspiration syndrome may also predispose to EIB.[6]

The association between atopic disease, cold exposure, and EIB was studied in a group of nonasthmatic elite distance runners. Those with atopic disease (but no chronic asthma) who exercised in sub-zero temperatures developed mild bronchospasm sufficient to adversely affect athletic performance but not severe enough to meet the definition of EIB. Runners without atopy developed no bronchospasm during exercise under identical conditions.[3] Additionally, serum levels of the markers for TH2 lymphocyte activation (CD25-bearing T-helper cells and CD23-bearing B-cells), which plays an important role in the development and continuation of the inflammatory response of asthma, increase linearly in individuals who develop EIB.[7]

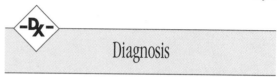

Diagnosis

Overview

An individual with suspected EIB should undergo a thorough medical history, physical examination, and resting pulmonary spirometry. To confirm the diagnosis of EIB, bronchospasm provocative testing (e.g., the exercise-challenge test and/or methacholine inhalation challenge test) may be necessary. The clinician should confirm the diagnosis of EIB by using appropriate testing, rather than simply treating a suspected case empirically with inhaled beta$_2$-adrenergic agonists. This approach helps to avoid overdiagnosing EIB and unnecessary pharmacologic treatment.

History and Physical Examination

The history and physical examination often provide strong evidence for the diagnosis of EIB. The medical history must include a careful inquiry of possible EIB attack signs and symptoms, predisposing stimuli, and provoking environmental conditions. Prior personal or family histories of asthma, allergic rhinitis, or eczema must also be identified.

Typically, the physical examination will be normal during evaluation in the medical office. Components of the physical examination should involve a thorough appraisal of the upper and lower respiratory tracts, including the nasopharynx and sinuses for signs of allergic disease and infection, and the chest and lungs for signs of wheezing, other abnormal breath sounds, coughing during deep inspiration, a prolonged expiratory phase, and abnormal chest configuration.

Diagnostic Testing

SPIROMETRY

Pulmonary function spirometry measurements useful in the evaluation of EIB include forced vital capacity (FVC), forced expiratory volume in one second (FEV_1), and the FEV_1/FVC ratio. The peak expiratory flow rate (PEFR) has less diagnostic accuracy than FEV_1, but is often easier to perform and thus may be useful to assess treatment responses. Reduced values for FEV_1 and FEV_1/FVC indicate the presence of obstructive airway disease. Normal resting PFTs do not exclude the presence of EIB.

EXERCISE-CHALLENGE TEST

The exercise-challenge test is the most frequent test used to confirm the diagnosis of EIB. To perform this test, asthma medications are withheld, and pre-exercise pulmonary function FEV_1 spirometry measurements are taken. The subject is then exercised on a treadmill or cycle ergometer using rapid incremental increases in exercise intensity to achieve and maintain 90 percent of the maximum predicted heart rate (MHR) for 5 to 8 min duration. Exercise intensity must be accelerated much more rapidly than in the standard Bruce exercise testing protocol. To elicit EIB, the typical routine used is stage I = 2 min at 50 percent of MHR; stage II = 2 min at 70 percent of MHR; and stage III = 2 min at 90 percent of MHR. This minimizes the potential effects of the refractory period and reduces the likelihood of a false negative test. Post-exercise spirometry values are obtained at 5-min intervals for 20 to 30 min and compared to the pre-exercise readings.

Reductions in FEV_1 of 20 percent or greater are considered consistent with the diagnosis of EIB. Mild EIB is defined by 20 to 30 percent reductions; moderate EIB by 30 to 40 percent decreases; and severe EIB by declines of greater than 40 percent. The sensitivity of the exercise-challenge test, which is less than that of the methacholine inhalation challenge or eucapnic voluntary hyperventilation tests, may be improved by performing the test in a cold and dry environment.

IN-THE-FIELD EXERCISE-CHALLENGE TEST

A modified exercise-challenge test may be performed "in-the-field" by using portable pulmonary function testing equipment such as a hand-held peak expiratory flow rate (PEFR) device. Although the PFT measurements obtainable in the field are more limited than in the pulmonary laboratory, the environmental and activity conditions that provoke suspected EIB attacks may be replicated.

For example, a runner or cross-country skier who develops pulmonary symptoms following exercise on a cold winter day may be tested directly under such conditions. Alternatively, a swimmer or rower may be evaluated after performing the specific activities that provoke symptoms. The sensitivity of the test may be increased by performing the evaluation in both cold winter air and during the pollen season, because many individuals will show positive results under only one of these conditions.[3]

A "free running" screening test for EIB was described in which in a group of high school students were instructed to run for 7 min while maintaining a heart rate of 160 beats per min. PEFR levels, measured 5 min after running, which declined by 15 percent or greater from pre-exercise values were considered positive. The sensitivity of the free running test was 94 percent, specificity was 64 percent, and the positive predictive value was 44 percent when compared to formal pulmonary function testing.[8]

Recent work has shown that field-testing may be far more sensitive and specific for EIB. A recent study compared laboratory-based versus field-based testing in 23 elite Nordic athletes with known EIB and 23 control subjects. Baseline spirometry was similar in both groups. Seventy-eight percent of those with known EIB were field-based positive while they had negative laboratory exercise-challenge tests.[9]

METHACHOLINE INHALATION CHALLENGE TEST

The methacholine inhalation challenge test (MIC) has been the gold standard for determining airway hyperresponsiveness (AHR). The MIC test is technically easier to perform than the exercise-challenge test, because exercise is not required. The testing protocol involves comparing pretest pulmonary spirometry measurements with those obtained after the inhalation of increasing concentrations of methacholine, a nonspecific cholinergic agent. A 20 percent reduction in PEFR or FEV_1 from pre-inhalation values is considered positive for AHR.[10] The MIC test, which is more sensitive but less specific than the exercise-challenge test, may be obtained when a patient has symptoms suggestive of EIB but has normal resting pulmonary spirometry and/or a negative ECT.

EUCAPNIC VOLUNTARY HYPERVENTILATION TEST

The eucapnic voluntary hyperventilation test (EVH) induces AHR secondary to the hyperventilation of exercise. The patient voluntarily hyperventilates a dry gas mixture composed of 5 percent CO_2, 21 percent O_2, and 74 percent N_2 to maintain eucapnia. Significant reductions in post-hyperventilation spirometry values when compared to baseline readings indicate AHR. Although the EVH test is more sensitive than the exercise-challenge test, it is not often used due to the special equipment and gas mixture requirements.

Differential Diagnosis

Chronic Asthma

The presence of nighttime asthma symptoms, daily symptoms, frequent exacerbations, provocation by respiratory infections, or incomplete control with inhaled beta$_2$-adrenergic agonists in individuals with EIB indicates that a complete medical work-up should be performed to identify chronic asthma. The NIH recently published a classification of asthma based on severity of disease and a stepwise approach to pharmacologic treatment.[11]

Vocal Cord Dysfunction

Vocal cord dysfunction (VCD) refers to a spectrum of psychogenic disorders of the larynx in which upper airway obstruction results from paradoxical closure of the vocal cords or prolapse of the supraglottic structures during inspiration. Previous terminology of VCD conditions included Munchausen's stridor, factitious asthma, laryngoneurosis, episodic laryngeal dysfunction, adult spasmodic croup, pseudoasthma, psychogenic stridor, and laryngeal edema.

The incidence of VCD is not known. Of 182 cases reported in the medical literature between 1965 and 1995, 83 percent were females, and the mean age was 24 years (range 4 to 74 years). Several adolescents who were thought to have EIB, but failed treatment, were subsequently diagnosed with VCD.[12,13] The clinical presentation of VCD involves symptoms of upper airway obstruction that are predominantly inspiratory, and appear earlier and evolve more rapidly than a typical EIB attack. Among the specific signs and symptoms of VCD are choking, throat or chest tightness, coughing, dyspnea, stridor with or without wheezing, tachypnea, and respiratory distress. Abnormal respiratory patterns often normalize when the patient becomes distracted with activities such as coughing, panting, or breath holding.

The diagnosis of VCD should be suspected if attack characteristics develop very early in exercise, lack consistency, and fail to respond to EIB medications.[14] Pulmonary function testing may reveal a flattening of the inspiratory limb of the flow-volume curve. The diagnosis is confirmed by flexible fiberoptic rhinolaryngoscopic visualization of vocal cord adduction during inspiration.

The athlete with VCD is typically an adolescent or young adult, and exercise is the sole trigger of attacks. Symptoms occur most frequently during competitions and intense physical training, and often impede performance by causing a "choking" phenomenon. Many subjects are high academic achievers, and have personal or parental intolerance of failure. Treatment options for VCD include speech therapy, psychotherapy, relaxation techniques, and breathing the special helium-oxygen gaseous mixture Heliox (70 percent He/30 percent O_2).

Other

A number of other medical conditions must be considered in the evaluation of the patient with suspected EIB. Several causes of sudden cardiac death in young athletes such as hypertrophic cardiomyopathy, anomalous coronary artery disease, Marfan's syndrome, aortic stenosis, atherosclerotic coronary artery disease, and viral myocarditis may present with signs and symptoms that may be indistinguishable from EIB. Hyperventilation syndrome, spontaneous pneumothorax, and pulmonary embolus are additional possibilities. Further, congenital right aortic arch anomaly, which may cause exercise-induced dyspnea as a result of severe tracheal narrowing, has been reported.[15]

Treatment

Non-Pharmacologic

Counseling athletes about appropriate sport selection is important when treating patients with EIB. In general, sports that involve brief, repetitive, unsustained athletic efforts such as sprint running, gymnastics, baseball, and weightlifting are better tolerated than prolonged endurance activities. Additionally, sports that are played in a warm, moist environment are preferable to those occurring in cold, dry conditions. Swimming and aquatics sports performed in a heated swimming pool are particularly well suited to those with EIB because the air lying just above the water is warmed and fully humidified (Table 13-2).

The athlete can also reduce the risk of EIB further by maintaining aerobic conditioning and by using nasal breathing or wearing a scarf or mask over the mouth and nose during exercise in cold, dry environments to help warm and

Table 13-2

Specific Sports and the Risk of Exercise-Induced Bronchospasm (EIB)

HIGH RISK SPORTS	LOW RISK SPORTS
Ice skating	Sprint running
Ice hockey	Gymnastics
Cross-country skiing	Baseball
Distance running	Riflery
Soccer	Archery
Bicycling	Weight lifting
Rowing	Swimming*
Football	Water polo*

*The EIB protective effects of the warm, humidified air that these aquatics athletes typically breathe may be overridden by the sustained efforts that the sports require.

humidify air before it reaches the lungs. An adequate warm-up with gradual progression in the intensity of exercise may also protect against EIB.

Pharmacologic

Numerous pharmacologic agents are available to prevent EIA. The relative effectiveness and duration of action of a variety of these agents appears in Table 13-3.[16]

BETA$_2$-ADRENERGIC AGONISTS

MECHANISM OF ACTION   The inhaled beta$_2$-adrenergic agonists are the most effective pharmaceutical agents for prevention of EIB. The selective beta$_2$-adrenergic receptor agents, such as albuterol and salmeterol, are preferred over the non-selective adrenergic agonist, metaproterenol. Albuterol, the most commonly used beta$_2$-adrenergic agonist, prevents EIB in up to 90 percent of cases. The beta$_2$-adrenergic agonists exert their actions through adenyl cyclase, which increases intracellular concentrations of cAMP to inhibit smooth muscle contraction by sequestration of calcium resulting in bronchodi-

lation. These drugs also inhibit inflammatory mediator release from mast cells.

ALBUTEROL AND SALMETEROL   Inhaled albuterol is the drug of choice for the prevention of EIA due to its efficacy and rapid onset of action. The normal dose is two puffs taken 15 min before exercise, and the duration of action is 2 to 6 hrs. The aerosol (180 μg) and powder (200 μg) forms of albuterol demonstrate similar therapeutic efficacies.[17] Inhaled salmeterol is taken as two puffs 30 to 45 min before exercise, and exerts its therapeutic effects for up to 12 hrs.[18] The selective beta$_2$-adrenergic receptor properties of these medications reduce the incidence of adverse effects such as tremor, palpitations, agitation, and insomnia. A serious reported side effect of albuterol inhalation is ventricular tachycardia due to a hyperexcitable cardiac conduction system or the long QT syndrome.[19]

DEVELOPMENT OF TOLERANCE   Chronic use of beta$_2$-adrenergic agonists—for example, albuterol taken four times daily versus only before exercise—may lead to the development of tolerance, in which the medication becomes less effective in preventing EIB.[20] Although decreases in therapeutic efficacy may not be subjectively

Table 13-3

Relative Effectiveness of Common Anti-Asthma Medications in the Prevention of Exercise-Induced Asthma*

AGENT	EFFECTIVENESS**	DURATION OF PROTECTION (HRS)
Salmeterol aerosol	+++	10–12
Albuterol aerosol	+++	2.0–2.5
Cromolyn sodium	++	1.5–2.0
Nedocromil sodium	++	1.5–2.0
Theophylline	±	?
Anticholinergics	±	?

*Table data modified from McFadden and Gilbert.[16]
**Effectiveness is rated as follows: +++ = ablation or substantial reduction in obstructive response; ++ = marked reduction in obstructive response; ± = questionable efficacy.

apparent to the patient, they may be identifiable by formal pulmonary function testing.

CLENBUTEROL Clenbuterol is a long-acting oral beta$_2$-adrenergic agonists available as a veterinary drug (Spiropent™), which has been widely abused by body builders and strength sport athletes for its purported anabolic effects. Although animal studies have demonstrated muscle mass gains of 13 to 65 percent associated with clenbuterol administration, no controlled studies have documented such results in humans. Clenbuterol causes frequent side effects of tremor, headache, insomnia, and cardiac arrhythmias. Chronic usage also results in the development of tolerance. The International Olympic Committee (IOC) and National Collegiate Athletic Association (NCAA) banned clenbuterol and all oral formulations of beta$_2$ agonists (including albuterol in the form of Proventil Repetabs™) due to possible anabolic effects.

POTENTIAL ERGOGENIC EFFECTS In addition to the possible anabolic effects on skeletal muscle of the long-acting oral beta$_2$-adrenergic agents, concern has been expressed over a possible ergogenic effect related to bronchodilation. Recent anecdotal observations of elite competitive swimmers and triathletes at international competitions suggests usage of "asthma inhalers," which far exceeds estimates for the prevalence of EIB. Scientific studies to date, however, have failed to demonstrate any artificial increase in ventilatory capacity or "supra physiologic" bronchodilation that can be induced by using the inhaled beta$_2$-adrenergic agonists.

MAST CELL STABILIZERS

The mast cell membrane stabilizers—cromolyn and nedocromil—inhibit the release of mast cell inflammatory mediators that play a role in the pathogenesis of EIB. Although generally not as effective as the beta$_2$-adrenergic agonists, the mast cell membrane stabilizers prevent EIB in 70 percent of cases. These agents have a synergistic effect when used in combination with the beta$_2$-adrenergic agonists and are most commonly used when inhaled beta$_2$-adrenergic agonists are not effective in controlling symptoms of EIB when used alone. The mast cell membrane stabilizers have few adverse effects and are administered by inhalation 15 to 45 min before exercise. The relatively short duration of action necessitates that they be repeated often during prolonged athletic endeavors. These drugs are generally more effective in children and atopic individuals.

GLUCOCORTICOSTEROIDS

Inhaled and systemic glucocorticosteroids are widely prescribed to control chronic asthma and acute asthma exacerbations. The glucocorticosteroids exert their therapeutic effects by reducing inflammation and thus inhibiting bronchospasm. Adverse effects may be minimized by using the inhaled form of glucocorticosteroids or brief oral systemic "burst" courses when necessary. Although the pre-exercise administration of glucocorticosteroids has no known immediate preventive effects on EIB, these agents are most effective in reducing EIB when taken chronically in those with AHR.

THEOPHYLLINE

Theophylline is used primarily to control chronic asthma, but also has a protective effect on EIB when taken orally 30 to 60 min before exercise. In addition to the direct smooth muscle bronchodilation effects of theophylline, it also has mucolytic and anti-inflammatory properties. The use of theophylline is limited by frequent adverse effects, the need to monitor serum levels, and interactions with other drugs.

LEUKOTRIENE ANTAGONISTS

The leukotriene antagonists are oral medications used to control chronic asthma symptoms and prevent EIB. The agents exert their pharmacologic effects by blocking mast cell release of leukotrienes, which are inflammatory mediators that contribute to asthma by causing mucous production, bronchoconstriction, and eosinophil infiltration. The increased excretion of leukotriene E4 has been reported after exercise in patients with EIB. Treatment with the leukotriene antagonist montelukast caused a 50 percent mean reduction in the postexercise FEV_1 decline in adult asthmatics.[21] Similar preventive EIB effects were reported by zileuton, a leukotriene antagonist which inhibits 5-lipoxygenase, and the leukotriene D_4-receptor antagonist cinalukast.[22,23] These agents are best utilized in conjunction with an inhaled beta$_2$-adrenergic agonist in individuals who have poorly controlled symptoms when using an inhaled bronchodilator alone.

ANTIHISTAMINES AND INTRANASAL CORTICOSTEROIDS

Allergic rhinitis should be treated aggressively because exacerbations may provoke EIB.[24,25] The antihistamine terfenadine was shown to cause bronchodilation and block EIB in a dose-related response.[26] Intranasal corticosteroids are often highly effective in the treatment of allergic rhinitis and thus may also help to control EIB—especially in individuals with atopy.

ATROPINE AND IPRATROPIUM

Atropine and ipratropium, which are both competitive antagonists of acetylcholine, cause nonspecific bronchodilation. Ipratropium is a quaternary ammonium derivative of atropine that prevents it from readily crossing the blood-brain barrier. This results in fewer atropine-like side effects of dry mouth, tachycardia, visual problems, and psychological changes. Although ipratropium is effective in controlling chronic bronchitis when administered via inhalation, it has questionable efficacy in the prevention of EIB.

OTHER PHARMACOLOGIC AGENTS

The following agents, although not typically used for the management of EIB, have been shown to be effective in altering the bronchospastic response to exercise in individuals with EIB. In most instances, their use should be considered to be investigational.

HEPARIN   Although not approved by the FDA for this indication, inhaled heparin has been demonstrated to be effective in preventing EIB by modulating the release of inflammatory mediators from mast cells and counteracting histamine. The therapeutic effect in EIB is not related to its anticoagulant properties. Inhaled heparin has been shown to be more effective in preventing EIB than cromolyn.[27]

FUROSEMIDE   The diuretic furosemide has been shown to be effective in preventing EIB in children when taken in nebulized form. Although not approved by the FDA for this indication, pre-exercise nebulized furosemide was shown to limit mean reductions in FEV_1 after exercise to only 5 percent, as compared to 34 percent with pre-exercise nebulized saline in a series of children.[28] Higher doses of furosemide provide a longer duration of protection from EIB but also resulted in increased urine output, which could consequently predispose to dehydration.[29]

INDOMETHACIN   Indomethacin is a non-steroidal anti-inflammatory agent used primarily in its oral form to treat rheumatologic conditions. The inhaled form of indomethacin—which is not approved by the FDA—has also been shown to be effective in reducing the severity of EIB. Indomethacin exerts its therapeutic effects by inhibiting local prostaglandin synthesis and ion transport. A mean postexercise reduction in FEV_1 of 18 percent was measured in a group of children who were pre-exercise treated with inhaled indomethacin, compared to a reduction of 36 percent in a control group who received inhaled normal saline.[30]

CALCIUM CHANNEL BLOCKERS Calcium channel blocker (CCB) medications are widely used to treat hypertension, cardiac conditions, and prevent migraine headaches. The pharmacologic effect of CCBs stems from an ability to maintain a 10,000-to-1 extracellular-to-intracellular calcium concentration gradient, by blocking the cellular influx of calcium ions that inhibit muscle contraction. Through this mechanism, CCBs may cause bronchodilation, which may be responsible for the observed small, brief reductions in EIB severity that have been reported after pretreatment with both inhaled gallopamil and oral diltiazem.[31]

VITAMIN C (ASCORBIC ACID) A recent study discovered that 2 g of vitamin C taken 1 hour before exercise blocks EIB in 45 percent of young asthmatics.[32] The pharmacologic mechanism may be the antioxidant effect on the lung airway liquid surface, in which ascorbic acid

Table 13-4

The Status of Common Anti-Asthma Medications on USOC and NCAA Drug Lists

AGENT	USOC	NCAA
Theophylline	OK	OK
Mast cell membrane stabilizers	OK	OK
Leukotriene antagonists	OK	OK
Atropine	OK	OK
Ipratropium	OK	OK
Antihistamines	OK	OK
Corticosteroids—topical (e.g., aural, dermatologic, ophthalmologic)	OK	OK
Beta$_2$-adrenergic agonists—inhalation (albuterol, salmeterol, terbutaline)	OK*	OK
Corticosteroids—inhalation, local and intraarticular injections	OK*	OK
Sympathomimetic amines/OTC cold medications and decongestants other than ephedrine (e.g., phenylpropanolamine, pseudoephedrine)	Banned	OK
Corticosteroids—intravenous, intramuscular, oral, rectal	Banned	OK
Ephedrine	Banned	Banned
Beta$_2$-adrenergic agonists—oral (e.g., clenbuterol, albuterol sulfate as Proventil Repetabs or Volmax Controlled-Release Tablets)	Banned	Banned

*Permitted only with physician's written notification submitted prior to the competition.

shifts the cyclooxygenase pathway from synthesis of the bronchoconstrictory prostaglandin F_2 to the bronchodilator prostaglandin E_2.

ASTHMA MEDICATIONS AND DOPING

Concern about the potential ergogenic effects of various anti-asthma medications has prompted the International Olympic Committee (IOC), United States Olympic Committee (USOC), and National Collegiate Athletic Association (NCAA) to restrict or ban certain agents. Table 13-4 lists common anti-asthma medications and whether therapeutic use is permitted, restricted, or banned.[33]

PRE-COMPETITION EXERCISE-INDUCED BRONCHOSPASM PREVENTION PROCEDURE

To minimize the risk of developing EIB during competition, the athlete should premedicate with an inhaled beta$_2$-adrenergic agonist, such as albuterol or salmeterol, and/or a mast cell membrane stabilizer, such as cromolyn or nedocromil, 15 to 45 min before the pre-competition warm-up. The warm-up should start 30 to 60 min before the competition with 10 to 15 min of stretching exercises, followed by 5 to 15 min of light aerobic exercise at 50 to 60 percent of the maximum heart rate to induce the "refractory" period. The athlete should then perform a 10 to 30 min cool-down period that includes stretching and walking or other light activity. If necessary, the athlete may then repeat the preventive medication prior to competition, and have the inhaler available for use during prolonged athletic events.

More severe cases of EIB may require that the athlete take inhaled corticosteroids for at least 2 weeks prior to competition to reduce airway inflammation and hyper responsiveness. Allergic rhinitis symptoms should also be controlled with antihistamines, intranasal corticosteroids, and/or intranasal mast cell membrane stabilizers.

Table 13-5

Stepwise Approach for Managing Asthma in Adults and Children Older than 5 Years

SEVERITY OF ASTHMA	LONG-TERM CONTROL	QUICK RELIEF
Step 4 Severe persistent	High-dose inhaled CS* **AND** Long-acting bronchodilator** **AND** Oral CS	Short-acting inhaled B2AA*** for symptoms
Step 3 Moderate persistent	Medium-dose inhaled CS **OR** Low-medium inhaled CS **AND** Long-acting bronchodilator	Short-acting inhaled B2AA for symptoms
Step 2 Mild persistent	Low-dose inhaled CS **OR** Cromolyn/nedocromil (may alternatively consider theophylline or leukotriene antagonist)	Short-acting inhaled B2AA for symptoms
Step 1 Mild intermittent	No daily medication needed	Short-acting inhaled B2AA for symptoms

*CS = corticosteroid.
**Long-acting bronchodilator, e.g., long-acting inhaled beta$_2$-agonist, sustained-release theophylline, or long-acting beta$_2$-tablets.
***B2AA = beta$_2$-adrenergic agonist.
SOURCE: Adapted with permission from NIH National Asthma Education and Prevention Program. Expert panel report 2: Guidelines for the diagnosis and management of asthma.

Conditions to Refer

Patients should be referred to an asthma specialist for consultation or to assist with patient management if there are difficulties achieving or maintaining control of asthma, in the presence of severe persistent asthma (NIH Pharmacologic step 4 treatment), or, possibly, for moderate persistent asthma (NIH Pharmacologic step 3 treatment) (Table 13-5).[33] Individuals with severe atopic disease that is inadequately controlled with antihistamines and/or intranasal corticosteroid therapy may require referral to an allergy specialist to consider immunotherapy desensitization. Patients with suspected vocal cord dysfunction by clinical history or failure of improvement with EIB treatment should be evaluated by a specialist using flexible fiberoptic rhinolaryngoscopy to visualize the vocal cord function. Persons with symptoms consistent with possible cardiovascular disease may need cardiovascular consultation and evaluation.

References

1. Sly RM: History of exercise-induced asthma. *Med Sci Sports Exerc* 18:314, 1986.
2. American Academy of Pediatrics: Exercise and the asthmatic child. *Pediatrics* 84:392, 1989.
3. Helenius IJ, Tikkanen HO, Haahtela T: Occurrence of exercise induced bronchospasm in elite runners: Dependence on atopy and exposure to cold air and pollen. *Br J Sports Med* 32:125, 1998.
4. Kukafka DS, DM Lang, S Porter, et al: Exercise-induced bronchospasm in high school athletes via a free running test: Incidence and epidemiology. *Chest* 114:1613, 1998.
5. Hofstra WB, Sterk PJ, Neijens HJ, et al: Prolonged recovery from exercise-induced asthma with increasing age in childhood. *Pediatr Pulmonol* 20:177, 1995.
6. MacFarlane PI, Heaf DP: Pulmonary functioning children with neonatal meconium aspiration syndrome. *Arch Dis Child* 63:368, 1988.
7. Hallstrand TS, Ault KA, Bates PW, et al: Peripheral blood manifestations of T(H)$_2$ lymphocyte activation in stable atopic asthma and during exercise-induced bronchospasm. *Ann Allergy Asthma Immunol* 80:424, 1998.
8. Randolph C, Fraser B, Matasavage C: The free running athletic screening test as a screening test for exercise-induced asthma in high school. *Allergy Asthma Proc* 18:93, 1997.
9. Rundell KN, Wilber RL, Szmedra L, et al: Exercise-induced asthma screening of elite athletes: Field versus laboratory exercise challenge. *Med Sci Sports Exerc* 32:309, 2000.
10. Mahler DA: Exercise-induced asthma. *Med Sci Sports Exerc* 25:554, 1993.
11. National Institute of Health (NIH): *National Asthma Education and Prevention Program. Expert Panel Report 2: Guidelines for the Diagnosis and Management of asthma.* Publication No. 974051. April 1997; 8,13,31.
12. Kayani S, Shannon DC: Vocal cord dysfunction associated with exercise in adolescent girls. *Chest* 113:540, 1998.
13. Landwehr LP, Wood RP, Blager FB, et al: Vocal cord dysfunction mimicking exercise-induced bronchospasm in adolescents. *Pediatrics* 98:971, 1996.
14. McFadden ER, Zawadki DK: Vocal cord dysfunction masquerading as exercise-induced asthma. A physiologic cause for "choking" during athletic activities. *Am J Respir Crit Care Med* 153:942, 1996.
15. Bevelqua F, Schicchii JS, Haas F, et al: Aortic arch anomaly presenting as exercise-induced asthma. *Am Rev Respir Dis* 140:805, 1989.
16. McFadden ER, Gilbert IA: Exercise-induced asthma. *New Engl J Med* 330:1362, 1994.
17. Bronsky EA, Spector SL, Pearlman DS: Albuterol aerosol versus albuterol Rotacaps in exercise-induced bronchospasm in children. *J Asthma* 32:207, 1995.
18. Blake K, Pearlman DS, Scott C, Wang Y, et al: Prevention of exercise-induced bronchospasm in pediatric asthma patients: a comparison of salmeterol powder with albuterol. *Ann Allergy Asthma Immunol* 82:205, 1999.
19. Finn AF, Thompson CM, Banov CH, et al: Beta$_2$-

agonist induced ventricular dysrhythmias secondary to hyper excitable conduction system in the absence of long QT syndrome. *Ann Allergy Asthma Immunol* 78:230, 1997.

20. Inman MD, O'Byrne PM: The effect of regular inhaled albuterol on exercise-induced bronchoconstriction. *Am J Respir Crit Care Med* 153:65, 1996.

21. Reiss TF, Hill JB, Harman E, et al: Increased urinary excretion of LTE4 after exercise and attenuation of exercise-induced bronchospasm by montelukast, a cysteinyl leukotriene receptor antagonist. *Thorax* 52:1030, 1997.

22. Meltzer SS, Hasday JD, Chon J, et al: Inhibition of exercise-induced bronchospasm by zileuton: A 5-lipoxygenase inhibitor. *Am J Respir Crit Care Med* 153:93315, 1996.

23. Adelroth E, Inman MD, Summers E, et al: Prolonged protection against exercise-induced bronchoconstriction by the leukotriene D4-receptor antagonist cinalukast. *J Allergy Clin Immunol* 99:210, 1997.

24. Corren J: Allergic rhinitis and asthma: how important is the link? *J Allergy Clin Immunol* 99:S781, 1997.

25. Roizin H, Reshef A, Katz I: Atopy, bronchial hyper responsiveness, and peak flow variability in children with mild occasional wheezing. *Thorax* 51:272, 1996.

26. Pierson WE, Furukawa CT, Shapiro CT, et al: Terfenadine blockade of exercise-induced bronchospasm. *Ann Allergy* 63:461, 1989.

27. Garrigo J, DantaI, Ahmed T: Time course of the protective effect of inhaled heparin on exercise-induced asthma. *Am J Respir Crit Care Med* 153:1702, 1996.

28. Melo RE, Sole D, Napspitz CK: Comparative efficacy of inhaled furosemide and disodium cromoglycate in the treatment of exercise-induced asthma in children. *J Allergy Clin Immunol* 99:204, 1997.

29. Novembre E, Frongia G, Lombardi E, et al: The preventive effect and duration of action of two doses of inhaled furosemide on exercise-induced asthma in children. *J Allergy Clin Immunol* 96:906, 1995.

30. Shimizu T, Mochizuki H, Shigeta M, et al: Effect of inhaled indomethacin on exercise-induced bronchoconstriction in children with asthma. *Am J Respir Crit Care Med* 155:170, 1997.

31. Massey KL, Harman E, Hendeles L: Duration of protection of calcium channel blockers against exercise-induced bronchospasm: Comparison of oral diltiazem and inhaled gallopamil. *Eur J Clin Pharmacol* 34:555, 1988.

32. Cohen HA, Neuman I, Nahum H: Blocking effect of vitamin C in exercise-induced asthma. *Arch Pediatr Adolesc Med* 151:367, 1997.

33. Fuentes RJ, Rosenberg JM (eds). *Athletic Drug Reference '99*, 8th ed. Durham: Glaxo-Wellcome Inc; 1999;225.

Daniel V. Vigil

Heat Illness

Introduction

The production of heat by exercising muscle goes hand-in-hand with aerobic exercise. This production of heat can sometimes lead to elevation in core body temperature that can impair athletic performance or even jeopardize health. With more people taking part in traditional sports such as bicycling and running, participants of all levels should be aware of these heat-generating effects. Medical personnel who care for these athletes must also be able to recognize the warning signs of heat injury and intervene properly.

While runners and cyclists have become faster and stronger in their traditional disciplines, a new wave of athletes, in their quest for greater athletic challenges, has established new and increasingly popular sports such as triathlon and adventure racing. The level of participation inthese new sports reflects the emergence of a new generation of sports enthusiasts who seek athletic achievement in the form of highly demanding endurance and ultra-endurance competitions.

The demand created by this new breed of athletes has not only led to a greater number of marathons, ultra-marathons, and triathlons, but these competitions have also evolved in the physical demands they place on the athlete. Once regarded as inadvisable and perhaps even dangerous, participation in the Ironman Triathlon World Championship, with its 90° heat and accompanying humidity, is now regarded by many as the pinnacle of competition in triathlon and the privilege of competing in this event is highly sought. This is only one example in the growing number of events being conducted in extreme conditions.

Athletes training for these events are faced with a unique challenge: the quest for athletic achievement while balancing physiologically detrimental heat *accumulation* with performance-sustaining heat *dissipation*.

Temperature Homeostasis During Exercise

Human beings are homeotherms, whose normal physiologic functions depend on a core body temperature that varies only 1° to 2°C, even when ambient temperature fluctuates widely. During exercise, excess heat is generated, which leads to elevated core body temperature. However, at any single level of activity, the range of core body temperature variability is consistently small (Fig. 14-1).[1] During exercise, this means that the body must effectively dissipate both heat produced by muscular contraction and that acquired from the environment. Thermoregulation of this precision requires a delicate balance of heat production, heat accumulation, and heat dissipation.

Figure 14-1 shows how core body temperature responds to two of these parameters. As workload increases, more heat is produced. As ambient temperature increases, more heat is accumulated. Hyperthermia can result from an increase in either parameter, or from a combination of the two. The graph in Fig. 14-1 also illustrates the core body temperatures achieved during exertion that are well tolerated by the exercising individual (39° to 40°C). Highly trained athletes are able to tolerate higher core body temperatures, and for longer periods of time, than less well trained individuals.

If core body temperature rises above these tolerable levels, however, performance will suffer and health may become jeopardized. Therefore, this excess heat must be dissipated. The major mechanism of heat loss is through sweat evaporation, and depending on the ambient

Figure 14-1

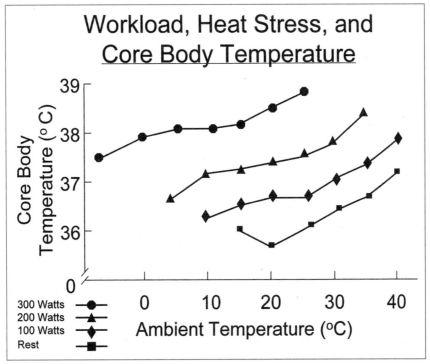

Workload, heat stress, and core body temperature. Esophageal temperature after 2 h of exercise at different exercise intensities. *(Adapted with permission from data in Nielsen B, Kaciuba-Uscilko H. Temperature regulation in exercise. In: Blatteis CM (ed): Physiology and Pathophysiology of Temperature Regulation. Singapore: World Scientific Publishing Co. Pte. Ltd., 1998; 128.)*

conditions, heat may be gained or lost through conduction, convection, and radiation. These mechanisms are considered individually.

Conduction

Heat transfer through a non-moving material is a property of physics known as conduction. Conduction is important during exercise because metabolic heat produced by physical activity must be transferred from the core to the skin surface. This form of heat dissipation occurs as heat energy is transferred directly from tissues and organs deep within the core to more superficial tissues nearer to the skin. This requires that the energy be transferred between tissues that are in direct contact with one another. Once the heat reaches the skin surface, conductive heat loss may continue if the temperature of the skin is greater than the motionless environment with which it is in contact. Therefore, as soon as ambient temperature exceeds skin temperature, conductive heat loss becomes ineffective as a means of warding off hyperthermia during exercise.

Once excess heat has reached the skin surface, its dissipation by conduction becomes highly dependent on whether the environment is air or water. Air has a very low thermal conductivity. This means that conduction of heat energy through air occurs at a very low rate. In contrast, water has a thermal conductivity more than 20 times that of air, resulting in a much higher rate of heat transfer at the same temperature. This is why running in an air temperature of 65°F is quite comfortable, while swimming in 65° water is not. (Loss of heat to 65° water occurs quickly and efficiently, leading to excessive body cooling). An understanding of this principle allows one to readily recognize why immersion in cool water is a highly effective means of treating the severely hyperthermic athlete.

Convection

Like conduction, convective heat exchange requires direct contact. In contrast to conduction, however, convective heat dissipation involves the transfer of heat between two bodies that are in motion relative to one another. One of the heat-exchanging bodies is typically fluid.

During exercise, heat exchange by convection is readily recognized as a cool breeze or cool water current that passes over the athlete's skin. As the fluid of lower temperature passes over the warmer surface, heat moves along a temperature gradient and is carried away. Also operating is the convection occurring within the body of the athlete. Cooled blood returning from the skin surface circulates through exercising muscles and the body core. This perfusing blood acts as the cooler fluid that accepts heat as it passes over and through metabolically active structures. Upon its return to the skin surface, this heated blood may transfer its heat energy to the environment by a combination of conduction and convection.

Radiation

Radiation refers to heat transfer from warmer to cooler areas along a gradient. Radiation does not require direct contact as heat moves from one object to another. Even in a vacuum heat will move along a temperature gradient in the form of short-wave solar radiation and infrared radiation. On a clear, sunny day human skin is estimated to absorb approximately 60 percent of the sun's shorter wave, ultraviolet radiation while the other 40 percent is reflected. Longer wave, infrared radiation is almost totally absorbed by the skin. This phenomenon does not necessarily work against the athlete because infrared heat exchange is an equilibrating process in which heat may be generously liberated *from* the athlete *to* the environment if such a temperature gradient is present.

Evaporation

As a group, conduction, convection, and radiation are referred to as mechanisms of non-evaporative or "dry" heat transfer. In a thermoneutral environment, a person at rest might experience up to 75 percent of his or her environmental heat exchange as dry heat transfer; the other 25 percent is through evaporation of perspiration and evaporation from the humidified air of the respiratory system (insensible fluid losses). During exercise, however, heat dissipation by dry heat transfer is quickly overwhelmed by the large amount of heat energy emanating from the body core. Furthermore, if exercise is undertaken in an environment with a temperature that is greater than skin temperature, evaporation of sweat is the body's only means of heat dissipation.

The vaporization of water leads to the liberation of 580 calories per mL. This large potential for heat dissipation allows conditioned athletes to tolerate large amounts of heat production within their active muscles, even when exercising in hot environments. As skin and core temperature rise, eccrine sweat glands are activated which secrete sweat onto the skin surface. Well-conditioned athletes may produce in excess of 2 L of sweat per hour. As this water evaporates, more than 1100 kcal of heat energy is liberated from the body.

DEHYDRATION

As sweat evaporates from the body in response to environmental heat stress, a state of dehydration results. This is characterized by serum hyperosmolality and hypernatremia. Physiologically, a state of hypovolemia results, which leads to hypotension and decreased cardiac output. These physiologic changes are unavoidable consequences of the body's absolute requirement for excess heat dissipation. Therefore, thermoregulation and fluid homeostasis are intrinsically related. The physiologic responses to dehydration include activation of the renin-angiotensin-aldosterone (RAA) system, secretion of antidiuretic hormone (ADH), and stimulation of thirst.

The RAA system remedies dehydration by first, stimulating systemic vasoconstriction. This leads to augmentation of blood pressure, which enhances cardiac output. Secondly, cardiac output is enhanced by the RAA system's effect on the kidneys, which is to stimulate sodium reabsorption, thereby augmenting circulating blood volume. Physiologically speaking, this system is a sensor of volume status and is sensitive to very small fluctuations in fluid balance. As such, it becomes active during the earliest stages of dehydration.

Hyperosmolality and hypernatremia are sensed by the hypothalamic-pituitary axis. The response is secretion of ADH, also known as arginine vasopressin, from the posterior pituitary. Also a potent vasoconstrictor, ADH acts on the kidneys' distal collecting tubule to stimulate water reabsorption. As a result, blood pressure and circulating blood volume are directly augmented. Like the RAA system, sensitivity to changes in sodium concentration and osmolality by the ADH secretion system is quite high and response to these changes is very rapid.

Thirst is much less efficient in responding to, and correcting, fluid loss. The thirst center is located in the hypothalamus and is sensitive to changes in osmolality. However, the individual may not sense thirst until more than 5 percent of body mass has been lost as evaporated sweat. One evolutionary reason for this might be the fact that ingested fluid requires several minutes to hours to equilibrate throughout the body. Delayed thirst might be a protective mechanism against inadvertent over-hydration. For the athlete, this presents the problem of trying to maintain a state of euhydration without the input of "physiologic information." Furthermore, the athlete must have access to water in order to make use of thirst. This is not always immediately possible during practice and/or competition.

Acclimatization

When an individual native to a cool, temperate environment moves to a hotter and perhaps more humid environment, heat intolerance is quickly observed. Difficulty staying cool, decreased energy level, and more rapid onset of fatigue with exercise are common findings. After a period of time this intolerance decreases and exercise capacity approaches its level in the cooler environment. This phenomenon has been shown not to be a training effect but rather an adaptation to the hot environment that occurs over a predictable amount of time. This process is referred to as acclimatization if it occurs in a natural environment and acclimation if observed in a controlled setting such as a laboratory.

Because skin temperature is elevated in a hotter environment, a smaller gradient for heat exchange exists which requires higher cutaneous perfusion to dissipate the excess heat. This stress accounts for the higher heart rate and higher core body temperature seen in the unacclimatized individual. The response to this stress is a higher sweat rate and a lower threshold for the onset of sweating. The secreted sweat is also modified, becoming lower in sodium content and more hypotonic. Renal sodium conservation is also seen, which contributes to expansion of plasma volume. These changes account for the lower heart rate, enhanced sweating response, and overall improved thermoregulation seen in the heat-acclimated individual. The process is usually complete within 7 to 10 days in the trained athlete and up to 75 percent of the process is complete within 5 days.[2]

High levels of physical fitness can lend some degree of acclimation to the heat, but exposure to heat induces the adaptation most effectively. By simply resting in the new hot environment, heat acclimatization can occur to a small extent. The process is certainly accelerated by repeated bouts of exercise in the heat. Daily bouts of 60 to 90 min of moderate aerobic exercise seem to be the most effective. For athletes preparing for competition with expected high heat conditions, acclimatization training beginning at least 5 days prior to the event is recommended.

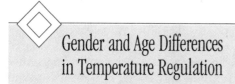

Gender and Age Differences in Temperature Regulation

Because protection against hyperthermia during exercise is highly dependent on the ability to secrete adequate quantities of sweat, individuals with different sweating capabilities will have correspondingly different tolerances to heat stress. The young, athletic, adult male serves as our point of reference in this discussion because most available scientific data represents this population. Individuals thought to have different heat tolerances are children, women, and the elderly.

Children

The most obvious difference between a child and an adult is the difference in body size. Two important measurements, body surface area and mass, describe this size difference. The relationship between these two measurements is known as surface area-to-mass (SAM) ratio. When considered individually, each of these measurements shows that children are smaller than adults. Their surface area, expressed in square meters (m^2), as well as their mass, measured in kilograms (kg), is smaller. The differences in these parameters between children and adults are not proportionate, however.

Until adolescence, children have a larger SAM ratio than adults. An athletic, adult male who measures 180 cm in height and 70 kg in weight might have a SAM ratio of 1.87 m^2 per 70 kg (.027 m^2 kg^{-1}), whereas a 10-year-old child measuring 140 cm in height and weighing 35 kg would have a ratio of 1.17 m^2 per 35 kg (.033 m^2 kg^{-1}). Because the rate of heat exchange between the body and the environment is proportional to body surface area, it becomes readily apparent that a child's body core is heated more quickly when exposed to warmer ambient temperatures, and similarly, is cooled more quickly when exposed to cooler temperatures.

In a hot environment, this detrimental characteristic is amplified by the fact that, for reasons still unclear, children generate more metabolic heat per kg body mass than adults during a given level of exercise. The difficulty in dissipating this excess metabolic heat is even more striking if the child is exercising in a hot environment for the first time. Whereas acclimatization to exercise in the heat is thought to take 7 to 10 days for adults, children may require twice as long.[3]

When environmental temperature is higher than skin temperature, the child's only defense against hyperthermia is the evaporation of sweat. The child's sweating mechanism is different than an adult's. Children have been found to have a higher number of heat-activated sweat glands per unit area of skin. However, each of these individual sweat glands has such a lower rate of sweat secretion that the total sweat rate per unit surface area is less than an adult's. Furthermore, the core temperature at which sweating begins is often higher in children than adults.

In theory, these characteristics would place children at a much higher risk of hyperthermia than adults, when in fact, children thermoregulate quite effectively. Moderate heat stress does not appear to impair performance of short duration, even when the activity is performed at high intensity. A protective mechanism, proposed by some investigators, hypothesizes that a child's lower sweat output may actually be more efficient. This may be due to smaller droplets of sweat, which are spaced closely together and evaporate more readily than an adult male's sweat. This sweat, which is typically seen as larger, more copious droplets, are as likely to drip off the skin as they are to evaporate.

Scientific research regarding the effects of prolonged exercise in extreme heat in children is sparse. Given a child's limited physiologic reserve, risk of hyperthermia is thought to be higher. Because sweat evaporation, with resultant dehydration, is the only operative mechanism for heat dissipation under these conditions, children must hydrate adequately before exercise and they must be encouraged to drink fluids to replace their losses during exercise. This practice should be actively implemented because children's thirst, as in adults, has a significant time delay relative to actual onset of dehydration. Even when thirsty, children given free access to fluids do not consume enough to correct their dehydration.

Women

It is well known that, controlling for body mass and surface area, women do not sweat as much as men. This is true despite the observation that women have an equal number of heat-activated sweat glands as men. At first glance, one is tempted to quickly dispense with this observation as another physiologic difference attributable to the effects of testosterone and estrogen.

A study in 1960 strengthened this hypothesis by demonstrating that exogenous testosterone had a sudorific (sweat-producing) effect, whereas supplemental estradiol had an inhibitory effect on sweating.[4] In studies of women during various phases of the menstrual cycle, however, this same estrogenic trend has not been documented.

The hypothesized variation in sweat rate during the menstrual cycle stems from the fact that the normal menstrual cycle has a characteristic biphasic surge in estrogen secretion. When athletically fit women are exposed to neutral and hot environments during the follicular, luteal, and menstrual phases of the menstrual cycle, sweat rate and evaporative heat loss do not differ. Similarly, differences in peak elevations in rectal temperature and mean skin temperature have not been demonstrated. Elevation of basal body temperature during the luteal phase, associated with elevated progesterone levels, also has not been shown to impair thermoregulation in exercising women or in women exposed to hot environments. Women appear to thermoregulate with equal efficiency during the various phases of the menstrual cycle.[5]

Comparison of thermoregulation in women versus men is a methodologically difficult task. Inherent differences in strength require that the exercise protocol be standardized for either workload or level of exertion. Even if subjects are matched for age, height, weight, and athletic fitness, the same exercise bout cannot be used for a comparative study. For this reason, data are sparse. In the few available studies, it appears that men and women achieve similar absolute peak core body temperatures at various levels of environmental heat stress. Women also seem to acclimatize to a similar degree and over a similar period of time as men. An interesting difference however, is that men show a greater increase in oxygen uptake (VO_2) as they experience greater heat stress. This parallels the observation that men are generally more prolific sweaters than women. While the answer is not known, could it be that women sweat less because they are more efficient in dissipating heat by other cardiovascular mechanisms?

Elderly

Older individuals do not comprise a homogeneous population simply by virtue of being older than some arbitrary age. Chronologic age is easy to identify and is often used to categorize individuals. "Physiologic" age, however, might be a more useful, albeit more difficult to quantify, perspective from which to evaluate the mature athlete. This is a reasonable consideration because we often see "elderly" individuals who function as if they were much younger, and similarly, many people younger than 65 years of age who are debilitated as if they were much older. This inconsistency in the aging process makes study of thermoregulation in the older athlete difficult. Consequently, literature is sparse. Some of the individual modes of heat dissipation have been studied, however.

Sweat production is lower in older subjects compared to their younger counterparts. This is true despite the fact that the density of heat-activated sweat glands seems to be similar among people of various ages. This suggests a declining ability of each gland to produce sweat as people grow older. By extrapolation, older athletes may be more prone to heat stress as their mechanism for evaporative heat loss becomes overwhelmed.

With this in mind, these individuals should be made aware of strategies to reduce the risk of thermal stress.

Heat Illnesses

Heat Cramps

First described in the 1920s among heavy laborers, heat cramps have been defined as diffuse muscular tetany affecting the calves, thighs, and muscles of the abdominal wall. They seem to occur more often in athletes during the latter stages of a strenuous athletic event, often under hot conditions. Because of this association, the mechanism of this severe cramping historically has been thought to be related to dehydration, sodium loss, and muscle fatigue. As the athlete sweats to stay cool, water and sodium are lost, creating a state of hypovolemia and hypernatremia that affects electrical depolarization within myocytes. Recent studies in marathon runners, however, have shown no difference in serum electrolyte concentrations or changes in plasma volume among runners who develop cramps and those who do not.[6]

Because the mechanism of cramping remains ill defined, treatment of muscle cramps currently includes a wide variety of interventions. Stretch and massage of the affected muscle is a frequently employed sideline technique that often proves effective. Athletes who cannot immediately seek medical assistance, such as marathon runners or open water swimmers, have resorted to contraction of antagonistic muscle groups to impart elongation and stretch of the cramped muscle. Remedies, such as increasing dietary salt in the days prior to an athletic event, or even drinking a dilute solution of salt water at the onset of cramping, have been advocated.[7] As a corollary, some believe that an intravenous infusion of saline is indicated in the treatment of severe cramping. The use of intravenous benzodiazepines, such as diazepam, in the treatment of refractory muscle cramps has also been reported.[8] Success with these practices is purely anecdotal and conclusive scientific evidence for their efficacy is lacking. Their efficacy is based on the experience of the individual practitioner.

Clinical experience tells us that muscle cramps certainly occur during prolonged physical activity, but we also see them during shorter bouts and even among individuals at rest. Clinically, identical cramping has been seen in swimmers emerging from a cold ocean swim just as in athletes competing under hot, humid land conditions. This suggests that the cause of cramping is more fundamental and due to something inherent within the muscle. Further research is needed to address this hypothesis. In the meantime, prevention of cramps continues to include proper stretching, adequate hydration, and maintaining a high level of physical fitness.

Heat Exhaustion and Heat Strain

Of all heat illnesses, this group of conditions is the most difficult to define. Some authorities believe heat exhaustion to be a predecessor of the certainly dangerous condition, heat stroke. Others find the description of heat exhaustion so arbitrary that its very existence is questioned.

The heat-exhausted athlete has postural hypotension, tachycardia, and a moderately elevated (38° to 40°C) core body temperature. Clinical signs and symptoms include hyperventilation, piloerection, loss of coordination, headache, paresthesias, dizziness, nausea, and confusion. The key point that makes understanding this condition difficult is the fact that core body temperature is usually not significantly higher than in asymptomatic athletes undergoing the same intensity of exercise.[9,10] Because dehydration has often been thought to be a contributing factor, athletes presenting with this constellation of findings should be removed from participation, evaluated for evidence of heat illness, placed in a cool environment, and given free access to chilled oral fluids.

The suspicion that heat exhaustion or its experimentally induced relative, heat strain, will progress to heat stroke if not treated, has not been demonstrated. A published report of 12-years experience at the Twin Cities Marathon shows that athletes evaluated for exhaustion and collapse were not substantially more dehydrated than their well counterparts, and neither were they more hyperthermic.[9] After prolonged competition, most athletes will become dehydrated to some degree. If this is not sufficient to cause the previously mentioned findings, then some other mechanisms must be operative. Some pos-

sibilities include lack of an available energy source such as glycogen, or a transient central nervous system dysfunction such as autonomic dysfunction or a hypothalamic temperature dysregulation. Further research is needed to test these hypotheses.

Exercise-Associated Collapse (Heat Syncope)

Athletes who collapse during the course of exercise or shortly after the cessation of exercise are said to suffer from exercise-associated collapse (EAC). EAC does not include cardiopulmonary failure, insulin reaction/hypoglycemia, seizures, or other commonly identified medical etiologies. Historically, this clinical entity has been termed heat syncope when it occurs in a hot environment. The problem with this terminology is the observation that collapsed athletes are not always hyperthermic. Because it describes the phenomenon more accurately, *exercise-associated collapse* is the preferentially used term.

As a result of the seminal paper by Wyndham and Strydom in 1969, sports medicine physicians have traditionally been taught that EAC is secondary to hypovolemia that is a direct consequence of dehydration.[11] This school of thought also suggests that dehydration leads to impaired heat dissipation such that EAC is a disorder that occurs along a spectrum of thermal injury that culminates in potentially lethal heat stroke if left untreated. For these reasons, a central component in treating EAC is rapid cooling plus aggressive rehydration, usually with oral fluids, but often with intravenous fluids. Recent research, however, suggests that this physiologic explanation is flawed, and that this treatment approach may be inappropriate or even dangerous in some athletes.

Athletes who collapse in association with exercise most often do so at the end of the exercise bout or shortly after its conclusion.[12] The timing of such episodes requires that postural hypotension be considered as a possible etiology. When an athlete makes that final push for the finish line or goal line then suddenly stops, blood immediately begins to pool in the dilated venous beds of the lower extremities. Since the lower limb musculature is no longer forcefully contracting, cardiac preload is acutely decreased. The resultant decreased cardiac output may manifest as syncope. Because presyncopal, or frankly syncopal, athletes often fully recover after assuming a horizontal (or Trendelenburg) position, this physiologic phenomenon is likely the cause of many cases of EAC.

The role of hyperthermia in EAC continues to spark debate among experts. It is plausible that mild to moderate hyperthermia (38 to 40°C) could cause central nervous system dysfunction resulting in incoordination, confusion, and/or muscular weakness resulting in a syncopal event. Although this is often suspected anecdotally, the current literature does not support this association in the majority of cases. Consider again the Twin Cities Marathon data. This is an event held in an environment with an ambient temperature range from 41° to 68°F as many runners are crossing the finish line, yet clinical EAC among these athletes is similar to that reported at the Two Oceans Ultramarathon, which is con-

tested under much warmer conditions. In fact, the majority (85 percent) of EAC cases reported in the Two Oceans data occurred after the affected athletes crossed the finish line (and began the cooling down process). The 15 percent who collapsed before finishing the event all had readily identifiable medical conditions that ruled out a diagnosis of EAC.[10]

EAC is a multifactorial clinical entity, which usually occurs upon the cessation of exercise. The clinician evaluating an affected individual must keep an open mind regarding the differential diagnosis and must not assume that every collapsed athlete is dehydrated and hyperthermic. Arriving at an accurate diagnosis begins with a rapid yet thorough physical examination, which includes measurement of vital signs, assessment of hydration status, and evaluation of mental status and neurologic function. Roberts developed a classification system for EAC that helps direct management based on the severity of these clinical findings (Table 14-1).[8]

From a practical standpoint, the system begins with evaluation of cognitive function, motor ability, and ability to take oral fluids. At endurance

Table 14-1

Classification of Exercise-Associated Collapse

CLASS	MILD	MODERATE	SEVERE
Hyperthermic	Temp ≥ 103°F, CNS normal, walks with or without help	Temp ≥ 105°F, CNS normal, or no oral intake, or dehydrated, or unable to walk, or severe muscle spasm	Temp ≥ 106°F, + CNS changes
Normothermic	Temp < 103°F, CNS normal, walks with or without help	97°F < Temp < 103°F, CNS normal, or no oral intake, or dehydrated, or unable to walk, or severe muscle spasm	97°F < Temp < 103°F, + CNS changes
Hypothermic	Temp ≤ 97°F, CNS normal, walks with or without help	Temp ≤ 95°F, CNS normal, or no oral intake, or dehydrated, or unable to walk, or severe muscle spasm	Temp ≤ 90°F, or CNS changes

competitions, this evaluation is initiated by event volunteers stationed in the finishing area who are responsible for greeting athletes as they complete their competition. If EAC appears imminent, assistance should be given to prevent injury from falls. Evaluation of mental status may begin simultaneously as the athlete is assisted through the finishing area or off the playing field. Engaging the athlete in simple conversation usually allows rapid assessment of cognition. If mental status changes are noted, such as confusion, disorientation, agitation, or frank loss of consciousness, transfer of the athlete to the medical area for evaluation should be expedited. If the athlete has no presyncopal symptoms, such as lightheadedness or dizziness, he or she should be encouraged to continue walking so that lower extremity muscle contraction can continue to help maintain cardiac preload and cerebral perfusion. This walk should continue at least to the medical tent where, if necessary, the athlete can assume a recumbent or Trendelenburg position in an area of cool shade and adequate observation. When EAC presents as muscle spasm or tetany, walking may not be possible. In this instance, the athlete should be assisted to the medical tent where supine positioning will help maintain cerebral perfusion while medical personnel attend to the muscle spasms.

Once the athlete has arrived at the medical tent, EAC must then be categorized as either hyperthermic, normothermic, or hypothermic. This must be determined by measurement of rectal temperature. Oral temperature is notoriously unreliable due to the athlete's difficulty with maintaining proper thermometer position, and to the effect of cold beverages on the temperature of the oral cavity. Axillary and tympanic membrane temperatures are also unreliable because they are measurements of shell temperature and not core body temperature. Because hypothermic athletes competing in relatively warm weather have been described, it cannot be assumed that a victim of EAC is hyperthermic. In

warm environments, these chilled athletes may be effectively warmed with lightweight, foil-like wraps known as space blankets. To complete the documentation of vital signs, orthostatic measurement of pulse rate and blood pressure should be done.

Classification of signs and symptoms in this fashion allows for a more precise diagnosis. Tailored treatment may then address temperature correction, fluid replacement, fuel replacement, muscle cramp treatment, and finally, a decision regarding transfer or discharge from the medical area. Fig. 14-2 schematically illustrates the management of the athlete presenting with EAC. As in any clinical setting, medical documentation should be meticulous. Fig. 14-3 depicts an easily applied encounter form that documents the pertinent aspects of an athlete's clinical course in the medical tent.[8]

Heat Stroke

Exertional heat stroke (EHS) must be considered when an athlete manifests significant changes in mentation in association with a rectal temperature in excess of 41°C. By definition, affected individuals are profoundly hyperthermic. Neurologic symptoms may vary, however. Many of these athletes present with exercise-associated collapse, but the continuum of suspicious changes in mental function include irritability, confusion, stupor, seizure, and coma. Since increasing core body temperature and declining mental function occur over a period of time, various combinations of signs and symptoms may be seen. Dehydration may or may not be present, and affected athletes are often sweating on presentation.

Since the hallmark finding in EHS is a markedly elevated core body temperature, rectal temperature must be measured in anyone suspected of the disorder. Prompt diagnosis is of paramount importance because morbidity is directly proportional to peak core temperature and the length of time spent in the severely

Figure 14-2

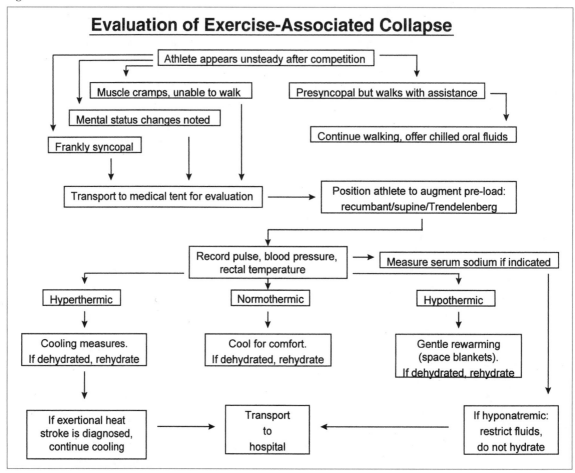

Evaluation of Exercise-Associated Collapse

Evaluation of exercise-associated collapse (EAC). Suggested algorithm illustrating the sequential assessment of the athlete with EAC.

hyperthermic state. Widespread cellular damage resulting in rhabdomyolysis, disseminated intravascular coagulation, and multisystem organ failure may be seen. To minimize these potential complications, treatment must be initiated immediately on-site.

Due to the much higher thermal conductivity of water compared to air, cool water immersion is thought to be the most effective method of rapid cooling.[13] This may not be practical if seizure activity is noted or if the athlete is unco-

operative due to confusion. In these instances, other useful methods include application of ice packs to the neck, axillae, and groin. Evaporative techniques such as fanning and wet towel wrapping may be helpful but are slower and much less effective in humid environments.

Aggressive cooling measures should be continued until the rectal temperature falls to 38°C, in order to prevent over-cooling. Once heatstroke is diagnosed and cooling measures have begun, transport to an emergency department is

Figure 14-3A

Medical Record

Event Name: _____ Date: _____

Uniform/Race Bib No. _____ Arrival time: _____

Name: _____ Discharge time: _____

Age: _____ Sex: ☐ Male ☐ Female

Finish time: _____ ☐ Did not finish Best previous time: _____

Previous marathons: Entered: _____ Finished: _____

Weekly mileage: _____

Premarathon injury or illness? ☐ Yes ☐ No

Describe: _____

Skin, Bones, and Joints

Complaint: ☐ Blister ☐ Pain ☐ Bleeding
           ☐ Other: _____

Tissue: ☐ Skin ☐ Muscle ☐ Ligament ☐ Tendon ☐ Bone
        ☐ Other: _____

Location: Foot ☐ R ☐ L Thigh ☐ R ☐ L
           Ankle ☐ R ☐ L Hip ☐ R ☐ L
           Calf ☐ R ☐ L Back ☐ R ☐ L
           Knee ☐ R ☐ L Other: _____

Diagnosis: ☐ Blister ☐ Hematoma
           ☐ Sprain ☐ Abrasion
           ☐ Strain ☐ Stress fracture (suspected)
           ☐ Bursitis ☐ Other: _____
           ☐ Fasciitis

           Notes: _____

_____

_____

_____

_____

Casualty encounter record. Medical record for documentation of casualties seen in an athletic event medical tent. *(Adapted with permission from Roberts WO: Exercise-associated collapse in endurance events: a classification system. Phys Sport Med 17:49, 1989).*

usually indicated. Cooling should continue during transportation.

The endogenous production of heat during exercise added to environmental heat stress makes EHS a distinct entity. The resulting variability in presenting signs and symptoms distinguishes EHS from classic heatstroke, which is characterized by the triad of hyperthermia, anhidrosis, and altered mental status. Classic heatstroke most commonly affects the frail and

Figure 14-3B

Time of admission: _____

Signs and	☐ Exhaustion	☐ Headache	☐ Vomiting
Symptoms:	☐ Fatigue	☐ Nausea	☐ Diarrhea
	☐ Hot or Fever	☐ Stomach cramps	☐ Unconscious
	☐ Cold/chilled	☐ Leg cramps	☐ CNS changes _____
	☐ Lightheaded	☐ Rapid heart rate	
	☐ Confused	☐ Leg spasms	
	☐ Other: _____		

Mental status: ☐ Alert ☐ Lethargic ☐ Responds to:_____

Orientation: ☐ Person ☐ Place ☐ Time

Walking status: ☐ Alone ☐ With assistance ☐ Unable

☐ Other: _____

Vital signs and Treatment:	Time	Rectal Temp	Blood Pressure	Pulse Rate	IV Solution Infused	Medications Prescribed

Notes:				
	IV Fluid	☐ Yes	☐ No	☐ Other:_____
	D50W IV	☐ Yes	☐ No	
	Transfer to ER	☐ Yes	☐ No	
	Discharge to home	☐ Yes	☐ No	

Diagnosis

EAC		Mild	Moderate	Severe
Category:	Hyperthermic	☐	☐	☐
	Normothermic	☐	☐	☐
	Hypothermic	☐	☐	☐
	Other: _____			

Time of discharge: _____

Casualty encounter record. Medical record for documentation of casualties seen in an athletic event medical tent. *(Adapted with permission from Roberts WO: Exercise-associated collapse in endurance events: a classification system. Phys Sport Med 17:49, 1989).*

elderly during summertime heat waves in urban areas.

Exertional heatstroke has also been compared to the syndrome of malignant hyperthermia (MH). MH is a pharmacogenetic muscular disorder in which muscular rigidity and hypermetabolism lead to hyperthermia and its sequelae. Anesthetic gases and curare are the usual pharmacologic triggering agents. Dantrolene sodium is used as an effective treatment. Although profound hyperthermia is seen in both EHS and MH, other metabolic similarities have not been consistently shown. Dantrolene sodium is ineffective in the treatment of EHS.[14]

The Role of Hydration During Exercise

Athletes who experience a decline in performance during prolonged activity or who suffer from metabolic disturbances such as muscle cramps are often presumed to be dehydrated and hyperthermic. The association between dehydration and rectal temperature rise has been interpreted by many as a cause-and-effect relationship, and is now widely accepted and incorporated into the management of exercise in the heat. These athletes are typically offered copious oral rehydration, and if their symptoms are more advanced, intravenous rehydration has been advocated. This approach is based on two scientific beliefs: (1) dehydration leads to hyperthermia, and (2) dehydration impairs athletic performance. The first belief arose from a study of core body temperature rise in elite marathon runners.

In 1969, Wyndham and Strydom published their landmark paper titled, "The danger of inadequate water intake during marathon running."[11] They concluded that dehydration occurring during distance running is the main determinant of core body temperature elevation, which is the underlying problem in heat injury during exercise. This conclusion was based on the observed linear relationship between level of dehydration and the athletes' postexercise rectal temperatures. Ironically, the runners in the study with the highest rectal temperatures were those who performed best (i.e., the top finishers). These runners drank less and sweated more as they ran faster than their competition. No particular dangers were identified in these runners as the title suggests. In fact, the most dehydrated runners demonstrated an impressive tolerance to low fluid intake while exercising at a very high level. Similar rectal temperature elevations are seen in athletes exercising at higher aerobic levels but of

much shorter duration.[15] Athletes are quite capable of generating tremendous amounts of metabolic heat before significant dehydration is apparent. In other words, core body temperature is directly related to relative workload as measured by percent VO_{2max}, and indirectly related to percent dehydration.

Water loss has been more conclusively shown to be detrimental to exercise performance. A linear relationship between percent dehydration and work capacity has been shown. Dehydration of as little as 1 to 2 percent of body weight may result in performance decrease of up to 40 percent during high intensity exercise.[16] This is likely due to decreased circulating plasma volume, which leads to a diminished ability to deliver substrate to working muscle and an impaired ability to carry away excess heat. For this reason, oral rehydration during exercise is now widely accepted as a method for preserving optimal performance and limiting decline of work output.

The composition of the optimal rehydration solution has been studied. Since fluid loss during exercise is primarily due to the loss of hypotonic sweat, rehydration begins with replacement of this loss. Sweat is mostly water. Therefore, water is usually an adequate fluid choice during most activities lasting 1 hour or less. For longer events, solutions containing carbohydrates and electrolytes are preferred.

Electrolyte solutions have been shown to be beneficial during exercise. Although the presence of sodium, potassium, and chloride in a drink have no clear link to thermoregulation, or even to performance enhancement, they seem to enhance the process of rehydration. A dilute sodium solution of 25 to 50 mmol/L increases palatability and leads to increased voluntary ingestion. This is not a small point because thirst is known to be a poor indicator of dehydration because the desire to drink is often delayed. Similarly, thirst is often quenched before fluid loss is fully replaced.

Palatability is further enhanced by the addition of carbohydrate. The optimal concentration seems to be 6 to 7 percent (60 to 70 g/L), which provides palatability while promoting gastric emptying and intestinal absorption of both water and energy substrate.[17] Early studies suggested that gastric emptying and intestinal absorption were promoted by chilled fluids. The most recent investigations have not conclusively shown this; however, a cold drink on a hot day can be quite refreshing while offering a psychological boost.[18]

Because sweat rate may vary from 1 to 3 L/hr, athletes are encouraged to drink 500 to 1,000 cc/hr while exercising. It is best to ingest small amounts at frequent intervals, such as 100 to 200 cc every 10 to 20 min. For the "average sweater," this is sufficient to prevent significant dehydration. If one sweats in excess of 1.5 L/hr, the task of adequate fluid replacement becomes more difficult. Ingestion of more than 1,000 cc per hour leads to gastrointestinal distress in some athletes.

While dehydration is a far more common finding among athletes competing in the heat, it must be noted, however, that over-hydration resulting in hyponatremia has been reported in athletes competing in ultramarathons and triathlons.[12] As the emphasis on oral rehydration during endurance events has grown in recent years, some athletes have become overzealous in their fluid consumption during prolonged competition. The hyponatremia seen in these athletes is, therefore, thought to be secondary to water intoxication. Some investigators have postulated that a total body deficit of sodium due to sweat losses contributes to the hyponatremia, however, symptomatic athletes typically present with findings suggestive of volume overload, such as weight gain during the course of the event, and the voiding of dilute urine. Symptomatic athletes may present with altered mental status, EAC, or they may be frankly unconscious. If these symptoms are accompanied by a dilute urine and a rectal temperature that is not significantly elevated, symptomatic hyponatremia

should be considered. In this instance, serum sodium must be measured. Without this assessment, the care of such an athlete may erroneously include hydration, which could lead to further lowering of the serum sodium concentration, which could then increase the risk of neurologic complications. Athletes with symptomatic hyponatremia must be fluid-restricted and their transfer to a hospital expedited (see Fig. 14-2).[20]

Medical Management of Competition in the Heat

When organizing medical care for an event contested in the heat, knowledge of the environmental conditions is essential in estimating risk of heat stress among the competitors. Specifically, the wet-bulb globe-temperature (WBGT) is the most widely used index of thermal stress. Expressed mathematically:

$$WBGT = 0.7\ T_{wb} + 0.2\ T_g + 0.1\ T_{db}$$

T_{wb} (wet-bulb temperature) refers to the temperature measured by a bulb thermometer wrapped in a water-saturated cloth wick. T_{wb} is measured in direct sunlight and is a reflection of heat stress imparted by humidity. T_g (globe temperature) is measured by a dry bulb thermometer enclosed within a black copper sphere. Also measured in direct sunlight, T_g is a measure of radiant heat stress. T_{db} (dry-bulb temperature) is measured by a dry bulb thermometer exposed to ambient air but shielded from direct sunlight. T_{db} is a measure of ambient temperature. The large effect of humidity on heat stress can be readily seen, as it accounts for 70 percent of the index whereas ambient temperature accounts for only 10 percent. For this reason, ambient temperature alone is inadequate in assessing environmental heat stress.

Table 14-2

Suggested Applications of WBGT

WBGT RANGE	RECOMMENDATION
15–18°C (59–65°F)	Low risk of heat illness. Provide adequate hydration.
18–23°C (65–73°F)	Moderate risk of heat illness. Provide ample hydration. Inform competitors of conditions with general announcements before and during competition.
23–28°C (73–82°F)	High risk of heat illness. Provide ample hydration. Emphasize heat stress conditions in race registration packet if possible. Announce heat stress index and implications throughout event. Encourage hydration and heat illness prevention.
>28°C (82°F)	Very high risk of heat illness. Postpone event until conditions are favorable.

Although prevention of hyperthermia cannot be guaranteed, a WBGT range of 15° to 18°C (59° to 65°F) is associated with a low risk of heat illness. When WBGT is between 18° and 23°C (65° to 73°F), risk of heat illness is moderate. High risk for heat illness or even heat stroke is considered when WBGT reaches 23° to 28°C (73° to 82°F). With this degree of heat stress, competitors should be made aware of the risk and instructed on the importance of hydration and cooling during the competition. Water stops, aid stations, and event support should be reviewed with the athletes before the start of the competition. Individuals who are prone to heat illness probably should not compete under these high-risk conditions. If the WBGT exceeds 28°C (82°F), the risk of thermal injury and heat stroke is very high. Postponement of the event should be considered until more favorable conditions prevail (Table 14-2).[19]

If a WBGT measurement is not available at the start of competition, an estimation of heat illness risk may be made based on ambient temperature and relative humidity, two measurements that are usually readily available. Figure 14-4 illustrates the inverse relationship of heat stress tolerance between ambient temperature (dry-bulb temperature) and relative humidity.[19]

The best efforts at prevention of heat-related injury would not reduce the incidence to zero.

Therefore, on-site medical officers at athletic events must be prepared to evaluate and treat victims of heat stress. Because diagnosis begins with documentation of rectal temperature, facilities for making this measurement must be available. The triage area is easily adapted for this by the use of portable partitions or by the construction of a separate, temporary room that affords the necessary measure of privacy.[20] If cooling measures are indicated, equipment for the rapid initiation of treatment should be easily accessed. This includes water, ice, ice packs, and tubs for cool water immersion. Recall the very high thermal conductivity of water, which makes immersion an extremely effective method of cooling. Should an athlete require evacuation to an emergency medical facility, a mechanism should be in place for its efficient implementation. Activation of the local emergency medical service (EMS, 911) by cellular telephone may be sufficient, or an on-site ambulance may be arranged before the event begins. Cooling measures and rehydration should not be delayed while transportation is being arranged.

Chilled oral rehydration solutions should be offered to individuals who are conscious and alert. If the athlete is unable to drink or if significant dehydration is noted, intravenous (IV) access should be considered and proper equipment for IV therapy should be readily available.

Figure 14-4

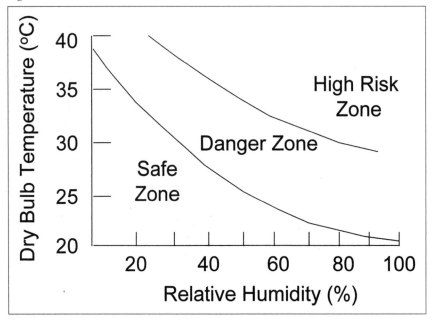

Environmental heat stress. Risk of heat illness while competing in hot environments may be estimated from ambient (dry bulb) temperature and relative humidity. *(Adapted with permission from data in Armstrong LE, Epstein Y, Greenleaf JE, et al: Heat and cold illnesses during distance running. American College of Sports Medicine Position Stand. Med Sci Sports Exerc 28:i, 1996.)*

Intravenous fluids commonly used include 5 percent dextrose in either 0.45 percent saline or 0.9 percent saline. Intravenous fluid therapy should be physician-supervised. Even when IV therapy is needed, the vast majority of athletes recover fully from heat illness without long term or permanent sequelae.

References

1. Nielsen B, Kaciuba-Uscilko H: Temperature regulation in exercise, In: Blatteis CM (ed): *Physiology and Pathophysiology of Temperature Regulation.* Singapore: World Scientific Publishing Co. Pte. Ltd., 1998;128.
2. Sawka MN, Wenger CB, Pandolf KB: Thermoregulatory responses to acute exercise-heat stress and heat acclimation, In: Fregly MJ, Blatteis CM (eds): *Handbook of Physiology: Environmental Physiology.* New York: Oxford University Press; 1996.
3. Bar-Or O: Children's responses to exercise in hot climates: Implications for performance and health. *Sports Science Exchange* 7:1, 1994.
4. Kawahata A: Sex differences in sweating, In: Yoshimura H, et al (eds): *Essential Problems in Climatic Physiology.* Kyoto, Japan: Nankada Publishing Company, Ltd.; 1960;169.
5. Bar-Or O:. Effects of age and gender on sweating pattern during exercise. *Int J Sport Med* 19:S106, 1998.
6. Noakes TD: Fluid and electrolyte disturbances in heat illness. *Int J Sport Med* 19:S146, 1998.
7. Eichner ER: Treatment of suspected heat illness. *Int J Sport Med* 19:S150, 1998.
8. Roberts WO: Exercise-associated collapse in endurance events: A classification system. *Phys Sport Med* 17:49, 1989.
9. Roberts WO: A 12-year summary of Twin Cities

Marathon injury. *Med Sci Sports Exerc* 28(Suppl):S123, 1996.

10. Holtzhausen LM, Noakes TD, Kroning B, et al: Clinical and biochemical characteristics of collapsed ultramarathon runners. *Med Sci Sports Exerc* 26:1095, 1994.

11. Wyndham CH, Strydom NB: The danger of an inadequate water intake during marathon running. *S Afr Med J* 43:893, 1969.

12. Noakes TD: Dehydration during exercise: What are the real dangers? *Clin J Sport Med* 5:123, 1995.

13. Armstrong LE, Crago AE, Adams R, et al: Whole body cooling of hyperthermic runners: Comparison of two field therapies. *Am J Emerg Med* 14:355, 1996.

14. Bourdon L, Canini F: On the nature of the link between malignant hyperthermia and exertional heatstroke. *Med Hypoth* 45:268, 1995.

15. Saltin B, Hermannsen L: Esophageal, rectal and muscle temperature during exercise. *J Appl Physiol* 21:1757, 1966.

16. Walsh RM, Noakes TD, Hawley JA, et al: Impaired high-intensity cycling performance time at low levels of dehydration. *Int J Sports Med* 15:392, 1994.

17. Murray R: Rehydration strategies—Balancing substrate, fluid, and electrolyte provision. *Int J Sport Med* 19:S133, 1998.

18. Brouns F: Gastric emptying as a regulatory factor in fluid uptake. *Int J Sport Med* 19:S125, 1998.

19. Armstrong LE, Epstein Y, Greenleaf JE, et al: Heat and cold illnesses during distance running. American College of Sports Medicine Position Stand. *Med Sci Sports Exerc* 28:i, 1996.

20. Holtzhausen LM, Noakes TD: Collapsed ultraendurance athlete: Proposed mechanisms and an approach to management. *Clin J Sport Med* 7:292, 1997.

John McShane
Eugene Hong
Jennifer M. Naticchia

Chapter
15

Concussion

Definition

In 1892, Sir William Osler, renowned as one of the most astute observers of the human condition, described a syndrome he referred to as "traumatic neurasthenia." He stated that this condition "succeeds a shock or concussion" and that "[a] slight blow, a fall from a carriage or on the stairs may suffice." He gave the following description:

> The patient complains of headache and tired feelings. He is sleepless and finds himself unable to concentrate his attention properly upon his work. . . . the entire mental attitude of the person may for a time be changed. He may complain of numbness and tingling in the extremities. . . . The reflexes are slightly increased . . . The pupils may be unequal . . ."[1]

This may be one of the first modern descriptions of concussion. Of note is how consistent Osler's description of the condition is with our current understanding of concussion. It is also interesting to see that he observed that it only takes "a slight blow" to produce the condition.

In terms of describing the effects of concussion, not much has changed since Osler's description in 1892. In fact, it is only in the past few years that there has come to be even the most basic understanding of the pathophysiologic effects of sustaining a concussion.

The definition of concussion has been modified only slightly over the years. In 1952, *The New Gould Medical Dictionary* gave this definition of concussion:

> A condition produced by a fall or blow on the head, and marked by unconsciousness, feeble pulse, cold skin, pallor, at times the involuntary discharge of feces and urine; this is followed by partial stupor, vomiting, headache, and eventual recovery. In severe cases, inflammation of the brain or a condition of feeblemindedness may follow.

In 1982, *Steadman's Medical Dictionary* defined concussion as:

> A clinical syndrome, due to mechanical forces, characterized by immediate and transient impairment of neural function, such as alteration of consciousness, disturbance of vision and equilibrium, etc.

Most recently, the American Academy of Neurology defined concussion as:

> Concussion is a trauma-induced alteration in mental status that may or may not involve the loss of consciousness. Confusion and amnesia are the hallmarks of concussion.[2]

It is interesting to note that each of these definitions describes a mechanism and symptoms, but none of them describes in any way the pathophysiology of the disorder. Whereas the signs and symptoms of the condition may be varied, perhaps the most important thing to understand about concussion, and which is implied in all of the above descriptions, is that it results from a traumatic injury to the brain.

Incidence

The true incidence of concussion is extremely difficult to determine. This is due to a variety of factors. To begin with, there is great inconsistency in the definition of concussion that is applied from one clinician to another. It is also impossible to know how many concussive injuries go unreported by athletes who either do not understand the significance of the injury or who fear being precluded from participation.

Concussion has been reported to be the most common head injury in athletics.[3] Higher-risk sports include football, ice hockey, boxing, wrestling, and soccer; incidence rates in one recent study of high school athletes ranged from 0.92 to 1.58 to 3.66 per 100 player-seasons for boys' soccer, wrestling, and football respectively.[4] Even some non-contact sports, such as gymnastics, baseball, and cycling, pose a risk for concussion.

In 1983, Gerberich et al surveyed Minnesota high school football players, and described a concussion incidence of 19 per 100 players over one season.[5] They also found that players with a prior history of loss of consciousness had a four-fold increase in risk of subsequent loss of consciousness, when compared to players with no prior history.

Extrapolating from their figures, Gerberich et al estimated that there are 250,000 concussions yearly in high school football players in the United States. Since the study was first reported, these figures have been cited in the majority of papers that have described concussion incidence in the United States. Unfortunately, these numbers may be flawed for the same reasons noted previously. Because the information was self-reported, rather than objectively observed, the athletes' abilities to accurately recall the injuries may have varied. In addition, their understanding of what events actually constituted a concussion may not have been fully accurate. Also, it is difficult to know if the definition that would be used today would change the incidence. Finally, the figure of 250,000 per year is based on the assumption that the rates in Minnesota are the same as in the rest of the country, a concept that has not been verified.

A recent study of high school athletes, polled from schools across the country, projected a yearly incidence of over 62,000 concussions for all high school players participating in 10 representative sports. Football accounted for more than 60 percent of all concussions in the study.[4] It has been estimated that 10 percent of college football players will have a concussion in a given season, and that 40 percent of all these athletes will have at least one concussion

in their high school and college careers combined.[6]

Regardless of whether the actual number of concussions is at the higher or lower end of these estimates, clearly this rate of mild traumatic brain injury in youth sports programs presents a significant public health concern.

Mechanism and Pathophysiology

Concussion does not require a direct blow to the head; it also can result from indirect forces to the brain. Indirect forces can be linear or rotational in nature because either can cause shearing forces to the brain; these are forces that are parallel to the surface plane of the tissue. Brain cells appear to be particularly susceptible to injury by shearing forces.

From a physiologic standpoint, the brain cells remain in a state of increased vulnerability after trauma has occurred. Depending on the severity of the injury, this state may last from several days to as long as a week or more. In animal models, this period of vulnerability is characterized by increased sensitivity to minor changes in the brain tissue environment (e.g., blood flow, pressure, or oxygenation). This state of metabolic dysfunction results in an increased demand for glucose by the brain, accompanied by an as yet unexplained reduction in cerebral blood flow. In later stages, there is an overall metabolic depression. The reduction in blood flow may be due to vasoconstriction from accumulation of Ca^{++} released in response to injury; this metabolic imbalance has also been observed in more severe human head injuries.[7] So, although the trauma causing a concussion may not result in direct anatomic change or damage to the brain, the post-traumatic state is one of heightened susceptibility to injury of the brain cells.

Signs and Symptoms

References to having one's "bell rung," or suffering a "ding" are common in sports. Athletes may not be aware that they have suffered a concussion. Amnesia is a hallmark of concussion. As part of the post-concussive symptoms, athletes may even forget the inciting traumatic event. It is up to the observer to be aware, and to look for the player whose only sign of head injury may be heading for the wrong huddle or seeming to have forgotten the plays.

Typical signs of a concussion are confusion, disorientation, change in speech or coordination, vacant stare, memory loss, emotional lability, and, occasionally, a loss of consciousness. The early symptoms that may be reported include headache, dizziness, nausea, difficulty with concentration, lack of balance, and vision disturbance. These symptoms may become persistent and be associated with decreased attention span, memory problems, depressed mood, irritability, sleep disturbance, changes in vision and hearing, and decreased libido.[8]

Diagnosis and Evaluation

Initial evaluation of a head injury begins with the A, B, C's—assessing airway, breathing, and circulation. An unconscious athlete will be obvious, but what may not be so evident is whether there was a brief loss of consciousness prior to assessment by the trainer or physician. Those nearby, such as teammates and officials, can be questioned regarding this issue, as it may make a difference in the assessment and management of the injured player. The head-injured player

may not be able to recall any loss of consciousness.

In any incident of head trauma, always evaluate for the possibility of an injury to the cervical spine. This evaluation should take place immediately after the "A, B, C's" and levels of consciousness are assessed. An unconscious player should always be assumed to have a neck injury, and the cervical spine is immobilized before the player is transported. Be wary of the player who is afraid or refuses to turn the head for the examination; this may indicate a cervical spine injury.

Once the cervical spine has been evaluated and it is determined that it is safe to move the athlete, further evaluation can take place off of the field of play. Sideline assessment includes further evaluation and observation over time. At this point, the examiner should perform a more thorough neurologic examination including assessment of the cranial nerves, gross motor strength, coordination, and Romberg testing.

Cognitive function should be evaluated including orientation, short- and long-term memory, and the ability to concentrate. Orientation can be assessed, not only by asking for person, place, and time, but also the score of the game, who the opponent is, what particular play was last called, and what period the game is in. Short-term memory may be tested by having the athlete repeat three words that are given, and then recalling them approximately 5 min later. Counting backwards from 100 by seven or reciting the months in reverse order are ways to assess concentration ability.

After the first assessment, the athlete should be re-evaluated at regular intervals, observing for improvement, persistence, or deterioration of the person's condition. During this period of observation and re-evaluation, the player may very likely want to return to the game. If this is the case, consider taking a necessary piece of equipment from the player, such as a shoe or helmet, to prevent premature return to play.

In those individuals whose signs and symptoms resolve quickly, further provocative testing should be performed before a final return-to-play decision is made. This should include some form of physical exertion, such as sprinting, doing push-ups, sit-ups, and deep-knee bends. Observe and re-examine for any signs or symptoms of concussion. If symptoms recur with this testing, then the player should continue to be monitored and withheld from play.

In any individual who has sustained a concussion, the possibility of other injury needs to be considered. This differential diagnosis of head injury includes, but is not limited to, skull fracture, epidural hematoma, subdural hematoma, intracranial hemorrhage, diffuse axonal injury, and second impact syndrome (described later in this chapter). These conditions should be considered during the time of evaluation to avoid missing a more emergent or severe traumatic brain injury. Immediate transport to a hospital should be considered for any player with sustained loss of consciousness, worsening mental status, suspected cervical spine injury, or physician discomfort with the player's condition on the sideline.

Grading Concussion

The medical literature contains as many as 20 different protocols for evaluating concussion. Each of these systems is based entirely on the presence of particular signs and symptoms and how long after the initial injury these signs and symptoms persist. There is no grading system that even attempts to correlate the actual pathophysiology of the injury with its severity. Instead, these systems are based on the particular author's attempt to interpret what has been observed clinically. In this regard, even the most respected grading systems available today are not much more advanced than Osler's initial description in 1892.

Torg and Nelson described grades of concussion in 1982 and 1984, respectively. Later, in 1986, Cantu proposed a grading system that was adopted by the American College of Sports Medicine. In 1991, the Colorado Medical Society described its own grading system; this was later modified and adapted by the American Academy of Neurology (AAN) in 1997, and published as a practice parameters summary statement. This latest grading classification by the AAN incorporates a conservative approach to cumulative advances in understanding concussions. Listed in Table 15-1 are the grades and the criteria for each grade of one of the most widely used classification systems, the AAN guidelines.[2]

Regardless of which classification system is used, there must be some assessment of the severity of a concussion as part of the evaluation of the player. The different systems all use an assessment of mental status (amnesia, confusion, or any change in sensorium), level of consciousness, and duration of symptoms to define the criteria for severity. Obviously, the importance of grading the severity is that the grade in turn will help to manage the injured athlete, including return-to-play decisions. Incorporating a classification system into the evaluation assists in making consistent clinical decisions based on evidence regarding diagnosis and management of the injured athlete.

Table 15-1

American Academy of Neurology (1997) Definitions of the Three Different Grades of Concussion

GRADE	DEFINITION
I	No loss of consciousness, concussion symptoms resolve in less than 15 min
II	No loss of consciousness, symptoms last longer than 15 min
III	Any loss of consciousness, subdivided into brief (sec) and prolonged (min)

Management and Return to Play

Just as there is no one universally accepted grading system, there is no definitive management algorithm based on the evidence of randomized controlled trials. There are, however, several principles in the management of a player with a concussion that most experts agree upon.

First and foremost is the almost universally shared opinion that no player should be allowed to return to play while still having symptoms from a concussion, including symptoms that recur after exertional testing on the sidelines. Second, it is felt by many that loss of consciousness generally indicates a more serious brain injury, and therefore should preclude permitting the injured player to return to play. Third, a period of rest for the brain is indicated in cases where the symptoms do not resolve within minutes. The importance of this has been observed by physiologic changes in animal models and in cases of severely head-injured humans.[7] The lack of consensus among guidelines reflects the fact that there is essentially no evidence indicating that outcomes are better using one protocol compared to another. There is expert opinion shaped by what is known about the diagnosis and management of concussion, but no conclusive outcome-based evidence. The management and return-to-play guidelines as outlined by the AAN can be reviewed in Table 15-2.[2]

There are several aspects of management that are left unclear by nearly all of the previously published guidelines, including those of the AAN. Cases of multiple concussions of varying grades are poorly addressed by most of them. Also, return to play is usually discussed within the time frame of a sports season. There is rarely a reference to situations of back-to-back or overlapping seasons. For example, a concussion occurring during the last week of football season may be of clinical importance to the athlete who starts wrestling the following week. The differences in guidelines, their incompleteness, and the lack of universal acceptance all highlight the fact that there is inadequate scientific evidence on which to base clinical decision making in the area of sports related concussions.

In spite of the fact that existing knowledge does not provide for clearly defined protocols, the clinician is still faced with the problem of treating athletes who suffer concussions. It seems prudent, therefore, to take what is known, combine it with those aspects of published guidelines that make the most intuitive sense, and formulate an approach that lends itself to consistency and is appropriately protective of the injured athlete. What follows then is one such approach. It must be emphasized that this is not intended to be a guideline; it is, rather, one of several reasonable ways to manage concussions in athletes.

When an athlete is identified as having had a concussion, he or she should be withheld from

Table 15-2

American Academy of Neurology (1997) Guidelines for Return to Play after Concussion

GRADE	GUIDELINE
I	Return to play if symptoms resolved in less than 15 min. If second grade I the same day, no return that day and for 1 asymptomatic week.
II	Return after 1 week asymptomatic at rest and with exertion. After second grade II, return after 2 weeks asymptomatic.
III	If briefly unconscious, then return after 1 week asymptomatic. If prolonged, return after 2 weeks asymptomatic at rest and with exertion. After second grade III, return after 1 month asymptomatic.

play and observed for at least 15 min. If symptoms resolve within that time frame (both at rest and with exertion) and there is a normal neurologic examination with no history of loss of consciousness, the injured player may be allowed to return to play that same day. Even if a player is allowed to return the same day, there should continue to be observation and re-evaluation of the player.

A player with any loss of consciousness or symptoms lasting longer than 15 min should be withheld from play that day. A deteriorating clinical condition needs immediate transport to a medical facility, preferably one with neurosurgical consultation and head imaging capability available.

Once withheld from returning that same day, the injured player should be followed and re-examined until all symptoms have resolved. There should be no return to play at least until the individual is entirely symptom free. There are many people who feel that return to play should not be allowed until there have been at least 5 to 7 days without any symptoms. Again, at present, it is not known exactly how long a period of rest is needed in the human brain until vulnerability to further injury is returned to baseline. There may be individual variability and age may have an influence, as well.

Head Imaging

The issue of when to obtain head imaging is clinically driven. As in the other aspects of concussion management, there is no universally accepted guideline. In the immediate time period following the concussion, the player's condition will dictate the need for imaging. Prolonged loss of consciousness, an abnormal neurologic examination, and a deteriorating clinical condition are all relative indications for head imaging with CT or MRI. At the very least, these conditions warrant further medical attention. More difficult is the situation when, a few days

after the traumatic event, the injured athlete still has symptoms—a headache, visual complaints, or poor concentration ability—and a normal physical examination. The American Academy of Neurology recommends that the persistence of symptoms for a week is an indication for head imaging.

Assessment of cognitive changes resulting from a concussion, and other potentially long-term effects, is discussed in the section on neuropsychological testing.

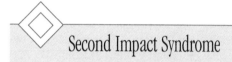

Second Impact Syndrome

There are several consequences of head injury that clinicians should think about when dealing with an athlete who has suffered a concussion. These syndromes can be divided into the acute, short-term, and long-term effects of the injury. Awareness of these conditions should be helpful in managing the injury at the time it occurs, as well as making treatment decisions in the days after the injury.

The first issue that should raise concern in the face of sports-related head injury is the possibility that there has also been an injury that could result in a catastrophic event. For example, attention should always be paid to the status of the cervical spine. This is particularly true when the athlete is unconscious. Any doubt as to the integrity of the cervical spine should lead to stabilizing the victim's neck and transporting to a hospital. Watch for signs of increased intracranial pressure, such as might occur with cerebral bleeding. Vomiting and increasing obtundation are signs that should raise concern.

One of the most alarming events described as being related to head injuries in athletes is the second impact syndrome. The second impact syndrome occurs when an athlete who has sustained an initial head injury, most often a concussion, sustains a second head injury before the pathophysiologic effects of the first injury have fully resolved.[10] As a result, there ensues a rapid onset of cerebral vascular congestion, brainstem herniation, and, ultimately, death. The "second impact" may be relatively minor, such as a light blow to a football helmet, or a push to the trunk that imparts accelerative forces on the brain. The outcome, however, is catastrophic.

The case reports of this syndrome have described a fairly typical clinical presentation.[10,11] After incurring what would otherwise seem to be a rather innocuous blow to the head, the athlete at first may appeared stunned, but remains conscious. Within a few minutes, however, the player collapses and becomes comatose. The pupils dilate and respiratory failure rapidly ensues. Once this has occurred, there is virtually no chance of recovery.

The true etiology of the second impact syndrome is not known. It is believed, however, to involve dysfunction of cerebral vascular autoregulation. This finely tuned system allows the brain to tightly control exactly how much intravascular fluid volume enters and exits the cranial cavity. When this autoregulatory ability is disrupted, fluid homeostasis is no longer maintained and pressure within the brain dramatically increases. Unless this process can be halted, death will ensue within a matter of minutes. Management, therefore, involves rapid intubation, hyperventilation, and administration of an osmotic diuretic.

The exact incidence of the second impact syndrome is difficult to determine, as there are only a handful of cases reported in the medical literature. Of note is the fact that the majority of these cases have been in adolescents. There has never been a case reported among professional football, soccer, or rugby players. In fact, the only cases reported to have occurred in individuals older than 21 years were in boxers and skiers. Given the nature of the brain impacts in these sports, it may be that these cases actually involved another injury altogether.

The reason that this syndrome occurs predominantly in adolescents is unclear. It may be that younger brains do not have the ability to recover from injury as well as those of more mature individuals; this may leave them vulnerable for a longer period of time. From a management perspective, this would then imply that extra caution should be used before returning an adolescent to play after a concussion.

Post-Concussion Syndrome

It is extremely rare for a catastrophic event to occur in association with sports-related head injury. It is, however, common for the athlete who has sustained a concussion to have symptoms lasting for several days after the injury. These symptoms may consist of such things as headache, difficulty concentrating, memory problems, fatigue, irritability, light sensitivity and visual difficulties, among others. In most cases these symptoms gradually subside, and within a matter of days to a couple of weeks, they are completely gone. In certain cases, however, symptoms can last beyond this time frame. When this occurs, the individual is said to be suffering from post-concussion syndrome. This syndrome is characterized by symptoms that result from a concussion, which persist, typically for longer than 4 weeks.[12]

Like concussion itself, and along with the second impact syndrome, the exact pathophysiologic mechanisms involved in the post-concussion syndrome are not well understood. The condition clearly involves an alteration of neuronal metabolic function within the brain. What these biochemical aberrations are, and why they lead to the symptoms described, have not been fully elucidated. It is interesting to note, however, that the spectra of symptoms that occur with this syndrome are relatively identical from one patient to another. This would imply that, regardless of the specific physiologic effects of concussion, the location of the injury within the brain must be fairly similar from one athlete to another.

The management of post-concussion syndrome is largely supportive. Other than rest and time, there is currently no treatment that can reverse the process. In individuals who have prolonged symptoms it is prudent to obtain some form of diagnostic imaging, such as a CT scan or MRI, to exclude intracranial bleeding. In most cases, however, these studies will be normal.

The most important aspect of treating this condition is to avoid another blow to the head. As has been noted, no athlete who has persistent symptoms should be permitted to return to sports until all of those symptoms have resolved.

In individuals who have suffered more significant neurocognitive deficits it may be helpful, if not necessary, for them to enter into formal rehabilitation programs. These programs can be helpful in teaching coping mechanisms, and perhaps can aid the individual in re-learning certain skills that have been lost.

Fortunately, it is quite rare for an athlete who has suffered a concussion to endure long-term difficulties as a result of a single injury. Several studies, however, have shown that repeated concussions may have cumulative effects, especially when these injuries occur close together in time. Using sensitive neuropsychological tests, Barth et al have found that subtle neurocognitive deficits, which would normally return to baseline after a single injury, persist for prolonged periods in those athletes who have had repeated injuries.[6] Occasionally, these deficits may be permanent. This may result in memory difficulties, trouble performing complex tasks such as balancing a checkbook or following lengthy directions, or an impaired ability to learn new skills, such as might be needed in a new job.

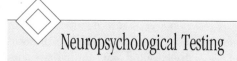

Neuropsychological Testing

Neuropsychological testing has received great attention in recent years as a means to evaluate the neurocognitive effects of a concussion. This testing uses a series of detailed evaluations to provide an assessment of an individual's cognitive abilities.

Neuropsychological testing has been used since World War I to assist in the diagnosis and treatment of traumatic brain injuries. Like most diagnostic testing, neuropsychological testing is best used as an adjunct to the history and physical examination, laboratory tests, and imaging studies when evaluating individuals with traumatic brain injury. Tests that have been developed in adherence with the American Psychological Association's Standards for Educational and Psychological testing have several advantages. These tests allow for a controlled method of examination with guidelines for scoring and interpretation. Because most of these tests are well standardized, clinical and statistical comparisons can be made. The standardization procedures and the reliability and validity of these tests allow investigators to compare observations; estimates of measurement error are provided so that changes in test scores can be interpreted appropriately.[13]

However, neuropsychological testing has some inherent weaknesses. Important variables, such as emotional or affective states, cannot be measured. Skilled interpretation is crucial, as the findings do not automatically indicate why a patient fails to perform a certain task. Another limitation is that neuropsychological tests are time-consuming to administer, and can be expensive. Finally, age, education, and cultural variables can influence a patient's performance.[13]

O'Brien recently published findings of a study

that compared a person's test results with that same individual's estimated level of premorbid intellectual functioning, rather than to age-normative data.[14] He hypothesized that this removed some of the within-group variance attributable to differences in premorbid level of cognitive functioning. In theory, it would be beneficial to have baseline testing prior to an athletic injury; the athlete can then act as his or her own control.

Chouinard and Braun performed a meta-analysis of the relative sensitivity of neuropsychological screening tests in 1993.[15] They determined that it is possible to use a brief battery of tests, a subset of neuropsychological tests, to diagnose early diffuse brain dysfunction; to do so, they concluded, such a test battery would need to assess a wide range of functions and have a high sensitivity.

One of the most widely used subsets of neuropsychological testing being used in athletes today has been pioneered by a group led by Lovell.[7,16] Lovell's selected set of psychological tests appear to demonstrate significant reliability, validity, and repeatability in athletes with concussions. The tests include the following: Trail Making Test—parts A and B, Stroop Test, Digit Span from the Wechsler Memory Scale—Revised, Symbol Digit Modalities Test, Controlled Oral Word Association Test, Hopkins Verbal Learning Test, Letter and Number Sequencing from the Wechsler Memory Scale-III, Grooved Pegboard Test, and Ruff's Figural Fluency Test. These tests assess memory, attention, concentration, mental processing speed, and motor speed.

In settings where neuropsychological testing is to be used, baseline evaluations should be obtained ideally on every player at the beginning of the season as individual performance can vary tremendously. Other factors that may influence neuropsychological testing are learning disabilities and previous concussion—an accurate past medical and injury history should be obtained from the athlete at the time of baseline testing. A

suggested timeline of testing is baseline testing at pre-season, 24 to 48 h after suspected brain injury, and then weekly until testing returns to baseline.[16]

The possibility of computerized versions of neuropsychological testing may make evaluations of brain-injured athletes quicker and less expensive. More research is needed in the area of combining neuropsychological testing with other diagnostic tools such as MRI, spectroscopy, and PET scanning.

Conclusion

A concussion results from a traumatic injury to the brain. Our current understanding of these injuries is currently quite limited; most definitions of concussion are based primarily on the mechanism of injury and the signs and symptoms that are present. The multiple classification systems for concussion described in the literature are based on an evaluation of mental status, the presence or absence of loss of consciousness, and the time course of symptoms. None are correlated with the pathophysiology because this is poorly understood, and there is little outcome-based evidence to determine the optimum management.

In spite of this, there are several principles of assessing and treating athletes with concussions that are nearly universally accepted and deserve highlighting. First, have a consistent approach to the evaluation and management of these injuries. Second, do not allow an athlete to return to play while still symptomatic. Finally, allow the brain the opportunity to rest after an injury.

Further investigation is needed in the areas of pathophysiology, evaluation, and outcome-based evidence for best treatment. As in other sports medicine injuries, prevention remains the best cure. Proper equipment, technique, and education of the athlete can greatly contribute to reducing the incidence of concussions. Health care providers caring for athletes who are involved in contact and collision sports should possess a solid understanding of the issues surrounding the diagnosis and management of concussions. Making an early diagnosis and taking a cautious approach to the management of athletes who have suffered concussions is the best advice. Remember, as has been often said, "you can't ice your brain!"

References

1. Osler W: *The Principles and Practice of Medicine.* New York: D. Appleton and Co., 1892; 981.

2. American Academy of Neurology. Practice parameter: the management of concussion in sports (summary statement). *Neurology* 48:581, 1997.

3. Harmon KG: Assessment and management of concussion in sports. *Am Fam Physician* 60:887, 1999.

4. Powell JW, Barber-Foss KD: Traumatic brain injury in high school athletes. *JAMA* 282:958, 1999.

5. Gerberich SG, Priest JD, Boen JR, et al: Concussion incidences and severity in secondary school varsity football players. *Am J Public Health* 73:1370, 1983.

6. Barth JT, Alves WM, Thomas VR, et al: Mild head injury in sports: neuropsychological sequelae and recovery of function. In: Levin HS, Eisenberg HM, Benton AL (eds): *Mild Head Injury.* New York: Oxford University Press, 1989;257.

7. Wojtys EM, Hovda D, Landry G, et al: Concussion in sports. *Am J Sports Med* 27:676, 1999.

8. Kelly JP, Rosenberg JH: Diagnosis and management of concussion in sports. *Neurology* 48:575, 1997.

9. Jennett B, Teasdale G: Predicting outcome in individuals after severe head injury. *Lancet* 1:1031, 1976.

10. Cantu RC: Second-impact syndrome. *Clin Sports Med* 17:37, 1998.

11. Saunders RL, Harbaugh RE: The second impact in catastrophic contact-sports head trauma. *JAMA* 252:538, 1984.

12. Wilberger JE: Minor head injuries in American football. *Sports Med* 15:338, 1993.

13. Prigatano GP, Redner JE: Uses and abuses of neuropsychological testing in behavioral neurology. *Neurol Clin* 11:219, 1993.

14. O'Brien LF, Godfrey HPD, et al: Determining clinically meaningful cognitive impairment following traumatic brain injury. *N Z Med J* 112:295, 1999.

15. Chouinard MJ, Braun CMJ: A meta-analysis of the relative sensitivity of neuropsychological screening tests. *J Clin Exp Neurol* 15:591, 1993.

16. Lovell M: Neuropsychological assessment of the college football player. *J Head Trauma Rehabil* 13:9, 1998.

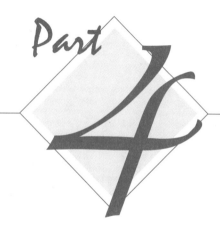

Part 4

Pediatric Problems

Sally S. Harris

Chapter 16

Developmental and Maturational Issues

Introduction

The concept that children are not merely small adults is particularly applicable to the field of pediatric sports medicine. The fact that children are skeletally immature and still growing makes them vulnerable to injuries not seen in adults. Children exhibit different physiologic responses to exercise training and conditioning. The obvious and dramatic physical changes of childhood and adolescence are also accompanied by a variety of developmental changes in other areas, such as motor skill acquisition, cognitive development, and social interaction, that have important implications for safe and appropriate sports participation. This chapter discusses these developmental and maturational changes of childhood and adolescence and their implications for developmentally appropriate sports participation, sports performance, training and conditioning, and injury risk.

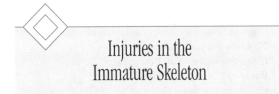

Injuries in the Immature Skeleton

Musculoskeletal injuries in sports typically fall into two categories: (1) acute traumatic injuries (macrotrauma) that occur as a result of a single event such as a fall, blow, or twist; and (2) overuse injuries (microtrauma) that occur insidiously as a result of repetitive musculoskeletal stress, such as occurs with rigorous training. Although overuse injuries used to be considered rare in children, they now account for the majority of sports injuries seen in children. The rise in overuse injuries is thought to be the direct consequence of the rise in organized sports and the repetitive training programs associated with these activities.

Children differ from adults with regard to susceptibility and patterns of sports injuries. Both the presence of growth cartilage and the growth process itself place children at risk for injuries not seen in adults. Growth cartilage occurs at three sites in the immature skeleton: (1) the epiphysis (growth plates); (2) the joint surface (articular cartilage); and (3) the apophysis (secondary growth centers around joints that are the attachment sites of muscles and their tendons) (Fig. 16-1). Both acute injury and overuse injury can occur at all three sites (see Chap. 17 and 18).

The musculoskeletal system appears to be most vulnerable to injury during the adolescent growth spurt, perhaps due to biochemical changes that occur during rapid growth. In addition, rapid bone growth, which occurs during the adolescent growth spurt, results in relative tightness of muscle-tendon units spanning the joints. The resulting diminished flexibility may place the adolescent at increased risk of overuse injury. For these reasons, it may be prudent to decrease the intensity of training during the periods of rapid growth and to place increased

Figure 16-1

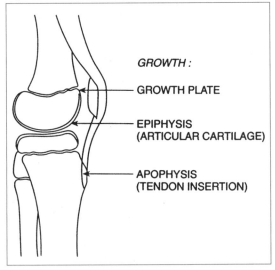

Growth cartilage. *(Reproduced with permission from O'Neill DB, Michele IJ: Overuse injuries in the young athlete. Clinics Sports Med 7:591–596,1988).*

emphasis on stretching exercises to improve flexibility.

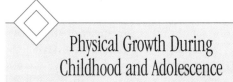

Physical Growth During Childhood and Adolescence

As height, weight, and strength change during childhood and adolescence, potential for sports performance also changes. Childhood represents a period of steady growth of approximately 2.0 to 2.5 in. per year and 5 to 7 lb. per year until the onset of the pubertal growth spurt. Puberty represents a period of accelerated growth, during which time the gain in height and weight may be more than double that of the previous year. Postpubertal growth represents a period of gradual decline in growth rate until final stature is attained at approximately age 15 in girls and age 17 in boys.

During childhood, growth of body dimensions occurs in a disproportionate fashion. In utero, the greatest component of longitudinal growth is growth of the head, whereas during infancy, it is growth of the trunk. After the first year of life through puberty, growth in the legs accounts for the majority of longitudinal growth. In fact, leg length accounts for two-thirds of the growth that occurs during this time. For this reason, late-maturing children have relatively longer limbs and, often, greater height potential, due to a prolonged period of prepubertal growth. Children in the midst of their pubertal growth spurt are often easily identifiable by their appearance of disproportionately long legs. After puberty, there is a period of ongoing slower growth, predominately in the trunk.

A temporary decline in coordination and balance may occur during puberty due to rapid growth. The marked physical changes year-to-year pose a particular challenge for children's participation in seasonal sports. For instance, children participating in baseball may have difficulty adjusting to the fact that their arms have grown several inches longer since last season when they last hit a baseball. Recognizing that children may be unable to perform a skill as effectively as the previous season and allowing them the opportunity for review and practice of previously learned skills can prevent unrealistic expectations, frustrating experiences, and injuries.

Just as growth of body dimensions occurs in a disproportionate fashion, changes in height, weight, strength, and endurance do not occur simultaneously. The adolescent growth spurt is characterized initially by a rapid gain in height. The period of peak height velocity (PHV) occurs on average at age 12 for girls (Tanner stage 2 to 3) and age 14 for boys (Tanner stage 3 to 4), with a standard deviation of 1 year. Menarche in girls is a relatively late pubertal event and occurs on average more than a year after PHV, and therefore serves as a convenient indication of near skeletal maturity. In boys, the period of peak height velocity is followed by a delay of approximately 6 to 14 months by the period of maximum gain in weight. Maximal increases in strength and endurance occur approximately a year after the period of peak height and weight gain. Therefore changes in height, weight, strength, and endurance occur in a serial fashion spanning a period of several years. It should be recognized that adolescent boys who are gaining height rapidly would take several years to fully develop the weight, strength, and endurance that would be expected based on their height. Expectations of sports performance should take these limitations into account.

Physical Mismatch

Since there is much individual variation in physical growth, there may be dramatic disparities in physical size among children of the same age. This disparity is particularly evident among adolescent boys, in whom the age spectrum across which puberty occurs as well as the magnitude of the associated physical changes are greater than they are for girls. Differences in growth and physical development are most evident in boys between the ages of 12 to 16 years. For instance, two 14-year-old boys on the same football team may differ by a foot in height, 100 lb. in weight, and 5 years in bone age. Some boys will enter puberty as young as 12 years old and be physically mature in high school, whereas others will not finish puberty until the end of high school or afterward. Because of the tremendous physical differences between boys of the same age, many authorities feel that participation in sports, particularly contact sports, would be more appropriately matched on the basis of size and maturational stage than on the basis of chronologic age. However, in most settings, it is impractical or considered unacceptable to separate boys of the same age and match boys by maturational stage. It may be prudent to counsel boys who are skeletally immature for their age with regard to the potential risks of injury in competing in contact sports against athletes who are physically more mature.

Gender Differences and Coeducational Sports Participation

Prior to puberty, there are no significant differences between boys and girls in height, weight, strength, endurance, or motor skill development. Therefore, coeducational participation prior to puberty is not thought to place girls at a competitive disadvantage or at increased risk of injury. Children throughout middle childhood can participate equitably in sports and other physical activities on a coeducational basis.

Significant gender differences become apparent at puberty. The pubertal growth spurt occurs 2 years earlier in girls and is less intense than for boys. The 2 additional years of preadolescent growth and the more intense growth spurt that occurs for boys explains their greater height

potential and the more dramatic physical differences seen among pubertal boys than girls. Because girls experience their growth spurts 2 years earlier than boys, there is a brief period, between ages 10 to 12 years, where girls may be temporarily a little taller and heavier than boys their age; however, these differences have little functional significance. During puberty, weight gain in boys is due primarily to an increase in muscle mass, whereas in girls, weight gain is due primarily to an increase in body fat. For instance, a physically mature female carries approximately twice the amount of body fat but only two-thirds the muscle mass per body weight compared to a male (Table 16-1). Therefore, after puberty, girls are at a physical disadvantage relative to boys regarding sports performance, and are unlikely to be able to compete on an equal basis with boys their age in most physical activities and sports requiring strength and endurance.

Pubertal Changes in Boys: Early versus Late Maturation

During the pubertal growth spurt, the physical differences between children, particularly boys of the same age, can be dramatic and have important implications for choice of appropriate sport activities. Early-maturing boys, who begin their pubertal growth spurt ahead of other boys their age, will have a transient physical advantage over their peers because they will be temporarily taller, heavier, and stronger. This should not be misconstrued as superior ability or talent. These boys often achieve the most success in preadolescent sports programs. This can lead to unrealistic expectations that they will continue to be outstanding athletes if it is not recognized that their success is due to advanced physical maturity, rather than exceptional athletic skills. The athletic potential of these boys should be kept in proper perspective, and attempts made for them to participate and compete with boys of similar maturational status. Similarly, late-maturing boys

Table 16-1

Body Composition: Gender Differences

	FEMALES	MALES
Percent body fat		
8-year-old child[40]	23	15
Average college student	25	15
Average college track athlete	10–20	5–10
Percent lean muscle mass		
Age 5[41]	41	42
Age 17[41]	42	53
Adult[40]	36	45

may experience a temporary physical disadvantage in sports that should not be misinterpreted as a lack of talent or ability. Late-maturing boys may have a more positive sports experience if involvement in sports with high priority on size and strength, such as football and basketball, is postponed, and participation is encouraged initially in sports with less emphasis on physical size, such as racquet sports, soccer, martial arts, wrestling, and certain track events.

Pubertal Changes in Girls

For girls, the onset of puberty is associated with physical changes that can lead to declining sports performance. Almost all the weight gain that occurs in girls at puberty is due to an increase in body fat, whereas there is no significant increase in muscle mass. It should be understood that decreased sports performance of girls entering puberty may be due to the pubertal increase in body fat, rather than a lack of motivation, effort, or talent. Girls, parents, and coaches should be counseled to understand and accept the physical changes of puberty. Attempts to prevent these physical changes can lead to excessive dieting and eating disorders. The term "female athlete triad" has been coined to

describe the association of disordered eating, amenorrhea, and osteoporosis, a condition for which female athletes are at increased risk.[1] Increase in body fat as well as the changes in leg alignment that occur during puberty may predispose girls to increased risk of overuse injuries, particularly of the lower extremities. Most of these injuries can be prevented or treated with appropriate evaluation and treatment. Girls entering puberty are at particularly high risk of dropping out of sports and other physical activities. Therefore, anticipatory guidance is particularly important at this time to prevent this attrition.

DELAYED MENARCHE

It is well recognized that athletic girls experience menarche at least 1 to 2 years later than other girls. This has raised the concern that training may adversely affect sexual development and reproductive function. Frisch reported a statistical association of 0.4 years delay in menarche per year of prepubertal training.[2] It remains controversial whether delayed menarche is a direct consequence of athletic activity. More likely, the relationship is a result of selectivity; girls with delayed menarche are perhaps more likely to engage and succeed in sports.[3] This may be due to the fact that girls with delayed menarche typically maintain a prepubertal body habitus longer, characterized by slender physique, narrow hips, long legs, and low body fat composition, that may be advantageous in sports such as track, gymnastics, ballet, and swimming. In boys, on the other hand, there is no evidence of delay of pubertal development associated with sports participation. Boys encounter a situation the opposite to that for girls because traditionally boys' sports, such as football, baseball, and basketball, seem to favor early maturers who are temporarily stronger, heavier, and taller than their later maturing peers.

Mild delays of 1 to 2 years in the onset of menarche are common among adolescent athletes and may be due to a selection process favoring naturally late-maturing girls. More extreme delays in menarche, out of context with family history of age at menarche, are likely to involve a component of nutritional deprivation or endocrinopathy. In the past, menstrual irregularities, such as delayed menarche or secondary amenorrhea (cessation of menstrual periods after menarche has occurred), were thought to occur as a direct consequence of intensive exercise training due to the failure of these girls to attain and maintain a critical level of body fat thought to be needed to initiate and maintain menses. However, research has failed to identify a critical level of body fat needed to initiate and maintain menstrual function. The etiology of these menstrual disorders is thought to be multifactorial and due to an overall "energy drain" situation, where energy intake is inadequate to meet energy demands, resulting in a hypothalamic amenorrhea that appears to be an adaptive response of the body to conserve energy. Contributing factors include low body fat, high training intensity, suboptimal nutrition, physical and emotional stress, history of previous menstrual irregularities, and eating disorders.

Delayed menarche has no effect on ultimate fertility; however, concern exists with regard to the effects on bone density. It is well recognized that athletes with secondary amenorrhea can experience progressive and irreversible loss of bone density due to the associated hypoestrogenic state (see Chap. 12). The loss of bone density places amenorrheic girls at increased risk of stress fractures in the short term, and increased risk of premature osteoporosis in the long term. It is unclear whether delayed menarche has similar long-term effects on bone density. However, studies in young ballet dancers have found that girls with delayed menarche have a delay in bone development and an increased risk of stress fractures and scoliosis.[5] It is unclear whether normal bone density accretion is merely postponed until menses begin, or whether an irreplaceable period of time is lost during which

bone density would normally be increasing. Failure to achieve normal bone density for age due to delayed menarche or amenorrhea is of particular concern for teenage girls because adolescence is a critical period of time during which nearly half of bone density is accrued.[6]

Sports Readiness

Sports readiness addresses the concept of appropriate sports activities for children at various stages of cognitive, social, and motor skill development. A child's readiness to participate in organized sports or structured training sessions depends on a combination of factors: (1) neurodevelopmental level (motor skills acquisition), (2) social development (interaction with coaches and teammates), and (3) cognitive level (ability to understand instructions).[7]

Appropriate sports activities are those for which the individual's cognitive, social, and motor skill development meet the demands of the sport. Just as the clinician should not expect children to run as fast or throw as far as adults, they should not be expected to respond to coaching, interact with teammates, or understand strategies the same way as adults would. In many cases, the developmental limitations of children are overlooked and children are placed in situations where they are expected to mimic adult models of sports participation.

Children who attempt to play sports at a developmental level that is beyond them may have frustrating and unsuccessful experiences. One of the risks of organized sports is that it imposes a structure under which the flexibility for children to play at their own developmental level may be lost. Understanding the developmental appropriateness of children's participation in sports can enable health care providers to advocate appropriate sports activities for children and appropriately advise parents, coaches, and community sports programs.

Motor Skill Development

In addition to appropriate cognitive and social skills, sports readiness requires that motor skill development match the task demands of the sport. Therefore, it is important to understand the pattern of motor skill acquisition in children as it pertains to recreational and sports activities. Nine fundamental motor skills have been identified that form the basic skills required for sports and dance activities.[8] The fundamental skills are throwing, kicking, running, jumping, catching, striking, hopping, skipping, and galloping (Table 16-2). By preschool age, children can perform some of these tasks, but by early elementary school, most children can perform most of these skills. For this reason, age 6 is thought to be an appropriate age for most children to begin organized sports activities, which require performing these skills in various combinations. Prior to age 5 or 6 years, most children do not have the motor skills necessary to perform the skills required for organized sports.

Like developmental milestones of infancy, such as rolling over, sitting up, crawling, and walking, most children follow the same sequence of acquisition of the fundamental

Table 16-2

Fundamental Motor Skills Required for Sports Activities

Throwing
Kicking
Running
Jumping
Catching
Striking
Hopping
Skipping
Galloping

motor skills required for sports. Motor skill acquisition at the most basic levels seems to be an innate process, independent of gender, disabilities, or stage of physical maturity. Like other childhood developmental milestones, the rate at which children master motor skills is highly variable. It cannot be predicted by the age, size, weight, or strength of the child on an individual basis. There is no evidence that a child's subsequent sports ability can be maximized by physical training at a very young age. For example, there is no proof that special training can groom a preschooler to become a future champion. Although it is possible to accelerate the acquisition and refinement of fundamental motor skills by early instruction and practice, children are unlikely to respond until they are developmentally ready.

Although most children will acquire the fundamental motor skills at a basic level naturally through play experiences, instruction and practice are necessary to fully develop fundamental motor skills to their most mature level. Each fundamental skill is comprised of a series of stages of development of that skill.[9] Specific skills can be refined through repetitive practice only after the relevant level of motor development has been reached. Failure to achieve progression through all the stages to the fully mature form can limit proficiency in physical activities that require putting together fully developed fundamental skills into the transitional skills required for most sports activities. "Throwing like a girl" is a common example of failure to acquire the fully developed stage of throwing, and can limit proficiency in a variety of physical activities requiring a throwing or serving motion.

Selection of Developmentally Appropriate Sports Activities

If readiness to participate in specific physical activities cannot be predicted on the basis of age or other specific parameters, how does one determine a child's readiness to learn certain skills or participate in certain sports activities? There is no scientific answer to this question from a neurodevelopmental standpoint. Common sense and experience suggest that sports readiness is best determined on the basis of the child's eagerness to participate and subsequent enjoyment of the activity. When given the opportunity, children will naturally select and modify activities so that they can participate successfully and have fun.

Many sports and physical activities can be tailored to match the developmental level of the child to maximize fun and participation by making simple modifications such as smaller balls, smaller fields, shorter duration of games and practices, reduced number of participants playing at the same time, frequent changing of positions, and de-emphasis on score keeping. An example of such an adaptation is the game of "T" ball, in which children hit a stationary baseball mounted on a stand, rather than a pitched ball, which would require more advanced visual tracking skills.

Selection of appropriate sports activities for children can be guided by an understanding of the developmental skills and limitations of specific age groups.[10] This information for early childhood (2 to 5 years), mid childhood (6 to 9 years), and late childhood (10 to 12 years) is discussed in more detail as follows.

EARLY CHILDHOOD (2 TO 5 YEARS)

Children in this age group are still learning the fundamental skills and attempts to master these basic skills take up most of the focus of their sports activities. Balance skills are limited because the children are just starting to integrate visual, vestibular, and proprioceptive cues. Vision is not fully mature before ages 6 or 7; children younger than this age are farsighted. Imprecise eye movements limit the ability to track and judge the speed of moving objects, and should not be misinterpreted as a lack of coordination.

Appropriate sports activities are ones that emphasize the fundamental skills that can be performed the same way repeatedly and do not require significant variation of these skills. Examples of such activities include running, swimming, tumbling, throwing, and catching.

Children in the age group learn best by trial and error. Emphasis should be on fun, playfulness, exploration, and experimentation. Instruction should be limited and follow a show-and-tell format. Competition should be avoided, as it does not add anything of value to the experience and may detract.

MID CHILDHOOD (6 TO 9 YEARS)

Children in this age group are continuing to improve the fundamental skills and are beginning to master transitional skills. Transitional skills are fundamental skills performed in various combinations and with variations, such as throwing for distance or accuracy. These are the types of skills required for participation in an organized sports activity. Posture and balance become more automatic and reaction times are quicker. However, limited development of memory and the capacity to make rapid decisions limit the ability to master complex strategies. Vision is almost mature but children still have difficulty determining the directionality of moving objects.

Sports activities for this age group should emphasize fundamental skills and beginning transitional skills. Organized sports that can be played without complex motor skills and strategies, such as entry-level baseball and soccer, are more appropriate than sports such as football that do not lend themselves as easily to adaptation to a more basic level.

Rules of sports should be flexible to promote success, action, and participation. Instruction time should be short. Emphasis should be on skill acquisition rather than winning; therefore, competition should be minimal. Because there are no significant differences between boys and girls in height, weight, strength, endurance, or motor skill development prior to puberty, children in this age group can participate equitably on a coeducational basis.

LATE CHILDHOOD (10 TO 12 YEARS)

Children in this age group have improved transitional skills and are able to master complex motor skills. They have the cognitive ability to understand and remember strategies and rules for sports such as football and basketball. Vision is fully mature. Children of this age are generally ready to participate in most sports activities that require more complex motor and cognitive skills. Emphasis should continue to be on skill development, but can begin to incorporate instruction on tactics and strategy. Most experts feel that skill development, fun, and participation should take priority over competition.

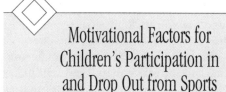

Motivational Factors for Children's Participation in and Drop Out from Sports

It is important for adults organizing sports activities for children to understand the motivational factors for children's participation to ensure that the children's goals and needs are being met. Multiple surveys have shown that the leading motivational factors for children's participation in sports are to have fun, to improve skills and learn new ones, and to be with friends and make new ones.[11,12] Other factors, such as family participation and enthusiastic leadership, are also important. Winning is usually the least important factor; for example, surveys have shown that 90 percent of young athletes would rather play on a losing team than sit on the bench on a winning team.

If the health care provider understands what motivates children's participation in sports, their reasons for dropping out of sports are not surprising. They include interest in other activities; not getting to play enough; skills not improving; boredom and lack of fun due to over-organization and regimentation; and not liking the coach because the coach yells, plays favorites, or is unfair.

It is estimated that by age 15, 75 percent of children who had been involved in organized sports have dropped out. This suggests that many youth sports programs are organized in ways that do not promote the interests of the children, but rather, those of the adults involved. Instead, game structures and adults' expectations for participation and performance should be revised to match the interests and developmental capabilities of the children to provide positive sports experiences during childhood to promote lifelong involvement.

Training and Conditioning

Endurance

Do children have the ability to improve endurance in response to training? For many years, the answer to this question was thought to be "no," because many training studies in children showed little or no improvement in endurance. However, cardiorespiratory profiles of child athletes are superior to those of non-athletic children.

Subsequent research and careful analysis of training studies shows that when training programs meet adult standards (in terms of the intensity, frequency, and duration of the training), most studies in children show improvements in endurance. In addition, children show other adaptations to training similar to those seen in adults, such as lower resting heart rate, decreased submaximal heart rate, increased left ventricular mass, and higher stroke volume with exercise.

However, the magnitude of response of children to endurance training is smaller than that seen in adults. For instance, an endurance training program in adults typically elicits a 25 to 30 percent improvement in $VO_{2\,max}$,[13] compared to an average improvement of 14 percent (range 7 to 26 percent) in children.[14] Certain physiologic factors may limit the response to endurance training in children, such as lower cardiac output, less efficient ventilation due to higher respiratory rate, and lower hemoglobin mass. It is particularly difficult to show a training effect in child athletes as opposed to untrained children, and to distinguish a response to training from the effects of growth alone.

In addition, improvements in endurance in children are not closely related to improvements in physiologic measures of endurance such as maximal aerobic capacity ($VO_{2\,max}$). For example, despite the fact that $VO_{2\,max}$ per kg remains essentially unchanged during childhood, there is a progressive improvement in endurance performance. For instance, a 15-year-old boy can run a mile twice as fast as a 5-year-old boy although their $VO_{2\,max}$ per kg is similar.[15] In children, improvements in endurance performance are due to a variety of other factors irrespective of improvements in $VO_{2\,max}$. These include improvements in economy of motion, technique,

skill, and motivation. In addition, the genetic contribution to endurance potential is significant, as it is estimated that heredity may account for 40 to 60 percent of the variation seen in aerobic capacity ($VO_{2\,max}$).[16] For these reasons, until puberty, endurance training is of limited value in terms of improving cardiorespiratory endurance. Excessive training may contribute to increased risk of overuse injuries, as well as burnout and withdrawal from sports participation. There is some evidence to suggest that the response to endurance training is enhanced during puberty, and that this may be a critical period for optimizing aerobic fitness.[17,18]

Gender differences in measurements of endurance become significant at puberty (Table 16-3). Whereas as absolute $VO_{2\,max}$ rises steadily for boys and girls with childhood growth, it plateaus in girls at menarche while continuing to rise in boys until adulthood. $VO_{2\,max}$ is typically 20 percent greater in males than females after puberty.[19] This gender difference is due in large part, but not completely, to the higher percent body fat and lower muscle mass of females after puberty. Therefore, in sports where the effects of body weight are less, such as swimming and cycling, the performance gap between males and females is narrower than in sports such as running. However, $VO_{2\,max}$ remains 6 percent greater in males even when expressed relative to lean body mass.[19] Other factors beside the differences in body composition, such as lower blood volume, fewer red blood cells, lower

Table 16-3

Strength and Endurance: Relative Gender Differences

MEASURE	AGE	GENDER DIFFERENCE
$VO_{2\,max}$ per body weight	Ages 12–17	Males 20% greater than females[19]
$VO_{2\,max}$ per body weight	High school runner	Males 12% greater[42]
$VO_{2\,max}$ per lean body weight	High school runner	Males 5% greater than females[42]
Grip strength	Age 17	Males twice that of females[43]
Upper body strength	Adult	Females 30–35% that of males[44]
Lower body strength	Adult	Females 70% that of males[44]

hemoglobin mass, and lower cardiac output, limit endurance performance in females.

Strength

Strength gains during childhood parallel growth because development of muscle strength is a function of the cross-sectional area of muscles. An individual is born with a fixed number of muscle fibers, and growth occurs as a result of hypertrophy and increase in fiber diameter. During childhood, muscle mass increases steadily with growth in boys and girls until puberty, at which time, muscle mass plateaus in girls and accelerates in boys. Therefore, prior to puberty, females and males have similar muscle mass and strength. At puberty, boys show marked acceleration in development of strength secondary to increased muscle mass, while in girls, strength and muscle mass do not change appreciably. Therefore, gender differences in strength and the potential for boys to improve absolute strength increase significantly at puberty (see Tables 16-1 and 16-3).

Traditional dogma held that prepubertal children were incapable of improving muscle strength. This belief was based on the fallacy that improvement in strength is dependent on the presence of androgens and associated increase in muscle mass. However, significant strength gains can occur independent of increases in muscle size. This is particularly true for prepubertal children, women, and even adult males during the early phases of a strength-training program, before any change in muscle size occurs. Neurologic factors, such as increased neural drive, synchronization of motor unit fibers, and improved motor skill coordination, appear to be important mechanisms for strength gains in these instances.

Studies of strength training in children show that both boys and girls demonstrate significant gains in strength (20 to 30 percent), similar to that seen in adults, without any significant increase in muscle mass.[20] Prepubescent children make similar relative strength gains (percent improvement) compared to older children and adults. In fact, evidence suggests that prepubertal children experience greater percent improvement of pretraining strength values compared to older children and adults, whereas postpubertal adolescents demonstrate greater improvements in absolute strength. Girls have the same capacity for strength gains as boys, controlling for body composition and size, and gender differences in strength disappear when determined on the basis of lean body mass. As is true for endurance, there appears to be a significant genetic contribution to muscle strength in children.[21–23]

Safety of Weight Training

Although the efficacy of strength training in children has been confirmed, concern has been raised with regard to the safety of this activity with regard to risk of injury to the immature skeleton. Although numerous case reports of epiphyseal fracture due to weight training in children have been reported, the majority occur as a result of improper technique, excessive loading, and ballistic movements, and therefore appear to be preventable. The majority of such injuries occur in the home setting where supervision may be inadequate.

Most injuries are neither epiphyseal nor acute injuries, but rather soft tissue injuries.[24,25] There are no reports of epiphyseal injury in supervised prospective studies of resistance training in children. There is no evidence that weight training is more risky in this regard than participation in other sports and recreational activities. There is no evidence that prepubertal children are more prone to injury during weight training than older children or adults. In addition, there is no evidence of subclinical injury based on markers of repetitive stress to bone (bone scan), collagen (urinary hydroxyproline), cartilage (keratin sulfate), or muscle (creatine phosphate).[26,27] Concerns that weight training might lead to muscle boundness and decreased flexibility that could predispose to injury appear unwarranted; numerous prospective studies show no change or show slight improvements in flexibility.[26,28,29]

In addition to improvements in strength, there may be other benefits associated with weight training in children and adolescents. Strength training appears to improve performance on selected motor fitness tests (vertical jump, standing long jump)[30,31] and may enhance performance in sports involving a substantial strength and power component. In addition, there is some evidence to suggest that strength training in adolescents may result in decreased rate and rehabilitation time of injuries during other sports activities.[32,33] Other possible health benefits include favorable changes in blood lipoproteins[34,35] and prevention of osteoporosis in girls.[36]

The term "weight training" should be distinguished from "weight lifting" and "power lifting." Weight training refers to a variety of resistance training modalities (free weights, weight machines) designed to increase muscle strength and endurance by performing multiple repetitions and sets of each exercise. Weight lifting and power lifting on the other hand are competitive sports emphasizing maximal lifts and ballistic maneuvers, such as the clean and jerk and the snatch (weight lifting) and the squat, dead lift, and bench press (power lifting). These activities are not recommended for children and adolescents prior to skeletal maturity (Tanner stage 5) due to a theoretical concern of increased risk of injury to open growth plates.[37] Weight training, on the other hand, is thought to be safe when closely supervised and appropriately designed. This would include emphasis on low resistance and high repetitions, no maximal lifts, and no competitive weight lifting or power lifting.

Heat Illness and Dehydration

Children are more prone to dehydration and heat intolerance than adults, due to a variety of physiologic differences. Children produce more metabolic heat during exercise than adults.

Although sweat gland density is higher in children, they produce less sweat to dissipate the heat. Children's larger surface area-per-mass ratio allows more heat uptake from the environment. Lower cardiac output leads to less peripheral perfusion and thereby lower capacity for heat transfer from body core to skin. In addition, children take longer than adults to acclimatize to new environments and also become fatigued sooner than adults during exercise in heat. Often children are less aware of early signs of heat stress and may fail to decrease their activity level. Voluntary hypohydration occurs frequently in children, and for a given level of dehydration, children experience a faster rise in core temperature than adults. Obese children and very young children may be at particular risk, due to the insulating effect of increased layers of adipose tissue. The most common cause of heat-related illness in healthy children is insufficient acclimatization. In this regard, heat-related illness is entirely preventable by taking appropriate precautions.

Dehydration and heat illness such as heat cramps, heat exhaustion, and heat stroke can be prevented by adequate fluid intake during and after exercise. In most situations, water is an adequate choice of fluid replacement to prevent dehydration and should be readily available during exercise. Sports drinks, which usually contain 6 to 8 percent carbohydrate, are beneficial only for exercise activities lasting longer than 90 min. However, children may voluntarily drink more of a flavored drink if they prefer the taste.

Children should be encouraged to drink before they feel thirsty because mild dehydration (2 to 3 percent) occurs before one feels thirsty. Approximately one cup of fluids is required for every 15 to 20 min of strenuous exercise to prevent dehydration. Young athletes should understand that even mild dehydration impairs performance and leads to fatigue. Salt tablets should be avoided because they can cause dangerous side effects and are unnecessary because salt loss is adequately replaced through a normal diet.

Cold Tolerance

Children do not appear to be at greater risk of hypothermia than adults except during exercise in water. In cold weather, children, like adults, generate adequate metabolic heat to maintain and usually increase body core temperature during moderate and intense exercise. However, in cold water, the greater thermal conductivity of the water and the larger surface area-to-mass ratio of the child allow for greater conductive heat loss. The smaller and leaner the child, the faster the cooling rate and the greater the risk of hypothermia in water.

Special Issues

The "Clumsy" Child

A minority of children may have difficulty achieving the expected level of motor skill development. These children are often considered clumsy or uncoordinated. These children should be evaluated to determine whether poor motor skills are simply due to a delay in motor skill development or whether there is any underlying physical abnormality that may be limiting motor skill performance.

In some cases, poor motor skill development may be due to a learning disability regarding motor skill development, termed "developmental coordination disorder."[38] Children with this disorder often have problems learning both gross and fine motor skills, and most often come to medical attention due to difficulty with fine motor skills, such as handwriting and tying their shoes. These children can be helped by appropriate interventions, such as appropriate selection of physical activities and physical therapy. These children will probably have the best experience in activities that do not require complex motor skills, such as walking, cycling, and swimming; individual rather than team sports; noncompetitive physical activities; and participation with younger children, whose skills may be of an equivalent level. Evidence suggests that children with developmental coordination disorder will not simply outgrow the problem.

The Talented Child Athlete

What about those children who appear to be truly exceptionally talented athletes? In this situation, it is particularly important to keep athletic potential in proper perspective. Statistically, very few outstanding high school or college athletes are able to succeed in sports at the professional level after their school career is over. Athletic success should not excuse talented young athletes from developing in other areas. In particular, if allowed to become academic underachievers, they may sacrifice other career opportunities. Intensive training in sports with extreme time commitments and rigid structures may foster dependence and emotional immaturity. Therefore, it is important for talented young athletes to maintain a well-rounded life style and have the opportunity for normal maturity experiences. Risk of overuse injuries and burnout may be minimized by care not to push a young athlete too hard too soon.

Contact Sports for Prepubertal Children

Is it acceptable for a 9-year-old child to participate in a contact sport such as football? In this situation, most parents are concerned about the risk of injury to young children participating in contact sports. However, young children actually have a lower risk of injury in contact sports such as football than older children because they do not have the size and strength to cause forces great enough to cause the more serious injuries seen in adolescents and adults. Fortunately, most injuries in this age group are minor injuries such as bruises, abrasions, strains, and sprains. A more important concern than injury risk would be whether this activity and the associated competition is appropriate or necessary at this age. It is probably okay for 9-year-old children to participate in contact sports if they enjoy the experience and the emphasis is on participation and skill development rather than winning and if other children in the game are of similar age and size.

The "Nonathletic" Child

Some children are not very interested in sports or feel they are not very good at sports. They prefer sedentary activities, such as watching television and playing computer games. How can these children be encouraged to be more physically active? There are many physical activities that a child can enjoy other than sports. In fact, some of these other activities are more likely to be sustainable throughout a lifetime. These activities include walking, cycling, hiking, dancing, rollerblading, and swimming. A child need not participate in organized or competitive sports to achieve the benefits of physical activity. Younger children will enjoy active games played with other family members, such as tag and hide-and-seek. Time spent watching television or doing other sedentary activities may need to be restricted and a specific period of time designated for physical activities. It is important to positively reinforce the child's behavior during physical activity.

Intensive Training at Young Ages

Is it safe for prepubertal children to participate in intensive training programs, such as programs that require daily practices of an hour or more and several hours of competitions on weekends? Is this too much? What are the effects of exercise training on the process of growth and maturation in children? It is reassuring that most studies of child athletes show no apparent adverse effect of regular training on growth or skeletal maturation. However, some studies of elite female gym-

nasts have suggested a growth-stunting effect on ultimate height associated with their intensive training.[39] In these cases, the impairment of height was thought to be primarily due to nutritional deprivation rather than the intensive exercise per se. Therefore, proper nutrition may be particularly important in growing children involved in intensive training. Another concern would be risk of overuse injuries. However, prior to puberty, children are at low risk for overuse injuries, whereas risk of overuse injuries increases during adolescence. However, evidence suggests that the risk of overuse injury increases with the number of hours spent training. Overuse injuries are generally preventable by obtaining appropriate coaching, training, and equipment, and treatable by appropriate modification and evaluation when symptoms develop. A greater concern would be whether the sport was requiring too much time, at the expense of time available for other experiences that comprise a well-rounded life style, such as school, friends, family, and unstructured time. If the coaching is appropriate for age, and the emphasis is on fun and skill development, and, most importantly, if the child enjoys the experience, then it is probably fine to participate.

Physical Education in the Schools

If children participate in a lot of sports, do they need to participate in physical education at school? There are several benefits of physical education that are not necessarily provided through participation in organized sports. These include education regarding the health benefits of exercise, development of a variety of motor skills, participation in activities that are sustainable throughout a lifetime, and development of physical fitness. The emphasis in organized sports is typically on the acquisition of sport-specific skills. Many children involved in organized sports may not be achieving adequate fitness levels or developing well-rounded motor skills needed to participate in other physical activities.

Choosing the Right Sport or Sports Program for Children

When choosing a program, parents or caregivers should look for a community sports program that encourages participation for everyone and emphasizes age-appropriate skill development rather than competition and winning. The program should address appropriate safety issues and ensure that coaching and structure are appropriate for the child's age. Levels of enjoyment and fun experienced by the children who are participating are some of the best indicators of a good program. There is no best sports activity. Any sport or physical activity that the child enjoys and is safe and developmentally appropriate will be beneficial. The most important goal is to encourage participation and enjoyment in physical activities in general. Physical activities that are sustainable over a lifetime are ideal, such as walking, hiking, cycling, rollerblading, dancing, and swimming.

References

1. Yeager KK, Agostini R, Nattiv A, et al: The female athlete triad: Disordered eating, amenorrhea, osteoporosis. *Med Sci Sports Exerc* 25:775, 1993.
2. Frisch RE: Body fat, menarche, fitness, and fertility. *Human Reprod* 2:521, 1987.
3. Malina RM: Menarche in athletes: A synthesis and hypothesis. *Ann Human Biol* 10:1, 1983.
4. Warren MP: The effects of exercise on pubertal progression and reproductive function in girls. *J Clin Endo Metab* 51:1150, 1980.
5. Warren MP, Brooks-Gunn J, Hamilton LH, et al: Scoliosis and fractures in young ballet dancers. Relation to delayed menarche and secondary amenorrhea. *N Engl J Med* 314:1348, 1986.
6. Matkovic V: Calcium metabolism and calcium requirements during skeletal modeling and consolidation of bone mass. *Am J Clin Nutr* 54(suppl): 245SS, 1991.
7. Dyment PG: Neurodevelopmental milestones: when is a child ready for sports participation? In: Sullivan JA, Grana WA (eds): *The pediatric athlete*. Baltimore, MD: Port City Press, Inc.; 1990;29.
8. Seefeldt V: The concept of readiness applied to motor skills acquisition. In: Magill RA, Ash MJ, Smoll FL (eds): *Children in Sport*, 2nd ed. Champaign, IL: Human Kinetics; 1982;31.
9. Seefeldt V, Haubenstricker J: Patterns, phases or stages. An analytical model for the study of developmental movement, In: Kelso JAS, Clark JE (eds): *The Development of Movement Control and Coordination*. New York: John Wiley; 1982;309.
10. Nelson MA: Developmental skills and children's sports. *Physician Sportsmed* 19:67, 1991.
11. *Joint Legislative Study on Youth Sports Programs: Phase II, Agency Sponsored Sports*. East Lansing, MI: State of Michigan; 1978.
12. Ewing ME, Seefeldt V: *American Youth and Sports Participation*. Youth Sports Institute of Michigan State University. North Palm Beach, FL: Athletic Footwear Association; 1990.
13. Hartley LH: Cardiac function and endurance. In: Shephard RJ, Astrand PO (eds): *Endurance in Sport*. London: Blackwell Scientific; 1992;72.
14. Rowland TW: Aerobic response to endurance training in prepubescent children: A critical analysis. *Med Sci Sports Exerc* 17:493, 1985.
15. American Alliance for Health, Physical Education, Recreation and Dance. *Youth Fitness Testing Manual*. Washington, DC: Author; 1980.
16. Bouchard C, Lesage R, Lortie G, et al: Aerobic performance in brothers, dizygotic and monozygotic twins. *Med Sci Sports Exerc* 18:639, 1984.
17. Kobayshi K, Kitamura K, Miura M, et al: Aerobic power as related to body growth and training in Japanese boys: A longitudinal study. *J Appl Physiol* 44:666, 1978.
18. Mirwald RL, Bailey DA, Cameron N, et al: Longitudinal comparison of aerobic power in active and inactive boys aged 7 to 17 years. *Ann Hum Biol* 8:404, 1981.
19. Kemper HCG, Verschuur R, de Mey L: Longitudinal changes of aerobic fitness in youth ages 12 to 23. *Pediatr Exerc Sci Sports* 1:257, 1989.
20. Rowland TW: *Developmental Exercise Physiology*. Champaign, IL: Human Kinetics; 1996;225.
21. Montoye HJ, Metzner HL, Keller JK: Familial aggregation of strength and heart rate responses to exercise. *Hum Biol* 47:17, 1975.
22. Szopa J: Familial studies on genetic determination of some manifestations of muscular strength in man. *Gen Polonica* 23:659, 1982.
23. Wolanski N, Kasprzak E: Similarity in some physiological, biochemical and psychomotor traits

between parents and 2 to 45 years old offspring. *Stud Hum Ecol* 3:85, 1979.

24. Brady TA, Cahill B, Bodnar L: Weight training-related injuries in the high school athlete. *Am J Sports Med* 10:1, 1982.

25. Brown EW, Kimball RG: Medical history associated with adolescent powerlifting. *Pediatrics* 72:636, 1983.

26. Rians CB, Weltman A, Cahill BR, et al: Strength training for prepubescent males: is it safe? *Am J Sports Med* 15:483, 1987.

27. Blimkie CJR: Strength training for the child athlete: The Institute Report. *Scholastic Coach* October 1989; 9.

28. Sewall L, Micheli LJ: Strength training for children. *J Pediatr Orthop* 6:143, 1986.

29. Servidio FJ, Bartels RL, Hamlin RL, et al: The effects of weight training using Olympic style lifts on various physiological variables in pre-pubescent boys. *Med Sci Sports Exerc* 17:288, 1985.

30. Nielsen B, Nielsen K, Behrendt-Hansen M, et al: Training of functional muscular strength in girls 7–19 years old, In: Berg Eriksson (eds): *Children and Exercise IX*. Champaign, IL: Human Kinetics; 1980;69.

31. Weltman A, Janny C, Rians CB, et al: The effects of hydraulic resistance strength training in pre-pubertal males. *Med Sci Sports Exerc* 18:629, 1986.

32. Cahill BR, Griffith EH: Effect of preseason conditioning on the incidence and severity of high school football knee injuries. *Am J Sports Med* 6:180, 1978.

33. Henja WF, Rosenberg A, Buturusis DJ, et al: The prevention of sports injuries in high school students through strength training. *National Strength and Conditioning Association* 4:281, 1982.

34. Fripp RR, Hodgson JL: Effects of resistance training on plasma lipid and lipoprotein levels in male adolescents. *J Pediatr* 111:926, 1987.

35. Weltman A, Janney C, Rians CB, et al: The effects of hydraulic-resistance training on serum lipid levels in prepubertal boys. *Am J Dis Child* 141:777, 1987.

36. Loucks AB: Osteoporosis prevention begins in childhood. In: Brown EW, Branta CF (eds): *Competitive Sports for Children and Youth*. Champaign, IL: Human Kinetics; 1988;213.

37. American Academy of Pediatrics, Committee on Sports Medicine and Fitness: Strength training, weight and power lifting, and bodybuilding by children and adolescents. *Pediatrics* 86:801, 1990.

38. Willoughby C, Polataijko HJ: Motor problems in children with developmental coordination disorder: Review of the literature. *Am J Occup Ther* 49:787, 1995.

39. Theintz GE, Howald H, Weiss U, et al: Canton University Hospital, Geneva: Evidence for a reduction of growth potential in adolescent female gymnasts. *J Pediatr* 122:306, 1993.

40. Behnke AR, Wilmore JH: *Evaluation and Regulation of Body Build and Composition*. Englewood Cliffs, NJ: Prentice-Hall; 1974.

41. Malina RM: Quantification of fat, muscle and bone in man. *Clin Orthop* 65:9, 1969.

42. Cunningham LN: Physiological comparison of adolescent female and male cross country runners. *Pedriatr Exerc Sci* 2:313, 1990.

43. Malina RM, Bouchard C: *Growth, maturation and physical activity*. Champaign, IL: Human Kinetics; 1991;115.

44. Wilmore JH: The application of science to sport: physiologic profiles of male and female athletes. *Can J Appl Sports Sci* 4:103, 1979.

Suggested Reading

1. Dyment PG (ed): *Health Care for Young Athletes*, 2nd ed. Elk Grove, IL: American Academy of Pediatrics; 1991.

2. Harris SS: The child athlete. In: Birrer, RB (ed): *Sports Medicine for the Primary Care Physician*, 2nd ed. Philadelphia, PA: FA Davis Company; 1994.

3. Martens R: *Joy and Sadness in Children's Sports*. Champaign, IL: Human Kinetics; 1978.

4. Micheli LJ: *Sportswise: an Essential Guide for Young Athletes, Parents, and Coaches*. Boston: Houghton Mifflin Company; 1990.

5. Nelson MA: Developmental skills and children's sports. *Physician Sportsmed* 19:67, 1991.

6. Rowland TW: *Exercise and Children's Health*. Champaign, IL: Human Kinetics; 1990.

7. Rowland TW: *Developmental Exercise Physiology*. Champaign, IL: Human Kinetics; 1996.

8. Seefeldt V (ed): *Handbook for Youth Sports Coaches*. Reston, VA: American Alliance for Health, Physical Education, Recreation, and Dance; 1987.

9. Sullivan AJ, Grana WA (eds): *The Pediatric Athlete*. Parkridge, IL: American Academy of Orthopedic Surgeons; 1990.

Paul R. Stricker
Cheryl Wasilewski

Chapter
17

Apophysitis

Introduction

Overuse injuries are becoming increasingly more common in children. In fact, they comprise as many as 30 to 50 percent of all pediatric sports injuries.[1] Most overuse injuries are more common in boys than girls, but with the increase in girls' participation in sports and in the number of sporting activities available for girls, the incidence will continue to approach that of boys. The increasing incidence of overuse injuries is due to a multitude of factors. Longer competitions for youngsters, including triathlons and half-marathons, that were unheard of years ago, are now activities for which many young athletes are training. Single-sport concentration is occurring at earlier ages, as are recruiting pressures. Outside forces, such as coaches, parents, and the media, can become sources of increased pressure to train. All too often adult training programs are implemented for children with few adjustments or variations to account for children's growing young bodies. Sports camps, youth leagues, year-round clubs, and backyard workouts with parents and personal trainers all add to the potential for overuse.[1] Excessive overload from overtraining or even just the simple biomechanics of a particular sport can lead to overuse injuries such as stress fractures, tendinitis, and apophysitis.

One of the unique characteristics of the young skeleton is the growth plate, or physis. This is located between the metaphysis and either the epiphysis or the apophysis. The epiphysis at the ends of long bones contributes to longitudinal bone growth. The apophysis appears where muscle-tendon units attach to bones via graded interdigitation into the cartilage of bone[2] and acts to buffer the tensile force transmitted to the underlying bone. Multiple epiphyses and apophyses exist throughout the skeleton and close at various times (Fig. 17-1). Injuries to the

apophysis can occur at any location, yet the primary areas affected are the knee, ankle, elbow, and pelvis. These areas are not only subject to chronic overuse, but can also be avulsed when subjected to abrupt forces. This chapter focuses on the locations, causes, and treatments of chronic overuse injury to the apophysis, which has been termed apophysitis.

Anatomy of the Apophysis

Anatomically, the apophysis is a cartilaginous secondary ossification center at the attachment site of a muscle-tendon unit. During early puberty, multiple forces contribute to the excessive pull on the apophysis. Elongation of bones often occurs more rapidly than the muscle-tendon units can stretch to accommodate. Increasing testosterone levels strengthen the muscle-tendon unit, increasing the force at the apophysis, which is much weaker than the connecting muscle-tendon unit. Flexibility is usually diminished, especially in boys, which leads to an increase in apophyseal tension. When these forces are combined with the mechanical loads of running, jumping, and throwing sports, the anatomic forces, such as foot pronation or genu valgum, and the possibility of improper training techniques, apophysitis can develop.

Pathophysiology of Apophysitis

The pathophysiology of apophysitis includes inflammation,[2,3] but primarily involves microfractures of the unfused apophysis.[4] Due to

Figure 17-1

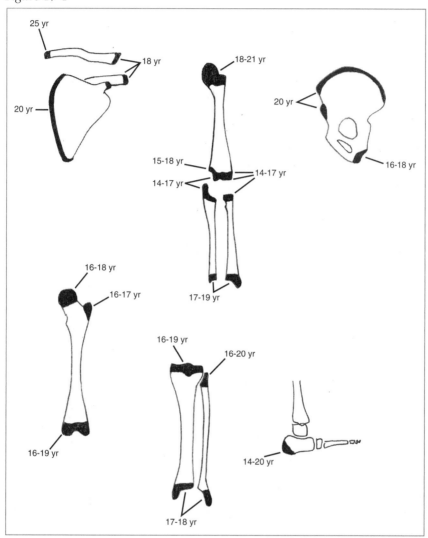

Ages of approximate closure of epiphyseal and apophyseal areas.

the repetitive forces at the site, apophysitis has also been viewed as a subclinical stress fracture of the apophysis.[5] Continuous tensile stress at the apophyseal site with resultant inflammation and microfractures of the underlying cartilaginous and bony structures leads to local swelling, pain, and even osteogenesis and callous formation. This process can present as a painful lump, such as that which occurs at the tibial tubercle of the knee, or simply as pain with activities, such as occurs at the iliac crest or ankle. Apophysitis is a unique condition involving tissue of the skeletally immature individual, and with closure of the apophysis usually comes a resolution of this painful condition.

Sites of Apophysitis

Young, active individuals can present with apophyseal tenderness in multiple areas. Depending on the activity demanded of the young, rapidly growing athlete, the location of apophysitis will differ. The following sections describe specific apophysitis entities followed by a treatment plan. However, to understand the treatment plans, it is first necessary to describe the general principles involved.

Because the mechanism that causes apophysitis is most often chronic overuse that results from repeated tensile stress at the apophysis, the basic repertoire of treatment and rehabilitation involves stretching of the muscle-tendon unit, local pain reduction with ice and occasional anti-inflammatory medications, and altering of activities to allow safe participation while reducing the stress at the apophyseal site. For example, if a young athlete has tibial tubercle apophysitis and participates in basketball, altering his or her activity during painful days would include concentrating on free throws and shooting, passing drills, and dribbling in place without much actual running and jumping. This alteration of activities is referred to as "relative rest."

Another very important concept is the fact that this is a problem encountered during rapid growth. Stretching exercises must be performed consistently in an attempt just to keep pace with skeletal changes. Because the adolescent growth process occurs over a matter of months, apophysitis will not disappear quickly. It has a reputation for being intermittently painful. This requires the athlete, parents, and coaches to understand that the condition may wax and wane in its severity with good days and bad days. Awareness of this oscillation will help everyone involved identify situations that will require adjustments in a youngster's athletic practice or participation without making him or her feel guilty. Apophysitis occurs most frequently in active and overly active children, who are more prone to want to participate too much rather than try to opt out of activities.

Tibial Tubercle

Apophysitis most frequently occurs at the insertion of the patellar tendon into the tibial tubercle. It is commonly referred to as Osgood-Schlatter's disease, but because apophysitis is not an actual disease, the sports medicine community describes these conditions more appropriately by their anatomic location (e.g., apophysitis of the tibial tubercle).

Tibial tubercle apophysitis occurs in running and jumping activities such as basketball, long jump, hurdles, and volleyball. Apophysitis of the tibial tubercle usually appears during ages 11 to 13 in girls and 13 to 15 in boys, and occurs bilaterally in 20 to 30 percent of both boys and girls.[6]

The large powerful quadriceps muscle complex induces a tremendous force on the patellar tendon, especially during landing or running downhill. Muscles lacking in flexibility exert more tension, especially if coupled with increased tension in an opposing direction from tight hamstring muscles. Other factors contributing to the abnormal forces on the tibial tubercle include patella alta, maltracking of the patella, and foot pronation, which rotates the tibia and thus alters the forces across the patella and patellar tendon.

Tibial apophysitis occurs both unilaterally and bilaterally. The history and presentation coupled with age and activity level are often classic for this diagnosis; thus radiographs are rarely indicated. If the condition is unilateral, there is often marked parental concern of the possibility of a tumor. High concern, nonclassic presentation, severe night pain, and pain persisting after skeletal maturity are conditions that support obtaining radiographs. On rare occasions, apophyseal fragmentation will result in a retained bony ossicle in the adult; this may be painful and require surgical excision. This condition occurs in approximately 10 percent of cases.[7]

Treatment focuses on increasing flexibility of

Figure 17-2

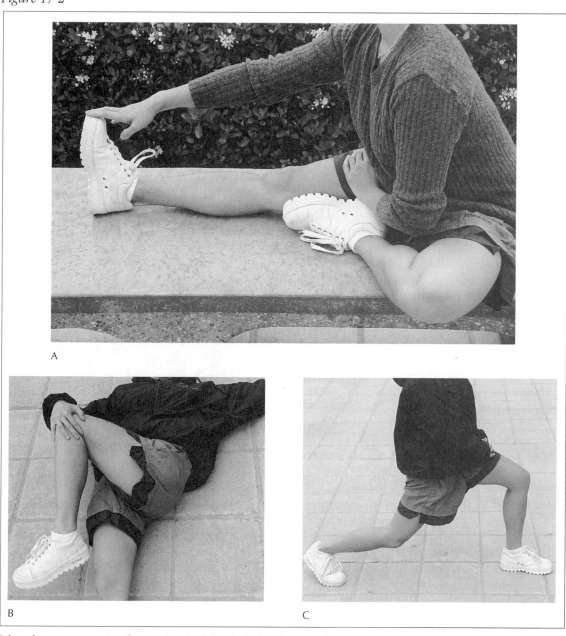

A

B   C

Selected treatment exercises for apophysitis of the tibial tubercle (Osgood-Schlatter's disease),
including **(A)** hamstring stretch, **(B)** hip stretch, and **(C)** quadriceps eccentric strengthening.

the quadriceps, hip flexors, hamstrings, adductors, and iliotibial band; progressive eccentric strengthening programs; local application of ice; judicious use of anti-inflammatory medications; orthotics if necessary; and altered activity levels. For a few representative therapy exercises, see Fig. 17-2.

Tension on the attachment of the other end of

the patellar tendon (i.e., on the distal pole of the patella rather than the tibial tubercle) can also cause irregular calcifications, pain, and swelling in active girls and boys 11 to 13 and 13 to 15 years of age, respectively. This condition is termed Sinding-Larsen-Johannson disease, and treated similarly to tibial tubercle apophysitis.[8]

Calcaneus

Calcaneal apophysitis, also known as Sever's disease, occurs at the base of the heel at the insertion of the Achilles tendon. In addition to repetitive loading during tension and shearing forces during contraction of the gastrocnemius, this apophyseal region is also subject to impact trauma, and both types of loads contribute to inflammation and microfractures of this apophysis.[9] In addition to repetitive microtrauma and rapid growth, tight gastrocnemius musculature, weak ankle dorsiflexors, and biomechanic abnormalities such as genu varum or subtalar and forefoot varus also contribute. Histologic studies of child autopsy calcanei with similar radiographs to those children with a diagnosis of apophysitis show disruption of perpendicular fibrous plates and reparative processes, consistent with a stress remodeling process.[10]

Apophysitis of the calcaneus is more common in runners and soccer players,[11] and the most common ages of presentation are 9 to 11 in girls and 10 to 12 in boys, with more predominance in boys.[12] The child presents with intermittent heel pain with activities, although it often dissipates once the athlete is warmed up. Cases with significant pain often cause the athlete to limp. Unlike tibial tubercle apophysitis, there is no real evidence of swelling or a painful lump on inspection. Palpation along the apophysis induces pain. It is important to know that the apophysis has a circumferential location around the posterior aspect of the calcaneus, and lies at approximately a 70° angle (Fig. 17-3); thus, squeezing along the sides of the posterior calca-

Figure 17-3

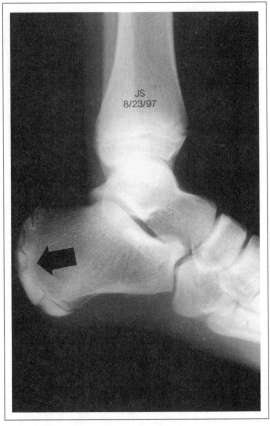

Calcaneal apophysitis (Sever's disease).

neus will be more painful than palpation directly on the posterior end of the calcaneus.

The apophysis is normally irregular in appearance even when asymptomatic.[9,13] Thus, radiographs do not contribute any further information and do not need to be performed unless there has been significant trauma, swelling and ecchymosis exist along with impaired gait, or if the history and presentation do not fit the clinical scenarios of calcaneal apophysitis.

Treatment includes increasing the flexibility of the gastrocnemius-soleus muscle complex, local application of ice after activities, and orthotics if

Figure 17-4

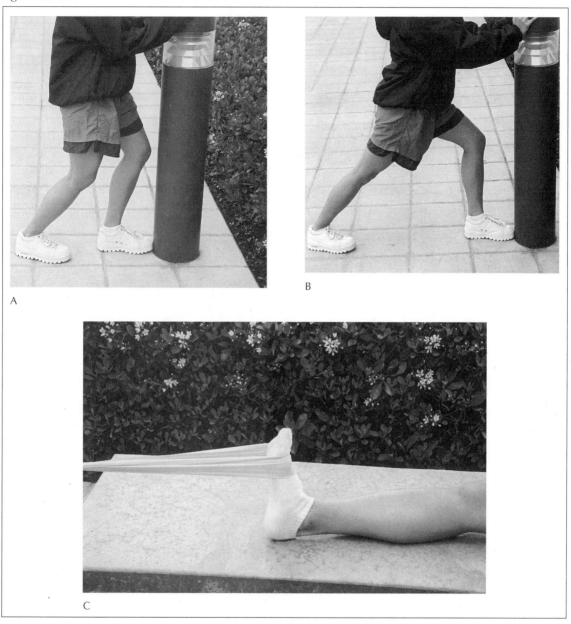

Selected treatment exercises for calcaneal apophysitis (Sever's disease), including **(A)** soleus stretch, **(B)** gastrocnemius stretch, **(C)** strengthening of dorsiflexors, and **(D)** calf stretch on a step.

Figure 17-4 (continued)

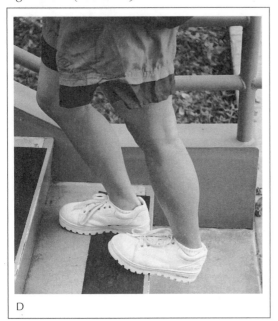

D

necessary. For a few representative therapy exercises, see Fig. 17-4. In very active youngsters, it may be necessary to further reduce tension of the Achilles tendon during activities with a small heel lift. This lift should then be removed after the activity has been completed, or the Achilles tendon will shorten over time, defeating the purpose of the stretching exercises. A progressive, eccentric-loading strengthening program may be beneficial, especially for those individuals in jumping sports.[14] Relative rest should be employed during bad days when pain is bothersome. If the athlete is a soccer player, time at practice could focus on drills and other foot skills, passing, and shooting, yet very little running.

Elbow

MEDIAL EPICONDYLE

Although there are many areas of the immature elbow that can be affected by abnormal stress forces, the area most affected is the medial epicondyle. This area of the elbow is most commonly stressed in youngsters participating in throwing sports, usually baseball pitchers. The term "Little League Elbow" has been coined to describe the insult to the apophysis of the medial epicondyle, and usually occurs in the 9- to 14-year-old age group.

The flexor muscle mass originates on the medial epicondyle; thus forceful wrist flexion at the end of the throwing maneuver, coupled with the valgus stress placed on the elbow during the cocking and acceleration phase of throwing, can place forces along the apophysis that are not well tolerated by the immature skeleton. Repeated valgus extension overload during the throwing maneuver places tremendous tensile stress on the medial side of the elbow and subsequent compression force on the lateral aspect (Fig. 17-5). Other factors additionally stress the medial apophysis, such as incorrect throwing technique, inappropriate types of pitches for the child or preadolescent, and a high volume of throws. More extension torque forces and prolonged valgus exists in younger throwers, and children who pitch in a side-arm style are three times more likely to have injuries than those who throw with an overhand technique.[15,16]

Repeated tension on the medial epicondyle can cause widening of the apophysis or even frank avulsion with a sudden, forceful event. These forces can also affect the lateral aspect of the elbow with repetitive compression of the radiocapitellar articulation. Painful swelling of the medial epicondyle is manifest on palpation, and pain is reproduced with resisted wrist flexion. Flexion contractures may exist, making full extension difficult. Valgus stress of the elbow can exacerbate the pain, and the amount of laxity and range of motion compared to the noninjured elbow should be noted. Hypertrophy of the medial epicondyle, microtearing of the flexor-pronator muscle group, and fragmentation of the apophysis can all occur with prolonged stress of the young elbow.[17] Radiographs are

Figure 17-5

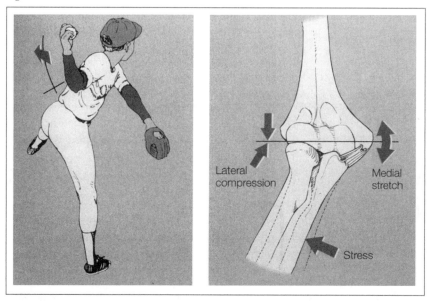

Forces placed on elbow during throwing. *(Courtesy of Joseph Congeni, MD, Sports Medicine Center and Children's Hospital Medical Center, Akron, OH.)*

necessary to observe the medial epicondyle and radial compartment. Comparison views are often required since there are many secondary ossification centers about the elbow.

Treatment of medial epicondyle apophysitis of the elbow focuses on decreasing the amount of force on the epicondyle. Flexibility exercises of the wrist flexors and extensors are important to aid in tension reduction. Pain can be addressed with anti-inflammatory medications, but ice should not be used due to the close proximity to the ulnar nerve. Once rest has allowed the pain to diminish and physical therapy is underway, a gradual return to throwing may begin. For a few representative therapy exercises, see Fig. 17-6.

In a throwing athlete, it is also important to determine the types and number of pitches being thrown. Curve balls or sliders place excessive valgus force on the elbow and should not be allowed until skeletal maturity has been reached. Proper technique should be stressed.

The number of pitches thrown must be limited to prevent many of the overuse problems associated with the elbow. In addition to avoiding certain types of pitches until skeletal maturity, overuse injuries may be reduced by following other general guidelines, such as pitching a maximum of 6 innings per week or pitching 4 innings per game followed by 3 days rest, throwing approximately 20 to 25 pitches per inning or 100 to 120 pitches per week. Easy warm-up throws should always be performed prior to significant throwing. It is important that parents, coaches, and athletes understand that the number of pitches also includes those done off the baseball field, such as in the back yard.

OLECRANON

Another area of the elbow that can be affected by tensile overload is the olecranon. Traction apophysitis from the triceps insertion on the olecranon is uncommon, although it has

Figure 17-6

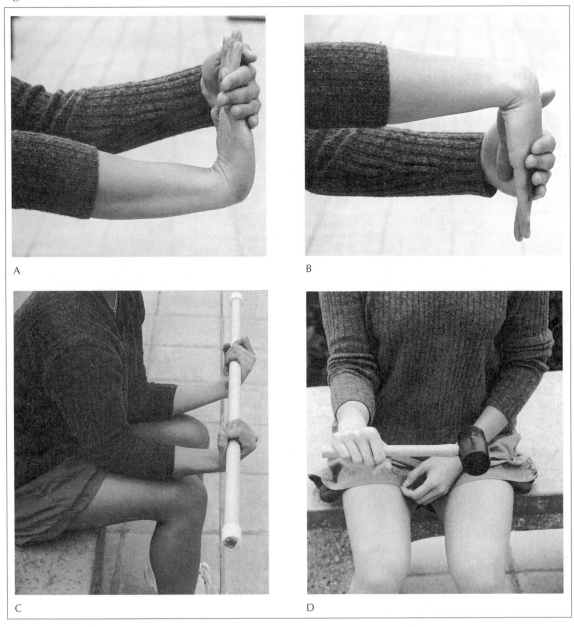

Selected treatment exercises for medial epicondyle apophysitis of the elbow, including **(A)** wrist flexor stretch, **(B)** wrist extensor stretch, **(C)** wrist flexor strengthening, and **(D, E)** strengthening of pronation/supination.

Figure 17-6 (continued)

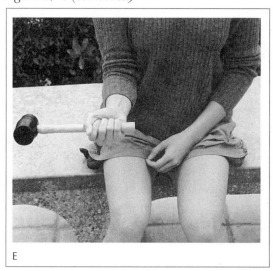

E

been reported to occur in young male gymnasts,[18] tennis players, and baseball players.[19] The growth center is vulnerable to traction during its maturation from about age 9 to 15. During this time, repeated forceful contractions from events such as extension in throwing, tennis serves, or tumbling, can induce pain at the triceps insertion. Pain can also be reproduced with

triceps resistance. Radiographs reveal varying degrees of fragmentation of the apophysis. Relative rest, improving throwing and serving techniques, and triceps flexibility are integral to treatment.

Foot

Apophysitis of the foot occurs at the base of the fifth metatarsal at the insertion site of the peroneus brevis tendon. Apophysitis in this area is referred to as Iselin's disease. This is a relatively uncommon area of apophysitis.[20] Youngsters affected are between 9 to 11 in girls and 12 to 14 in boys.[21] Painful swelling is noted upon palpation of the proximal fifth metatarsal, and pain is often exacerbated with resisted eversion of the foot. Pain also occurs with running, cutting, jumping, and inversion stress. Radiographs reveal a small linear apophysis at the most proximal aspect of the metatarsal, which may be wider than the non-affected side (Fig. 17-7). The thin apophysis should be distinguished from an avulsion fracture of the proximal tip of the metatarsal, the so-called "dancer's fracture" (Fig. 17-8).

Treatment of fifth metatarsal apophysitis is

Figure 17-7

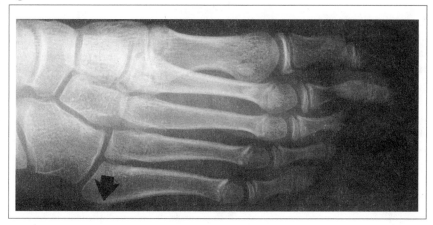

Iselin's disease.

Figure 17-8

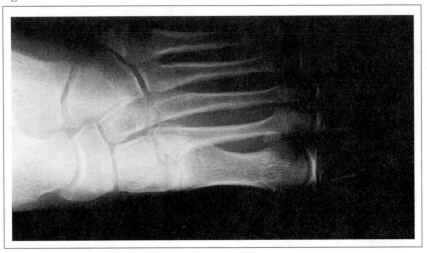

Avulsion fracture of proximal fifth metatarsal.

often minimal and conservative with avoidance of activities that cause pain. Local ice application, stretching of evertors/plantarflexors, and strengthening of invertors/dorsiflexors should also be included in the treatment regimen. For a few representative therapy exercises, see Fig. 17-9.

Pelvis

The pelvis contains multiple apophyses where various muscle-tendon groups are attached. These include the iliac crest (external oblique abdominal muscles, tensor fascia lata, transverse abdominus, and gluteus medius), anterior superior iliac spine (quadriceps), anterior inferior iliac spine (rectus femoris), ischial tubercle (hamstrings), and lesser trochanter of the proximal femur (iliopsoas). Of these sites, the iliac crest is more susceptible to overuse apophysitis, and the other locations are more prone to acute avulsion injuries.

Iliac crest apophysitis occurs most often from overuse among long-distance runners[22] and often during periods of increased skeletal growth velocity as well as with increases in mileage. It usually appears during 14 to 16 years of age, when the iliac crest apophysis remains open and is subject to the muscle contractions that are more powerful due to muscle enlargement after puberty. Iliac crest closure occurs around 14 to 18 years in females and 16 to 18 years in males.[23]

Repetitive pulling on the apophysis from lower abdominal muscles causes microfractures and inflammation and most often occurs in the anterior one-half of the apophysis.[2] Pain occurs with palpation, resisted hip abduction, and with sit-ups.

This self-limited entity resolves with stretching of the lower abdominal muscles, hip flexors, and hip abductor muscles, local ice application, and rest from active running with a gradual return over a 4 to 6 week period.[5] Conditioning by other means should be continued if possible. Radiographs are not indicated or helpful unless there has been an acute avulsion injury.

Figure 17-9

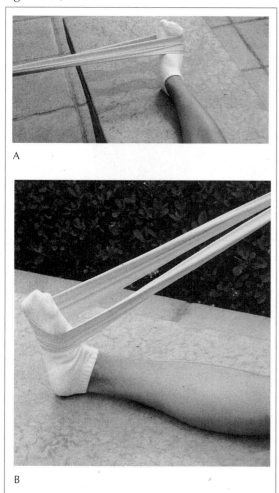

Selected treatment exercises for apophysitis of the fifth metatarsal of the foot (Iselin's disease), including **(A)** strengthening of evertor muscles, and **(B)** strengthening of invertor muscles and stretching of evertors.

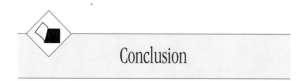

Conclusion

Rapid growth is one of the normal processes of puberty, yet it sometimes comes with a price—

the potential development of apophysitis. This usually manifests itself among physically active youth, either in the beginning or in the middle of their rapid skeletal growth phase. Increased bone growth coupled with decreased muscle flexibility, increased muscle strength, and repetitive loading activities all lead to microfractures and inflammation of the apophyseal growth plate and the manifestation of apophysitis. Due to the weakness of the growth plate compared to the attaching muscle-tendon unit, acute avulsion injuries can also occur.

Apophysitis is more common in those who are involved in athletics compared with those who are nonathletic.[4] The American College of Sports Medicine (ACSM) estimates that overuse injuries in young athletes are preventable in about 50 percent of cases.[25] Guidelines suggested by the ACSM include: emphasizing general fitness, avoiding excessive volume of training and early sport specialization, allowing children to participate in different activities, and gradually increasing intensity, frequency, and duration not more than 10 percent at a time.

Treatment of apophysitis involves reducing tension at the site with flexibility exercises, mild endurance and eccentric types of strengthening, and activity modification, or "relative rest." The process may recur until rapid growth starts to slow. Reassurance that this condition is temporary and education of which activities to continue during the painful episodes will allow the athletes to stay involved, understand the process of their condition, and weather this brief interference. Unnecessary stress and pressure on youngsters can be reduced by education of the athlete, parents, and coaches.

References

1. DiFiori J: Overuse injuries in children and adolescents. *Phys Sportsmed* 27:75, 1999.
2. Moreland MS: Special concerns of the pediatric athlete. In: Fu FH, Stone DA (eds): *Sports Injuries: Mechanisms, Prevention, Treatment.* Baltimore:

Williams & Wilkins; 1994;135.

3. Best TM: Muscle-tendon injuries in young athletes. *Clin Sports Med* 14:669, 1995.

4. Graf BK, Noordsij P, Reider B: Disorders of the patellar tendon. In: Reider B (ed): *Sports Medicine: The School-Age Athlete*. Philadelphia: WB Saunders Co; 1996;389.

5. Paletta GA, Andrish JT: Injuries about the hip and pelvis in the young athlete. *Clin Sports Med* 14:591, 1995.

6. Smith AD, Tao SS: Knee injuries in young athletes. *Clin Sports Med* 14:629, 1995.

7. Mital MA, Matza RA, Cohen J: The so-called unresolved Osgood-Schlatter lesion. *J Bone Joint Surg Am* 62:732, 1980.

8. Medlar RC, Lyne ED: Sinding-Larsen-Johansson disease: Its etiology and natural history. *J Bone Joint Surg Am* 60:11136, 1978.

9. Madden CC, Mellion MB: Sever's disease and other causes of heel pain in adolescents. *Am Fam Phys* 54:1995, 1996.

10. Liberson A, Lieberson S, Mendes DG, et al: Remodeling of the calcaneus apophysis in the growing child. *J Pediatr Orthop B* 4:74, 1995.

11. Micheli JG, Ireland ML: Prevention and management of calcaneal apophysitis in children: An overuse syndrome. *Pediatr Orthop* 7:34, 1987.

12. Outerbridge AR, Micheli LJ: Overuse injuries in the young athlete. *Clin Sports Med* 14:503, 1995.

13. Kaeding CC, Whitehead R: Musculoskeletal injuries in adolescents. *Primary Care* 25:211, 1998.

14. Stanish WD: Lower leg, foot, and ankle injuries in young athletes. *Clin Sports Med* 14:651, 1995.

15. Albright JA: Clinical study of baseball pitchers: Correlation of injury to the throwing arm with method of delivery. *Am J Sports Med* 6:15, 1978.

16. Micheli LJ: Sports injuries in special groups. In: Harris M, Williams C, Stanish WD, et al (eds): *Oxford Textbook of Sports Medicine*. New York: Oxford University Press; 1994;595.

17. Hannah GA, Whiteside JA: The elbow in athletics. In: Mellion MB (ed): *Sports Medicine Secrets*, 2nd ed. Philadelphia: Hanley & Belfus 1999;541.

18. Maffulli N, Chan D, Aldridge MJ: Overuse injuries of the olecranon in young gymnasts. *J Bone Joint Surg* 74:305, 1992.

19. Bryan WJ: Baseball and softball. In: Reider B (ed): *Sports Medicine: The School-Age Athlete*. Philadelphia: WB Saunders Co; 1996;491.

20. Lehman RC, Gregg JR, Torg E: Iselin's disease. *Am J Sports Med* 14:494, 1986.

21. Canale ST, Williams KD: Iselin's disease. *J Pediatr Orthop* 12:90, 1992.

22. Clancy WG, Martin SD: Running. In: Reider B (ed): *Sports Medicine: The School-Age Athlete*. Philadelphia: WB Saunders Co: 1996;691.

23. Peck K: Pelvis, hip and thigh injuries. In: Mellion MB (ed): *Sports Medicine Secrets*, 2nd ed. Philadelphia: Hanley & Belfus; 1999;461.

24. Kujala UM, Kvist M, Heinonen O: Osgood-Schlatter's disease in athletes. Retrospective study of incidence and duration. *Am J Sports Med* 13:236, 1985.

25. Current comment from the American College of Sports Medicine: The prevention of sport injuries of children and adolescents. *Med Sci Sports Exerc* 25(suppl 8):1, 1993.

Suzanne S. Hecht
Joseph P. Luftman

Chapter

18

Fractures in Pediatric Athletes

Introduction

Participation in organized athletics by the pediatric population continues to grow.[1] Unfortunately, increased participation in sports usually goes hand-in-hand with an increased incidence of injuries. The types of fractures suffered by pediatric athletes, and care of those fractures, often differ from their adult counterparts. Recognition and appropriate management of fractures seen in pediatric athletes is essential to avoid complications and allow for a safe and expedient return to athletics.

Bone Anatomy

Bones in growing children consist of four regions: epiphysis, physis, metaphysis, and the diaphysis. Secondary ossification centers are found on the ends of the long bones and are called epiphyses. As the epiphyses ossify, they appear visible on radiographs. Epiphyses are covered with articular cartilage. Separating the epiphysis from the metaphysis is the physis or growth plate. The physis is a wavy cartilagenous structure that is responsible for adding length and width to long bones. The physis contains four histologically distinct zones: reserve, proliferative, hypertrophic, and provisional calcification. Cells in the physis divide, grow, and, eventually, become calcified. This process of cell division, hypertrophy, and calcification begins along the epiphyseal side of the growth plate and progresses towards the metaphysis, such that the newly calcified cells are added to the metaphyseal border. The flared portion of the bone next to the physis is termed the metaphysis. The term diaphysis refers to the shaft of the bone.

A ring of fibrous tissue, the perichondrium, is found at the junction of the physis and the metaphysis. The perichondrium is attached to the metaphyseal periosteum and provides mechanical strength to physis.

Also found on growing bones are growth plates called apophyses. Apophyses add shape and contour to bones, but do not add length. Tendons and ligaments commonly attach on apophyses. The tibial tubercle is an example of an apophysis.

Blood is supplied to the physis from branches of the epiphyseal arteries. Since most epiphyses are located outside the joint capsule, the epiphyseal arteries reach the epiphysis via soft tissue attachments. Branches of the epiphyseal arteries penetrate the reserve and proliferative zones but terminate prior to the hypertrophic zone. Thus, the hypertrophic zone is avascular and depends on diffusion to supply nutrients to its cells. The metaphyseal circulation, which arises predominately from the nutrient artery, is entirely separate from the blood supply to the physis. Intermixing of these two blood supplies causes ossification of the growth plate.[2]

Pediatric Bones

The bones of children are different than the bones of adults (Table 18-1). Children's bones have greater remodeling potential and are able to tolerate greater fracture displacement than adults. The remodeling potential of a fracture in a child typically depends on three factors: age of the child, location of the fracture, and the type of fracture.

Age

The younger a child is, the greater the remodeling potential. Remodeling can be expected to occur if the child has at least 2 years of growth remaining.

Location

Location is important because fractures that are closer to the physis also offer greater remodeling capacity. Mild angulation, if it is in the same plane of motion of the nearest joint, is generally remodeled without residual deformity.

Type of Fracture

It is important to note that fractures that involve displacement and disruption of the articular cartilage or rotational deformities are not any better tolerated in children than adults. Growth plates are susceptible to injury because they are weaker than their associated tendons and ligaments. Children are more likely to suffer a growth plate injury than a sprain. In contrast to adults, the less dense bone in children is capable of bending (bowing) rather than breaking in response to a deforming stress. The thicker periosteum of children's bones help to protect from significant displacement, in addition to providing a bony bridge across fracture sites, which help the fractures to heal faster.[3,4]

Fracture Classification

Fracture Description

To fully evaluate and manage a fracture appropriately, it is important to understand how to describe a fracture. Proper fracture description allows for better communication between the primary care physician, radiology technician, radiologist, and consulting orthopedic surgeon. Correct description of a fracture includes the following seven components.

Table 18-1

Anatomic Differences in Pediatric versus Adult Bones

PEDIATRIC BONES
Greater remodeling potential
Growth plates
Less dense (greater deformation capacity)
Thicker and stronger periosteum

BONE(S) NAME

Often it is straightforward to name the bone(s) involved in a fracture. Reviewing anatomy from time to time can help the clinician to recognize some of the more subtle, smaller bone names, such as the carpal and tarsal bones, which can easily be forgotten.

REGION

Is it proximal, distal, or midshaft? Is it on the ulnar or radial side? Is it on the volar or dorsal aspect? Is it metaphyseal, diaphyseal, or epiphyseal? Is it medial or lateral? Is it at the base, head, or neck?

NUMBER OF FRAGMENTS

Usually self-explanatory, but very important to note. A fracture with multiple fragments is described as comminuted.

DIRECTION OF FRACTURE LINE

A single fracture line may be described as transverse, longitudinal, oblique, or spiral.

APPLIED FORCE

Compression, traction, and rotation are common forces and are determined by the mechanism of injury. It is crucial to consider child abuse or diseases of the bone if the mechanism of injury does not fit well with the fracture type.

Figure 18-1

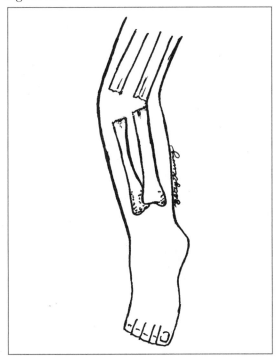

Apex lateral angulation. Note the point of the fracture angle pointing toward the lateral portion of the lower leg.

DISPLACEMENT

Displacement occurs when one fragment moves in relation to the other. Displacement can occur in the form of translation, shortening, rotation, or angulation. Typically, the amount of displacement is measured in millimeters (mm) or by the percentage of apposition of the fragments. For example, if the ends of two fragments have half of their shaft widths touching, this would be described as 50 percent apposition. Displacement of less than 3 to 4 mm is usually considered minimal, but this is also dependent upon the location of the fracture. Angulation is noted as the direction at which the apex of the fracture angle is pointing (Fig. 18-1). A goniometer is helpful to measure the degree of angulation seen on x-rays.

OPEN VERSUS CLOSED

An open fracture refers to a fracture that is associated with violation of the skin in the area of the fracture. Open fractures require prompt orthopedic consultation because the risk of infection is high, and they typically require surgical treatment in the operating room.

Fracture Types

Certain types of fractures can be stated in a single word, thus bypassing all of the descriptive terms (Fig. 18-2).

GREENSTICK

This fracture refers to a transverse fracture line through the shaft of a long bone with resultant break of only one cortex. This results from the plastic deformation ability of the bones in younger children, allowing the bones to fracture on only one side and bend on the other.

TORUS OR BUCKLE

Torus fractures involve a compressive and/or rotational force that causes failure of the bone at the junction of the metaphysis and diaphysis.[4] On radiographs, it appears as if the bone has been compressed such that part of the bone has collapsed and been pushed outward.

OBLIQUE

Oblique fractures run diagonally and are not in a coronal or sagittal plane. They usually have only one fracture line.

SPIRAL

Spiral fractures occur from the application of a rotational force. By definition, a spiral fracture line must be continuous and must traverse in two separate directions.

Figure 18-2

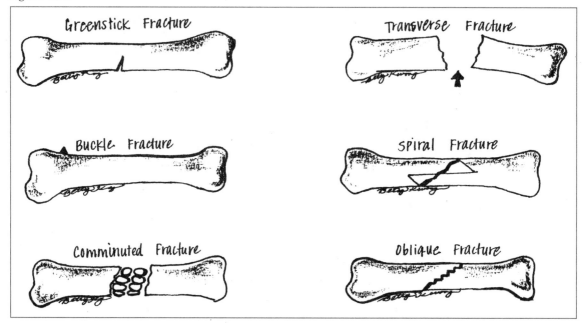

Fracture types.

STRESS

These fractures are very common and come in many sizes and shapes. They are usually due to chronic and repetitive forces across a specific area of bone, causing eventual cortical failure (see Chap. 20).

MISCELLANEOUS

Certain fractures are named after the physician that described them (i.e., Jones fracture, Tillaux fracture).

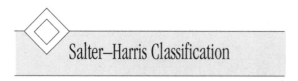

Salter–Harris Classification

Growth plate (physeal) fractures are unique to children and adolescents. Numerous classification systems have been proposed, but the Salter–Harris (SH) classification is the most widely used system.[5] This classification includes six types of growth plate fractures and is based on radiographic findings (Fig. 18-3). It is important to note that there are limitations of the SH classification because it does not consider important prognostic factors such as of the location of the fracture, blood supply, and the age of the child.

SH type I fractures involve only the physis. This fracture is located within the growth plate and does not involve the epiphysis or metaphysis. Because SH type I fractures only involve the physeal cartilage, radiographs will show no evidence of fracture unless there is displacement or widening of the growth plate. Clinically, however, the patient will be tender on the growth plate. It is unlikely to have growth arrest with this type of uncomplicated injury.

SH type II fractures involve the physis and the metaphysis. The epiphysis is not involved. Radiographs reveal a triangular-shaped metaphyseal

Figure 18-3

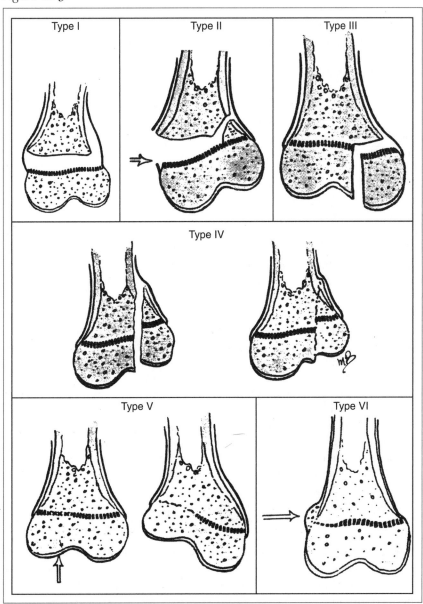

Salter–Harris classification of physeal fractures including type VI (perichondral ring injuries) as described by Rang. *(Reproduced with permission from Rang M: The growth plate and its disorders. Edingburgh E, Livingstone S. 1969.)*

fragment, which is known as a Thurston–Holland sign. Both SH type I and II fractures typically spare the germinal layer and its blood supply, so healing is usually rapid and without complications.

SH type III fractures extend vertically through the epiphysis and horizontally through the growth plate, but not through the metaphysis. This fracture is usually a result of vertical shearing forces through the articular surface. Because the joint surface is involved, it is critical that this fracture is reduced appropriately to prevent future joint degeneration. Orthopedic referral is necessary and open reduction and internal fixation (ORIF) may be needed to maintain an anatomic reduction.

SH type IV fractures represent a single oblique, or almost vertical, fracture line through the epiphysis, physis, and metaphysis. As with SH type III fractures, the most important elements to be wary of are growth plate and articular cartilage disruption. Orthopedic consultation is needed for this fracture. ORIF is often required for successful treatment.

SH type V fractures are the result of a crush injury to the growth plate. A large compressive force damages the growth plate by compromising the germinal layer and blood supply. Since radiographs are usually normal early on, the clinician must be suspicious of this injury based on the history and insist on careful follow-up. This injury is typically diagnosed retrospectively once growth arrest or angular deformity has occurred. SH type V fractures most commonly occur at the knee and ankle.

SH type VI fractures involve an injury to the perichondrium. This fracture may be complicated by an angular deformity if a bony bridge forms in the perichondrium.[2]

One of the most important complications of any SH fracture is the possibility of growth arrest. Radiographs have traditionally been used to monitor for evidence of growth arrest. It appears that magnetic resonance imaging (MRI) may be a valuable tool to assess for growth arrest in high risk areas because it can demonstrate changes of growth arrest before they are visible on plain x-rays.[6–8] Additionally, MRI may play a role in the diagnosis and management of acute SH injuries because it has been reported that MRI is able to detect occult SH fractures and, in some cases, upgrade the SH fracture classification as compared to x-rays.[9–11]

Upper Extremity Fractures

Clavicle Fractures

Clavicle fractures are the most common fractures seen in the general and athletic pediatric population.[4] Clavicle fractures are classified into one of three groups based on radiographic findings: distal third, middle third, or medial third fractures.[12,13] The two common mechanisms for this injury are direct and indirect trauma. A direct blow to the clavicle can cause different types of fractures based on the direction of the force. An inferiorly directed force may cause comminution and possible neurovascular damage to the underlying subclavian vessels and brachial plexus, whereas a posteriorly directed force may cause an uncomplicated transverse fracture. Stanley et al noted that 94 percent of clavicular fractures were from indirect blows.[14]

FRACTURES OF THE MIDDLE THIRD OF THE CLAVICLE

HISTORY AND PHYSICAL EXAMINATION   Up to 80 to 85 percent of clavicle fractures in the pediatric age group occur in the middle third of the clavicle.[15] This fracture typically occurs following a fall onto the shoulder with the forces being transmitted through the acromion to the clavicle. The resultant bone failure occurs at the s-shaped curve in the middle third of the clavicle (Fig. 18-4). The younger the child, the more likely the fracture will be greenstick-like with angulation but without displacement.

Figure 18-4

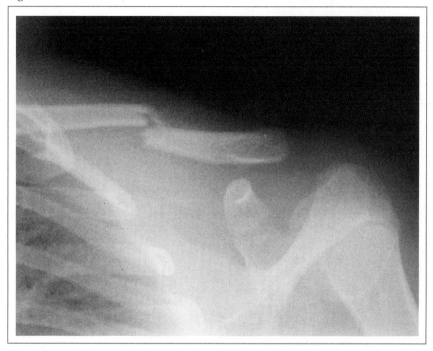

Mid-shaft clavicle fracture: although there is a marked degree of displacement, this fracture can easily be managed by a primary care physician. Proper healing is almost assured and the complication rate is very low. *(Radiograph courtesy of Michael Zucker, M.D., University of California at Los Angeles.)*

On physical examination, patients are often "splinting" the fracture by keeping their shoulder in a hyperadducted position with a downward and inward slump of the involved shoulder.[13] Due to the subcutaneous position of the clavicle, it is very easy to palpate the entire length of the bone. Swelling, tenderness, and, often, ecchymosis are usually visible at the fracture site. It is imperative that a comprehensive neurovascular examination is performed on the involved upper extremity. A thorough, but brief, neurovascular assessment includes palpation of bilateral radial and brachial pulses, sensory testing of the C5–T1 dermatomes, and strength testing (Table 18-2). Neurovascular warning signs include complaints of numbness in the upper extremity, venous distension, expanding hematoma, and diminished or absent pulses. Approximately 4 percent of clavicle fractures have associated injuries.[16]

IMAGING Radiographs should be obtained to assess the type and location of the fracture. Typically two views including an anterior–posterior (AP) view are sufficient, but requesting an apical lordotic view (AP position with tube directed 15° superiorly) can be helpful in presenting a more three-dimensional view of the fracture.

TREATMENT These fractures are located medial to the coracoclavicular ligaments, which give stability to the distal clavicle. Therefore, treatment generally consists of conservative management unless complications arise. For the child less than 12 years old, most investigators agree that

Table 18-2

Neurologic Examination of the Upper Extremity

	SENSORY	**MOTOR**	**REFLEX**
C5	Lateral upper arm	Deltoid	Biceps
C6	Lateral forearm	Wrist extension	Brachioradialis
C7	Middle finger	Triceps	Triceps
		Wrist flexion	
		Finger extension	
C8	Medial forearm	Finger flexion	
		Hand intrinsics	
T1	Medial upper arm	Hand intrinsics	
Axillary	Deltoid patch*	Deltoid	
Median	Index finger	Thumb opposition	
Musculocutaneous	Lateral forearm	Biceps	
Radial	Dorsal web space between thumb and index finger	Wrist extension	
Ulnar	Little finger	Little finger abduction	

*Deltoid patch: 2–3 cm circular area at the upper aspect of the lateral arm (deltoid insertion).

SOURCE: Adapted with permission from Hoppenfeld S: Physical Examination of the Spine and Extremities. Norwalk, CT: Appleton & Lange; 1976.

reduction is unnecessary, even with significant displacement. The "bump" of healing callus should be explained to the parents for anticipatory guidance.

For the older adolescent there is some controversy with regard to treatment of displaced middle-third fractures. If the clavicle is shortened 2 cm or greater as compared with the unaffected side, orthopedic consultation may be warranted to determine if closed reduction under local anesthesia is appropriate. An association between significant shortening of the clavicle and increased rates of nonunion has been demonstrated.[16] Complications of nonunion can include pain, parasthesias, and cosmetic deformity.

Middle-third clavicle fractures may be treated with either a figure-of-eight strap or a sling. A figure-of-eight strap pulls both shoulders posteriorly helping to align the two fracture ends. The splint must be tightened on a daily basis because it may loosen. If the splint is too tight, the child may complain of numbness, tingling, or cold extremities. Generally, the splint should be worn for 8 to 10 days, after which time a sling can be used. Immobilization can be discontinued when the child has good range of motion (ROM) without major discomfort in the affected shoulder. Primary care physicians can manage displaced and/or overlapping fractures, but more frequent follow-up is required to monitor for proper fracture healing. For the competitive athlete, it is imperative that active functional use of the affected extremity is started at an early stage. A program of cross training with cycling, running, or other lower-extremity aerobic exercise is crucial to keep the patient in "game-shape."

COMPLICATIONS Young athletes may present with inadequate healing of a clavicle fracture or no treatment at all. In these cases, nonunion of the fracture is a possible complication. If the patient is symptomatic with pain or lack of full shoulder ROM, orthopedic referral is indicated. Recently, it has been demonstrated that plating and bone grafting is an effective treatment option with minimal complications.[17] Abundant callus formation may cause brachial plexus compression and would be an indication for surgical consultation.

RETURN-TO-PLAY GUIDELINES   The patient should be non-tender at the fracture site with radiographic evidence of bony union. Additionally, the patient should have almost full shoulder ROM and good protective strength, including strong rotator cuff muscles prior to return to play.[18] Generally, 5 to 6 weeks is needed for return to noncontact sports, and 12 to 16 weeks for contact sports. In the younger child, the time frame is grossly 4 to 6 weeks, whereas in the older adolescent, 6 to 12 weeks are often needed.

FRACTURES OF THE DISTAL THIRD OF THE CLAVICLE

HISTORY AND PHYSICAL EXAMINATION   Distal-third clavicle fractures occur distal to the coracoclavicular ligaments and account for approximately 10 percent of all clavicle fractures in children (Fig. 18-5).[19] A fall directly onto the superior aspect of the shoulder is the classic mechanism. Neer has classified distal-third fractures into three types. Type I is a nondisplaced fracture with intact coracoclavicular ligaments. Type II fractures are displaced with rupture of the coracoclavicular ligaments. Type III fractures extend to the articular surface of the acromioclavicular (AC) joint. In children, these fractures are often difficult to distinguish from AC separation.[20]

Figure 18-5

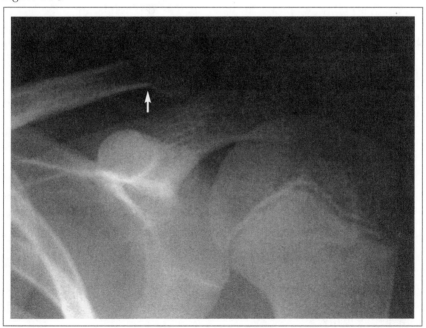

Distal clavicle fracture: this fracture is very subtle and easy to miss. If the examiner follows the inferior cortex from medial to lateral, there is an abrupt angulation (*arrow*) suggesting a torus fracture of the distal clavicle. (*Radiograph courtesy of James C. Puffer, MD, University of California at Los Angeles.*)

IMAGING   Although it is easy to diagnose type I and II fractures on routine x-rays, type III fractures are easily missed and may require special coned-down or stress views with weights if clinical suspicion is high.[19] Typically, the plain films show that the bone has been displaced superiorly out of the periosteal sleeve, which remains contiguous with the rest of the proximal clavicle. CT scanning is a good option for suspicious injuries with equivocal plain radiographs.

TREATMENT   Type I fractures of the distal clavicle are treated similar to middle-third fractures. Generally, these require 3 to 6 weeks of immobilization in a sling and 6 to 8 weeks of total healing time. Type II fractures require sling immobilization and prompt orthopedic referral. A figure-of-eight splint should not be used in these cases. Orthopedic referral is also indicated for type III fractures because AC joint involvement without proper healing can lead to early arthritis. Type III fractures often require ORIF for proper healing. Long-term studies have shown a less than 10 percent complication rate with all three types of distal-third fractures.[21]

FRACTURES OF THE PROXIMAL THIRD OF THE CLAVICLE

HISTORY AND PHYSICAL EXAMINATION   Proximal-third clavicle fractures involve the medial one third of the clavicle. These are fairly uncommon and usually sizable forces are needed to cause fractures in this area. The mechanism of injury is usually a direct blow to the medial clavicle or an indirect shoulder blow that causes compression of the clavicle against the sternum. Most injuries about the medial clavicle in children are SH I or II fractures. Shaft fractures are extremely rare in children.[20] Football and rugby are common sports for sustaining this injury.[21]

On physical examination, there is usually tenderness over or near the sternoclavicular (SC) joint. Due to the large forces needed to cause proximal-third clavicle fractures, a vigorous search for associated injuries is imperative. Intrathoracic injury must be considered and excluded with these fractures. Warning signs of intrathoracic injury include ipsilateral venous congestion, diminished pulse, shortness of breath, and difficulty swallowing.

IMAGING   Although AP and apical lordotic x-ray views are often sufficient to diagnose these fractures, a "serendipity" view may be needed. A "serendipity" view is taken with a 40° cephalad-directed beam that shows the clavicles above the rib cage.[22] A CT scan may be indicated if better visualization is needed to distinguish a fracture from an SC dislocation.

TREATMENT   Nondisplaced fractures can be managed conservatively with a figure-of-eight splint for 3 to 4 weeks. Displaced fractures or fractures with any suspicion of underlying vessel damage necessitate immediate referral. Due to the increased potential for remodeling at the medial clavicular physis, even substantial residual displacement is expected to heal without growth disturbance.

Proximal Humeral Physeal Stress Injury

A stress injury of the proximal humeral physis can develop in the young athlete from repetitive overhead activities. This condition is often called "Little Leaguer's Shoulder" because it typically occurs in high-level adolescent baseball pitchers. This injury has also been described in tennis and volleyball players and swimmers.[23]

HISTORY AND PHYSICAL EXAMINATION

The typical patient is an adolescent male, average age 11 to 16 years old, with the gradual onset of pain in the proximal humerus (near the level of the deltoid insertion) with throwing activities. Usually, there is no traumatic event noted. Most patients average 4 to 5 days/week of throwing, and are often the "best" and "hardest throwers" on their team. The average duration of symptoms, reported in one case series, was 7.7 months.[24]

The mechanism of injury involves the concentration of forces on the proximal humerus during the acceleration phase of throwing. During the acceleration phase, the arm is moving forward and is forcefully internally rotating. It is speculated that the force concentration on the proximal humerus from the internal rotators, adductors, and extensors causes repetitive microtrauma at the weakest link in the chain, which is the physis.[24]

On physical examination, almost 90 percent of patients will have tenderness to palpation over the proximal humerus, particularly on the lateral aspect. Strength testing of the shoulder is often normal, but close attention should be paid to the external rotators as they may be weak due to their insertion near the proximal humeral physis. Pain may be elicited with resisted abduction and external rotation due to the previously mentioned anatomy. Swelling is an uncommon finding and range-of-motion testing is usually within normal limits.

IMAGING

Radiographs are necessary if this injury is suspected as they are a very specific indicator of physeal injury. Proper radiographic evaluation should include external and internal rotation views and comparison views of the opposite shoulder. The diagnosis is made by radiographic evidence of physeal widening. It is also very common to see associated metaphyseal changes including lateral fragmentation, sclerosis, or demineralization.[24] It is important to be aware of the normal cone-shape appearance of the physis, which changes from external to internal rotation views. On the AP external rotation view, the widening is in the pointed portion of the physis, usually laterally. On the AP internal rotation view, the abnormal widening is seen as horizontally aligned radiolucent lines. The lateral aspect of the humerus appears to be more com-

monly involved, most likely due to thicker periosteum at the posteromedial border.

TREATMENT

Various treatment protocols have been reported. All investigators recommend rest, but the amount of time is variable. Some physicians prescribe a sling or other restrictive device to remind the athlete to refrain from overhead activities. The widened physis can take several months to completely remodel, and most experts believe that the fracture is clinically healed prior to resolution of radiographic findings. Therefore, progression in the treatment plan to throwing activities should be based on the resolution of symptoms and not on radiographic normalization. The average length of time for symptoms to subside is 3 months. Once the athlete is asymptomatic, a throwing program can be gradually reintroduced. The patient's throwing mechanics should be evaluated and corrected if there are errors. Rehabilitation programs designed specifically for the throwing athlete are available.[25]

RETURN-TO-PLAY GUIDELINES

It is imperative that when these athletes return to play, both the patient and their families are cautioned about throwing excessively at home or in practice, playing on multiple teams at the same time, and year-round throwing. Guidelines based on expert opinion have been published to address the above concerns.[26] Most case series have shown high success rates with return to asymptomatic, competitive overhead activities.

Humeral Shaft Fractures

Although fairly uncommon, it is important to make mention of the "ball throwers' fracture" or fracture of the humeral diaphysis resulting from an overhead throw without any external trauma.[27] The usual pattern is a spiral fracture in the middle to distal one-third of the diaphysis.

Angulation and severe displacement are rare.

The mechanism is thought to be a violent uncoordinated muscle contraction. It is speculated that this fracture occurs during rapid acceleration when contraction of the powerful internal rotators is initiated prior to full relaxation of the abductors and external rotators. This early firing of the internal rotators places tremendous torque on the mid-shaft of the humerus. Other theories include cumulative cortical fatigue (i.e., previous or current stress fracture site) and poor throwing mechanics.

Epidemiologically, these fractures occur in older-aged athletes, but there are reports in the literature of these fractures occurring in the late-adolescent age group. One series found four clear-cut risk factors including age older than 30 years, a prolonged lay-off from throwing, lack of an exercise program, and prodromal arm pain.[28]

Treatment is usually nonoperative, and for nondisplaced fractures consists of a posterior splint with the arm in a sling for 4 to 6 weeks. If there is complete displacement with marked angulation (more than 10°), referral to an orthopedic specialist is imperative for either specialized casting or operative intervention. Radial nerve palsy is a possible complication and is an indication for referral, but does not usually need operative intervention. There is evidence demonstrating that early nerve exploration does not improve functional outcome.[29] Pathologic fractures can also occur at this site, so it is crucial to take an appropriate history and examine the radiographs for signs of neoplasm.

Return to play is earlier with noncontact sports such as swimming and tennis. Return to collision sports should be delayed until the callus has developed a distinct cortex and all symptoms have resolved.

Supracondylar Fractures

Supracondylar fractures are generally considered the most common fracture in the first decade of life (3 to 11 years old). They are usually extra-articular and are associated with the highest rates of associated complications and poor outcomes.[3]

The classification system is somewhat complex, but it helps to differentiate the treatment regimens and overall prognosis (Fig. 18-6). Type I fractures occur from a fall on outstretched arm with the elbow in extension. The classic fracture pattern consists of a transverse fracture line just proximal to the condyles without associated dis-

Figure 18-6

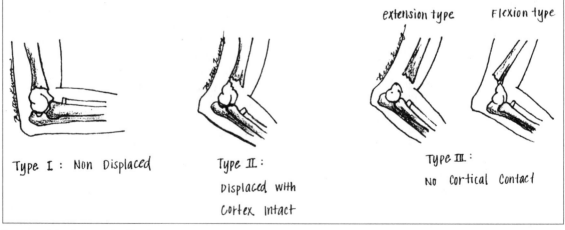

Supracondylar fracture classification.

placement and less than 20° of humerocapitellar angulation (i.e., anterior–posterior angulation). Type II fractures are caused by a direct blow to the posterior elbow while it is in flexion and results in anterior translation of the condylar fragment with respect to the humeral shaft. These fractures may have up to 15 mm of translation and over 20° of humerocapitellar angulation, but the posterior cortex is usually intact. Type III fractures have the same mechanism of injury as type II fractures, but represent a more severe injury with full loss of fracture surface contact and significant overlap.[29]

HISTORY AND PHYSICAL EXAMINATION

The young athlete can sustain a supracondylar fracture from either an indirect force (fall on outstretched arm) or, less commonly, a direct blow to the elbow. In one series, a fall from height accounted for 70 percent of supracondylar fractures.[30] The patient will complain of pain, swelling, and loss of ROM.

Physical examination typically reveals swelling with tenderness of the distal humeral condyles with palpation. A displaced fracture fragment may be palpable posteriorly. There may be significant loss of ROM as the child splints the injury. A thorough examination of the affected upper extremity is crucial because neurovascular injury and associated fractures are relatively common. The neurovascular structures most susceptible to injury are the median nerve and brachial artery. Five to ten percent of all supracondylar fractures have other associated fractures.[31]

IMAGING

Routine radiographs must include AP and lateral views with comparison views of the uninvolved side. There are four key features to look for on the x-rays: (1) abnormal fat pad signs, (2) abnormal anterior humeral line, (3) a carrying angle of more than 12°, and (4) subtle transverse

fracture lines along the cortices on the lateral border (Fig. 18-7).[32,33]

TREATMENT

The most important point for the primary care physician to understand is that the vast majority of these fractures need urgent orthopedic consultation. Most of these injuries, except for the very simple type I fractures, require close observation and usually some type of reduction with traction, percutaneous pinning, or ORIF.[32,33]

Figure 18-7

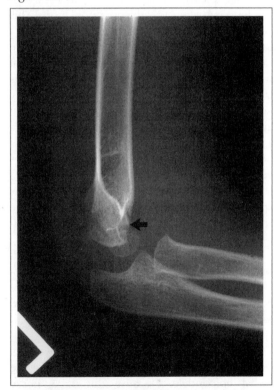

Type I supracondylar fracture: notice the loss of normal volar angulation and figure-of-eight formation of the distal humerus. There is a crack on the anterior cortical surface, but the posterior cortex is intact. Angulation in this example is less than 15°. (*Radiograph courtesy of Michael Zucker, MD, University of California at Los Angeles.*)

COMPLICATIONS

The overall risk of neurologic injury is 7 to 10 percent.[31] Vascular injury, although not as common, is another consideration. Some of the more common complications include Volkmann's ischemic contracture, ulnar nerve palsy, cubitus varus and valgus deformities, and loss of full elbow motion.[13]

Medial Epicondylar Apophyseal Avulsion Fractures

HISTORY AND PHYSICAL EXAMINATION

Medial epicondylar avulsion fractures occur in the 9- to 14-year-old athletic population. This fracture occurs as either an acute traumatic event associated with an underlying chronic overuse injury or as an acute injury without antecedent pain. The chronic overuse injury is referred to as "Little Leaguer's Elbow." The term is generally used to describe the traction apophysitis that can occur at the medial epicondylar apophysis in athletes that participate in throwing or racquet sports. Repetitive overhead throwing activities produce a valgus stress on the medial side of the elbow during the acceleration phase. This repetitive valgus stress places traction on the ulnar collateral ligament and the medial epicondylar apophysis. If there is a sudden, intense valgus stress across the elbow, the medial epicondyle can fracture and its fragment can be displaced. The athlete will complain of pain and swelling of the medial aspect of the elbow and may have heard or felt a "pop" at the time of injury.[32,34,35]

Examination usually reveals swelling, decreased elbow ROM, and tenderness over the medial epicondyle. Because the ulnar nerve courses in close proximity to the medial epicondyle, it is also susceptible to a traction injury from a valgus stress. Thus, it is important to assess the sensory and motor function of the ulnar nerve.

IMAGING

Elbow x-rays including AP, lateral, and oblique should be obtained. The AP radiograph is best for demonstrating a minimally displaced epicondylar fragment. Often contralateral radiographs are necessary to compare the degree of physeal separation. Younger children tend to have a larger fracture fragment with displacement and rotation as compared to adolescents, who tend to have a small fracture fragment with this injury.[32]

TREATMENT

Nondisplaced and minimally displaced (less than 3 mm) fractures are treated with immobilization in a posterior splint. Active ROM exercises are started 5 to 7 days after the acute injury to avoid chronic flexion contracture. Once the patient's pain and swelling are diminished, usually after 2 to 3 weeks, the splint can be discontinued.

Indications for referral are displacement greater than 3 mm, entrapment of an epicondylar fragment within the joint space, and/or any suspicion of neurovascular compromise. If the young athlete is very competitive, he or she may not tolerate even a small amount of displacement. Some investigators recommend surgical reduction of the fracture fragment in these cases.[36]

RETURN-TO-PLAY GUIDELINES

For cases managed conservatively or surgically, aggressive ROM and strengthening are started at approximately 4 to 6 weeks.[32] Throwing is allowed when full strength and ROM are achieved, which usually takes about 2 to 3 months.

Radial Head and Neck Fractures

Radial head and neck fractures can have serious consequences for athletes who require full elbow ROM. Anatomically, the ossification of the radial head begins at 5 years of age. In the skeletally immature patient, radial head or epiphyseal fractures are rare due to the large amount of cartilage present.

HISTORY AND PHYSICAL EXAMINATION

The three most common causes of a radial head or neck fracture are a fall on an outstretched arm (valgus stress to an extended forearm), a direct blow to the elbow, or an elbow dislocation.[37] The patient will complain of lateral elbow pain, swelling, and decreased ROM.

On physical examination, the patient will be tender over the radial head and have limited ROM due to effusion, loose bodies (fracture fragments), or severe pain. The radial head can be palpated on the lateral side of the elbow distal to the lateral epicondyle. Joint swelling, due to hemarthrosis, can be diffuse because the joint capsule attaches distal to the radial head.

IMAGING

Elbow x-rays including AP, lateral, and oblique views should be obtained (Fig. 18-8). It is imperative to check the lateral x-ray for abnormal fat pad signs. The presence of a posterior fat pad on x-ray reflects proximal displacement of the normal posterior fat pad by a bulging joint capsule and signifies a joint effusion. A posterior fat pad sign is 85 percent sensitive and 50 percent specific for subsequent fracture diagnosis.[38] A small anterior fat pad is seen on normal elbow radiographs, but a large sail-shaped lucency anterior to the distal humerus indicates an effusion and, possibly, a fracture. In this case, a radiocapitellar view (oblique view with forearm in neutral and beam directed 45° cephalad) is helpful to better visualize a radial head or neck fracture.

These fractures are classified into three types. Type I is a marginal fracture without displacement. Type II is a marginal fracture with dis-

Figure 18-8

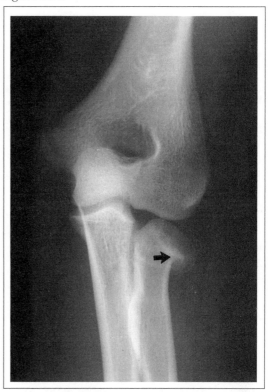

Type II radial neck fracture (*arrow*): note the significant overlap and modest angulation of the radial head. (*Radiograph courtesy of Michael Zucker, MD, University of California at Los Angeles.*)

placement greater than 2 mm, mechanical block, or involving a large portion of the radial head. Type III is a comminuted fracture of the radial head.[3]

TREATMENT AND RETURN-TO-PLAY GUIDELINES

Type I fractures are managed conservatively with the arm in a sling for 2 to 3 days and then early initiation of ROM exercises, first with flexion and extension, and later with pronation and supination. If there is greater than 30° of angulation, reduction is usually necessary, whereas if angulation is less than 30°, immobilization will suffice. Angulation is measured as a perpendicu-

Figure 18-9

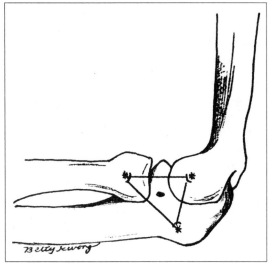

The center of the triangle, formed by the radial head, lateral epicondyle, and olecranon, marks the spot for needle entry when performing elbow joint injection or aspiration.

lar line to the articular surface of the humerus and a line through the midline of the radial metaphysis. If a large effusion is present, it is acceptable to aspirate the joint and inject a local anesthetic for pain control. The center of a triangle formed by the radial head, lateral epicondyle, and olecranon marks the spot for joint entry (Fig. 18-9). Dramatic pain relief is often provided with this procedure.[33]

Orthopedic referral is indicated for the following: (1) more than 2 mm displacement, (2) involvement of more than one third of the articular surface, (3) depression of greater than 3 mm, (4) comminution, or (5) mechanical block.[37]

ROM exercises must be initiated early in an athlete because an athlete's throwing will be adversely affected by a lack of full extension. Athletic participation is allowed when there is full, painless ROM, which usually takes 2 to 3 months.[33]

COMPLICATIONS

Permanent loss of 10 to 15° of extension is a common complication of radial head and neck fractures. This degree of extension loss is well-tolerated in daily living, but has the potential to negatively affect performance in a young athlete. Only minimal gains in ROM are expected 6 months after the fracture.

Distal Radial Fractures

Fractures of the radius are common in children. Seventy-five percent of all radial fractures occur in the distal third of the radius. Four types of fractures are commonly seen: physeal, torus, greenstick, and complete.[39] The most common site for a physeal fracture is at the distal radius.[2]

HISTORY AND PHYSICAL EXAMINATION

Distal radius fractures are usually caused by a FOOSH (fall on an outstretched hand) mechanism. Apex–volar angulation usually results from a FOOSH with the forearm in supination, whereas dorsal angulation results from a FOOSH with the forearm in pronation.[40] The athlete will complain of pain and swelling along the distal radius.

The distal radius will be tender to palpation and swelling will be noted in that area. ROM may be limited due to pain. A deformity may be present depending on the degree of displacement or angulation. The distal radial physis will be tender to palpation with a SH fracture. The neurovascular examination should be normal. A careful examination of the wrist and elbow is important to rule out associated injuries such as a radial head dislocation, disruption of the radioulnar joint, or scaphoid fracture.

IMAGING

Forearm x-rays are necessary to determine fracture type and to assess angulation, displacement, and rotation. Carefully evaluate the ulna, as well as the radius, for fractures or plastic deformation. Obtaining wrist and elbow x-rays, in addition to forearm x-rays, is prudent to avoid overlooking other injuries. For suspected physeal fractures, x-rays of the contralateral side may be helpful for comparison purposes.

TREATMENT

Distal radial fractures in children (up to the age of 12) with volar or dorsal angulation less than 20° to 30° do not require reduction.[1,39,41]

Figure 18-10

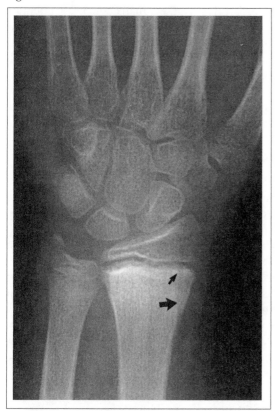

Salter–Harris type II fracture of the distal radial physis. Note the metaphyseal flag (*thick arrow*) that extends to the physis (*thin arrow*). (*Radiograph courtesy of Byron Patterson, MD, University of California at Los Angeles.*)

Figure 18-11

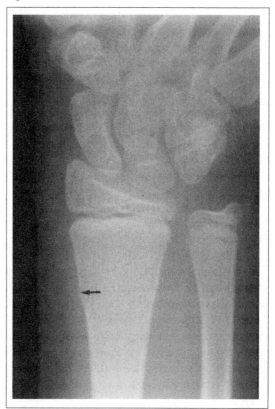

Torus fracture of the distal radius. Note the buckling of the cortex (*arrow*). (*Radiograph courtesy of Michael Zucker, MD, University of California at Los Angeles.*)

Nondisplaced and reduced SH I and II fractures (Fig. 18-10) require immobilization in a short-arm cast for approximately 3 weeks. Displaced SH III or IV fractures only need ORIF if greater than 2 mm of articular displacement remains after closed reduction attempts.[39,42]

Treatment of torus fractures (Fig. 18-11) consists of immobilization in a short-arm cast for 4 to 6 weeks in children over the age of 5. Children with a torus fracture who are less than 5 years old should be treated in a long-arm cast. Greenstick and complete fractures should be treated in a long-arm cast for 4 weeks, followed by a short-arm cast for 2 weeks.

COMPLICATIONS

One important complication of distal radial fractures is the loss of adequate fracture reduction. Young athletes should be followed closely in the first 2 weeks with weekly x-rays to monitor for this complication.[42] Growth plate arrest with resulting limb length discrepancy or angular deformity may result from physeal fractures. A limb length discrepancy of 9 cm or less is generally well-tolerated in the upper extremity.[2] Other rare complications of distal radial fractures include compartment syndrome, nerve injuries (i.e., acute carpal tunnel syndrome), fracture nonunion, and residual deformity.[41]

RETURN-TO-PLAY GUIDELINES

Athletes with distal radial fractures may return to play once the fracture has adequately healed. Football players may play with a short-arm cast as long as it is adequately padded to avoid injuring other players. Regaining full strength and ROM of the injured extremity is extremely important in some sports and for certain positions prior to return to play.

Distal Radial Physeal Stress Injury

In gymnasts, changes in the distal radial physis consistent with a chronic stress injury have been documented in the medical literature.[43–45] This overuse injury appears to be the result of using a non-weight-bearing extremity in weight-bearing positions.

HISTORY AND PHYSICAL EXAMINATION

The gymnast will complain of the gradual onset of dorsal wrist pain occurring during upper extremity weight-bearing positions.

Physical examination may reveal tenderness over the dorsal distal radial physis. Extension of the wrist may be decreased and may also reproduce the pain, particularly if coupled with an axial load.

IMAGING

Bilateral wrist radiographs should be obtained. Radiographic features consistent with stress injury to the distal radial physis include: widening and irregularity of the physis, beaking of the epiphysis, haziness of the physis, and cystic changes on the metaphyseal side of the physis.[43,46] An MRI may be necessary to further define the extent of the physeal injury or to diagnose the physeal injury if the plain radiographs are normal (Fig. 18-12).[47,48]

TREATMENT

If this diagnosis is suspected, it is probably best to refer these athletes to a sports medicine physician for further management. Generally, treatment of distal radial physeal stress injury consists of avoidance of upper extremity weight-bearing activities for 4 to 12 weeks, although longer times may be needed. Complete resolution of pain has been reported with and without the use of splint/cast immobilization.[46,47,49]

COMPLICATIONS

Various investigators have speculated that chronic stress injury to the distal radial physis can lead to premature closure of the physis and secondary growth inhibition of the radius. Growth inhibition of the radius and/or growth stimulation of the ulna could potentially result in positive ulnar variance. Positive ulnar variance refers to a condition where the ulna is longer than the radius (see Fig. 18-12). Positive ulnar variance in gymnasts has been associated with tears of the triangular fibrocartilagenous complex (TFCC), alterations in the radioulnar articulation, and degenerative changes of the triquetrum, lunate, and ulnar.[45,48,50–52]

RETURN-TO-PLAY GUIDELINES

Gymnasts may gradually return to upper extremity weight-bearing activities once their pain has completely resolved.

Figure 18-12

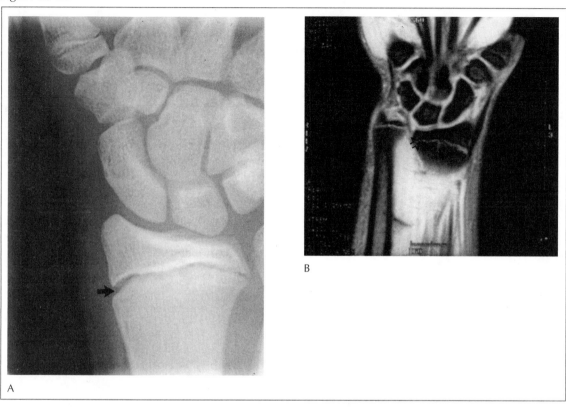

Chronic wrist pain in a gymnast. (**A**) Radiograph reveals widening of the radial portion of the distal radial physis (*arrow*). (**B**) MRI reveals physeal cartilage extension (*solid arrow*) and linear striation (*open arrow*) of the distal radial physis consistent with chronic physeal stress injury. Also note positive ulnar variance (length of ulna longer than the length of the radius).

Scaphoid Fractures

Scaphoid fractures in children under 10 years old are rare, although in adolescents it is the most common carpal bone fracture with a peak incidence seen between 12 to 15 years of age. The majority of scaphoid fractures in the pediatric population occur in the distal pole as compared to adults, where most occur in the waist of the scaphoid. Another notable difference between adult and pediatric scaphoid fractures is that fracture nonunion is not as common as in adults. In children, scaphoid fracture nonunion is usually due to a delay in diagnosis resulting in continued motion at the site of the fracture. For a complete discussion of scaphoid fractures, see Chap. 4.[42,53]

Physeal Fractures of the Hand

Thirty-four percent of hand fractures in children are to the physis, with almost 80 percent of those being SH type II fractures. The most common hand fracture in children is a SH type II fracture of the proximal phalanx of the little finger.

The thumb metacarpal and phalangeal growth plates are found in the proximal portion of the

Figure 18-13

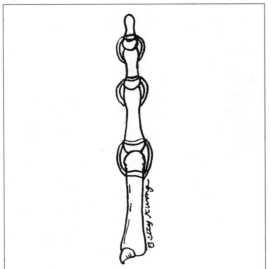

Growth plates and ligamentous attachments in the hand.

bone, whereas the growth plates in the remainder of the metacarpals are located distally (Fig. 18-13). These growth plates provide most of the longitudinal growth of the hand and usually close between 14 to 16 years of age.[53]

The attachments of the collateral ligaments, extensor tendons, and the volar plate on the phalanges all play an important role in determining fracture types in children. The collateral ligaments about the metacarpophalangeal (MCP) joints attach directly into the epiphysis of both the proximal phalanx and the distal metacarpal, in contrast to the collateral ligaments about the proximal and distal interphalangeal joints (PIP and DIP), which attach to the epiphysis and the metaphysis (see Fig. 18-13). The later configuration offers protection to the physis. This anatomic difference contributes to the higher incidence of SH fractures at the proximal phalanx. The central slip of the extensor tendon and the terminal extensor tendon insert on the epiphyseal portion of the middle phalanx and the distal phalanx, respectively. The volar plate also attaches only to

the epiphyseal portion of the PIP and DIP joints (Fig. 18-14). In adolescents who are near skeletal maturity, these anatomic relationships predispose to SH type III fractures.[53]

HISTORY AND PHYSICAL EXAMINATION

In the adolescent athlete, the most common mechanisms of injury involve either direct trauma to the hand from a moving object (i.e., a ball) or a fall. Crush injuries may also occur, but are more commonly encountered in the younger child. The athlete will complain of pain, swelling, and a loss of ROM.

The area of maximal tenderness and swelling helps to pinpoint the location of the fracture on physical examination. Ligamentous stress testing should be avoided until a periarticular fracture is ruled out by x-rays because stress testing can displace a periarticular fracture. Assessment of the fingers for a rotational deformity is done by having the patient flex the fingers. The fingers should point to the area of the scaphoid tubercle (Fig. 18-15). The scaphoid tubercle can be pal-

Figure 18-14

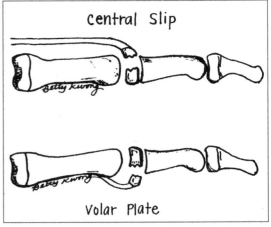

Attachment of the central slip and the volar plate on the epiphysis.

Figure 18-15

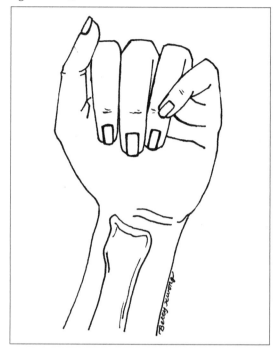

Malrotation of the little finger.

pated near the thenar crease along the base of the thumb. Any degree of rotational deformity is not acceptable. This test should be repeated following any reduction procedures. The neurovascular examination of the hand should be normal.

IMAGING

Radiographs of the hand, including anteroposterior, oblique, and lateral views, should be obtained. Comparison views of the uninjured hand may be helpful.

TREATMENT

PHYSEAL FRACTURES OF THE DISTAL PHALANX These fractures usually occur following a hyperflexion injury to the DIP joint and may present with a mallet finger. Patients with mallet fingers cannot

actively extend their DIP joint, although the DIP joint can be extended passively. Nondisplaced SH type I, II and III fractures of the distal phalanx can be treated with the DIP joint in an extension splint for 4 to 6 weeks.[42,53] Displaced SH fractures are reduced by gently extending the distal phalanx after adequate analgesia is obtained with a digital block.

Splinting of fractures treated with closed reduction is the same as a nondisplaced fracture. Post-reduction films should be obtained to document anatomic reduction. If closed reduction fails or if the fracture is large and significantly displaced, ORIF with Kirschner wire fixation is indicated.[53] Patients should be told to avoid any flexion to the DIP joint while this fracture is healing.

If full active extension of the DIP joint is regained at 6 weeks, the athlete is released for full sports participation, but should wear the extension splint for protection during sports activities for another 4 weeks. If an extension lag remains at 6 weeks, then the patient is placed back into the extension splint, to be worn 24 h per day, for another 4 weeks. If 10 weeks of treatment in an extension splint fails to restore full active DIP extension, the athlete should be referred to a hand surgeon for consideration of surgical treatment.[42,54]

PHYSEAL FRACTURES OF THE MIDDLE PHALANX Dorsal and volar physeal fractures of the middle phalanx are usually the result of an avulsion injury at the insertions of the central extensor tendon slip or the volar plate on the epiphysis, respectively. These are usually SH type III or IV fractures and occur in adolescence.

Treatment of dorsal physeal fractures depends on the size and displacement of the fracture. Closed treatment is acceptable if the fracture involves less than 25 percent of the articular surface and is displaced less than 2 mm. The fracture is treated in full extension with either a splint or a short-arm gutter cast for 3 to 6 weeks. The adjacent finger should be included in the cast with the hand casted in a position of function (30° of wrist extension, 50° to 70° of MCP flexion, and 0 to 10° of IP flexion). If an extension splint is used for treatment, the patient must be cautioned to not allow any flexion of the PIP to occur. ORIF is indicated if the fracture involves greater than 25 percent of the joint and is displaced greater than 2 mm.[42,53,54]

Volar physeal fractures are treated with a dorsal splint placed over the PIP joint with the joint in 20° to 30° of flexion for 3 weeks.[42,53] If the physeal fracture is large enough to cause the PIP joint to sublux, then ORIF is needed.[42]

PHYSEAL FRACTURES OF THE PROXIMAL PHALANX The most common type of fracture at this site is an SH type II of the little finger. Closed reduction is required because the little finger is typically displaced into an abducted position. Two reduction techniques are commonly employed. One method involves placing the MCP joints in 90° of flexion and applying traction to the little finger while it is adducted across the ring finger. Although discouraged by some authors,[53] the second technique involves using a pencil/pen as a fulcrum in the web space between the little and ring fingers while the little finger is adducted into a normal position. Dorsal or volar angulation of up to 30° is acceptable.

The little and ring fingers should be buddy-taped and then placed into an ulnar gutter cast (hand in position of function) for 3 weeks. Reduction should be confirmed with x-rays. After 3 weeks, the cast may be removed and the fingers buddy-taped for 1 more week to complete the treatment.[42,53,54]

PHYSEAL FRACTURES OF THE METACARPAL These are unusual fractures and require ORIF if they are displaced. Consultation with an orthopedic surgeon is usually best for metacarpal physeal fractures, even if they are nondisplaced, because avascular necrosis of the metacarpal head may complicate this fracture.

Physeal fractures of the thumb metacarpal occur proximally (at the carpometacarpal joint). They are best managed by an orthopedic surgeon.[53]

PEDIATRIC SKIER'S THUMB In athletes with open growth plates, a hyperabduction injury to thumb MCP joint often results in a SH fracture (usually type III in adolescents and type I or II in children) rather than an avulsion or sprain of the ulnar collateral ligament as seen in adults (Fig.18-16). If this fracture is nondisplaced, the patient can be treated in a short-arm thumb spica cast for 4 to 6 weeks with athletic participation allowed in the cast. If no fracture is seen on x-rays, then the thumb MCP joint can be stressed to assess the integrity of the ligament. Anesthesia may be necessary to accurately assess the stability of the ligament. It is not necessary to stress the ligament if a fracture is seen because this may displace the fracture. Displaced fractures (greater than 2 mm) or complete disruption of the ulnar collateral ligament require ORIF.[42,53,54]

Figure 18-16

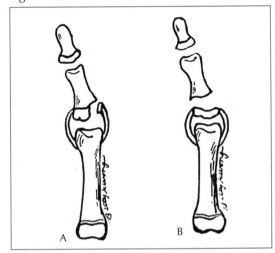

Pediatric skier's thumb. (**A**) Salter–Harris type III fracture. (**B**) Salter–Harris type I fracture.

COMPLICATIONS

Common complications include residual deformity, loss of hand function, and post-traumatic arthritis. Because any loss of hand function can be detrimental to an athlete who competes in a sport that requires exceptional hand mobility and strength, it is imperative to treat hand fractures with cautious concern and obtain expert consultation if the management is in question.[42,53] When treating physeal fractures of the hand, it is important to keep in mind that growth arrest is a complication of any growth plate injury (although is typically rare in the hand).

RETURN-TO-PLAY GUIDELINES

Most athletes will be able to return to full participation within 3 to 6 weeks following most physeal hand fractures that are treated with closed reduction. Cross training and maintaining or improving strength and flexibility in uninjured areas should be encouraged while the fracture is healing.

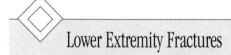

Lower Extremity Fractures

Distal Femoral Physeal Fractures

The distal femoral growth plate is considered the largest and fastest growing physis in the body.[55] Mechanically, the physis is shaped like a large W, and is, therefore, better able to tolerate most of the shearing forces that propagate up the femur. Most injuries are SH II fractures,[56] but the age of the patient, magnitude of displacement, and adequacy of reduction give a more accurate picture of the severity and prognosis of this injury rather than just the SH classification alone.[57,58] The importance of proper diagnosis

and treatment cannot be overemphasized due to the high risk of complications with injury to this growth plate.

HISTORY AND PHYSICAL EXAMINATION

Injuries to distal femoral physis can occur in all sports, but are most frequently seen in adolescent football players. The most common mechanism of injury is a hyperextension force with slight valgus or varus direction. Patients will complain of pain, swelling, and difficulty bearing weight.

On physical examination, the knee is usually held in a flexion position due to hamstring spasm. Tenderness of the distal femoral physis to palpation will be present along with swelling. If the fracture is displaced, the affected thigh may appear angulated. A common error on examination is the detection of valgus instability with medial collateral ligament (MCL) testing and then attributing the instability to an MCL injury as opposed to a growth plate injury. Careful neurovascular assessment of the lower extremity distal to the injury is crucial because the neurovascular bundle (popliteal artery, tibial nerve, and common peroneal nerve) lies just posterior to the femoral metaphysis (Table 18-3). Assess for signs of compartment syndrome signs such as massive swelling, marked tenseness of the limb compartments, and distal neurovascular insufficiency.

IMAGING

On radiographs, the typical SH type II fracture separation passes through the physis exiting laterally at the metaphysis in an oblique fashion. SH type I injuries are more difficult to identify because the fracture line does not travel through cortical bone. Often, the only identifiable feature is a slight asymmetry or irregularity of the physeal plate; this may only be seen with comparison views of the opposite femur. Radiographs with

Table 18-3

Neurologic Examination of Selected Lower Extremity Peripheral Nerves

NERVE	SENSORY	MOTOR
Deep peroneal	Area between first and second toes (dorsal aspect)	Toe extension
		Foot inversion
Superficial peroneal	Dorsum of foot	Foot eversion
Sural	Lateral aspect of foot	Plantar flexion
Tibial	Plantar aspect of foot	Toe flexion
		Foot inversion

SOURCE: Adapted with permission from Hoppenfeld S: Physical Examination of the Spine and Extremities. Norwalk, CT: Appleton & Lange; 1976.

valgus stress applied to the knee may also be necessary to make the diagnosis (Fig. 18-17). SH type III and IV fractures through the epiphysis to the articular surface are rare. SH type V compression fractures are extremely rare in athletes.

TREATMENT

Treatment is fairly straightforward in the nondisplaced, nonangulated fractures. The patient should be placed in a hip spica cast for 2 to 3 weeks and then a long-leg cast for another 2 to 3 weeks until the fracture is healed. Nondisplaced SH type I fractures generally heal well without significant sequelae. Fractures that are displaced more than 2 to 3 mm, or with more than 5° of angulation, need orthopedic referral for either closed reduction or ORIF. Displaced SH type I and II fractures are treated with closed reduction under anesthesia. Type III and IV displaced fractures are generally treated with ORIF.[57]

COMPLICATIONS

Complications include neurovascular injury, leg-length discrepancy, and decreased knee ROM. Angular deformity and leg-length discrepancy are probably the most common complications and occur in up to half of all cases.[56,58] Close follow-up for evidence of growth arrest is crucial with any injury to the distal femoral physis because it contributes 70 percent of final femur length. Fractures displaced more than half of the diameter of the bone have an increased risk for growth disturbance and leg-length discrepancy.[59]

RETURN-TO-PLAY GUIDELINES

Physical therapy is usually needed to restore full strength and mobility prior to return to sports. Full return to sports is typically in the range of 4 to 6 months.[60]

Acute Tibial Tubercle Avulsion Fractures

Avulsion fractures of the tibial tubercle are fairly uncommon, but very dramatic in presentation. Ninety percent of these fractures occur in sports-related activities. The male-to-female ratio is 5:1 and the average age for this injury is 17 years old. The tibial epiphysis and tibial tubercle apophysis arise from separate growth plates that fuse near the end of adolescence. The tibial tubercle is able to withstand substantial tensile forces because it is mostly fibrocartilage prior to ossification.[55]

It is unclear whether a previous diagnosis of Osgood–Schlatter's condition is a risk factor for an acute tibial tubercle avulsion fracture because the incidence of an antecedent Osgood–Schlatter's diagnosis ranges from 10 to 60 percent. Osgood–Schlatter's condition represents a

Figure 18-17

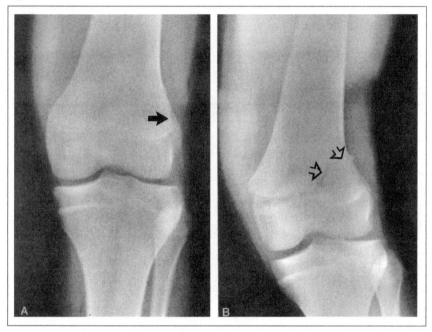

Distal femoral physeal injury. (**A**) The AP view shows a subtle fracture line laterally, just superior to the epiphysis (*solid arrow*). (**B**) An AP view with a valgus stress applied reveals a type II SH fracture with a large metaphyseal flag laterally (*open arrow*). (*Reproduced with permission from CL Stanitski et al (eds): Pediatric and Adolescent Sports Medicine. Philadelphia: WB Saunders, 1994.*)

chronic avulsion injury of the anterior ossicle of the tibial tubercle and thus, it is unknown whether this previously modified tibial tubercle cartilage somehow leads to an increased risk of fracture.[55] Some researchers believe that children with severe, disabling pain from chronic Osgood–Schlatter's condition should limit sports-related heavy eccentric loads to the quadriceps mechanism due to this possible increased risk of acute avulsion fracture.[61]

HISTORY AND PHYSICAL EXAMINATION

The classic case involves a late-adolescent male who sustains an acute avulsion of the tibial tubercle from the tibial shaft while performing leaping or jumping activities. The mechanism is thought to involve counteracting knee flexion and extension forces, which result in eccentric overload on the patellar tendon attachment on the tibial tubercle.[55] (Eccentric loading occurs when a muscle is forcefully contracting but elongating at the same time.) The type of fracture that ensues appears to be dependent on the amount of knee flexion at the time of the injury. For example, with the knee in flexion, both the anterior tubercle and the proximal tibial physis are prone to injury. Whereas with the knee in extension, usually only the anterior tubercle is fractured.[62]

The patient will have edema and tenderness at the tibial tubercle, often with associated eccyhmosis on examination. Patients with mild injury can actively extend the knee, but not against resistance. Patients with more severe injuries usually cannot extend the knee at all.[55]

A knee effusion may also be present due to intra-articular extension of the fracture or associated anterior cruciate ligament (ACL) injury.

IMAGING

This fracture is classified into four types based on radiographic findings (Fig. 18-18). The lateral x-ray provides the best view of this fracture. Type I is a nondisplaced fracture and is usually diagnosed by history and physical examination alone. Type II is a displaced tubercle fracture without tibial physis extension. A type III fracture involves both the proximal tibial epiphysis and tubercle apophysis. Extension of the fracture into the intra-articular space is classified as a type IV fracture.[61]

TREATMENT

If the fracture is nondisplaced or minimally displaced (less than 2 to 3 mm), long-leg cast immobilization with the knee in full extension for 3 to 4 weeks usually allows for adequate healing. For any other fractures, ORIF is necessary to restore proper anatomic alignment and normal knee extension. This needs urgent, but not emergent, consultation. The patient can be placed in a non-weight-bearing, long-leg splint with the knee in full extension while waiting for orthopedic evaluation, which should occur within a few days. If the joint space is involved, emergent orthopedic consultation should be obtained.[57]

RETURN-TO-PLAY GUIDELINES

Return to play is permitted when the patient has pain-free, full knee ROM, along with full strength of the quadriceps, hamstrings, and calf muscles. The usual time frame is 2 to 3 months for the nonsurgical cases and 3 to 4 months for the surgical cases.[61]

Tibial Eminence Avulsion Fractures

HISTORY AND PHYSICAL EXAMINATION

The ACL attaches to the tibia at the tibial eminence just anterolateral to the anterior tibial spine; it also has a small attachment to the anterior horn of the lateral meniscus.[63] In children, acute ACL injuries frequently result from avulsions of the ACL insertion at the tibial eminence,

Figure 18-18

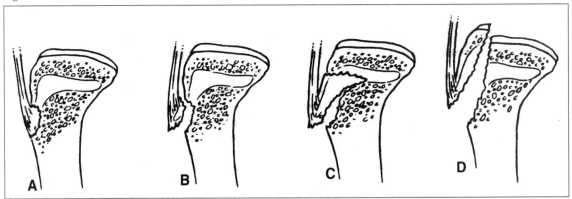

Tibial tubercle avusion fracture classification. (**A**) Undisplaced. (**B**) Displaced without physeal involvement. (**C**) Displaced with extension into the physis. (**D**) Displacement with extension through physis into the joint space *(Reproduced with permission from CL Stanitski et al (eds): Pediatric and Adolescent Sports Medicine. Philadelphia: WB Saunders, 1994.)*

Figure 18-19

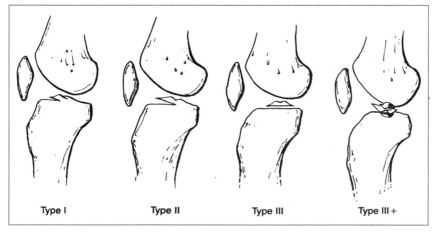

Type I   Type II   Type III   Type III +

Tibial eminence avulsion fracture classification. *(Reproduced with permission from CL Stanit-ski et al (eds): Pediatric and Adolescent Sports Medicine. Philadelphia: WB Saunders, 1994.)*

as compared to adults where midsubstance tears are more common. The probable mechanism of injury is tibial rotation relative to the femur during forced knee hyperextension.[64] The patient will typically complain of knee pain, swelling, decreased ROM, and, possibly, knee instability or mechanical symptoms.

Physical examination findings include generalized tenderness, effusion, and an antalgic gait. Lachman and anterior drawer testing may reveal AP laxity. Injuries to collateral ligaments and menisci are common with tibial eminence avulsion injuries. Thus, it is crucial to do a thorough knee examination to assess for associated injuries.[63]

IMAGING

AP and lateral x-rays are usually sufficient to diagnose this fracture. Acute tibial eminence fractures are classified into 4 types (Fig. 18-19): (1) nondisplaced, (2) slight elevation of the tibial eminence, (3) tibial eminence elevation with displacement, and (4) complete displacement with rotation.[63] MRI may be helpful to evaluate for associated injuries.

TREATMENT

Treatment of these injuries has been traditionally based on the degree of separation. Nondisplaced and slightly elevated fractures (type I and II) can be treated with immobilization in a long-leg cast with the knee in full extension for about 6 weeks.[57] Any displaced fractures should be immobilized and orthopedics should be consulted for ORIF. Prognosis of these injuries is generally very good with most children regaining excellent ROM. Most studies have shown that functional instability and/or joint deterioration does not occur frequently, despite residual laxity on knee examinations.[65]

RETURN-TO-PLAY GUIDELINES

Most patients require 4 to 6 weeks of rehabilitation following immobilization, with particular emphasis on knee ROM and quadriceps and hamstring strengthening. Patients may return to play when they demonstrate the ability to perform the functional skills required for their respective sports. Sports with a large degree of cutting (i.e., sudden side-to-side movements), acceleration, and deceleration, such as soccer, football, and basketball, may require a longer period of functional rehabilitation.

Osteochondritis Dissecans (OCD) of the Knee

OCD has become one of the most controversial topics in the sports medicine and orthopedic literature due to its numerous possible etiologies, intricate underlying pathoanatomy and pathophysiology, and complex treatment options. Although multiple etiologies, including ischemic, infectious, and genetic, have been proposed to explain the OCD lesion, traumatic injury is the most widely accepted theory.[66]

OCD is usually defined as a separation of subchondral bone and cartilage from the underlying vascularized bone.[67] The lesion is usually unilateral and rare before age 10 and after age 50. Forty to fifty percent of patients with OCD of the knee have some recollection of a significant traumatic event, which may have been the initial insult. Upward of 80 to 90 percent of all cases occur in active youngsters with or without trauma. The male-to-female ratio is 2:1. Seventy percent of the OCD lesions are found at the posterolateral aspect of the medial femoral condyle. Approximately 15 percent occur on other areas of the medial condyle and 15 percent occur on the lateral condyle.[68,69]

HISTORY AND PHYSICAL EXAMINATION

Clinically, patients present with vague knee aching that is worsened by activities. Intermittent effusion is not uncommon. Patients may describe mechanical symptoms such as locking, catching, or painful popping.

The physical examination is often nonspecific. ROM may be diminished due to loose bodies within the joint. Quadriceps atrophy may be present due to chronic effusion and/or to relative underuse of the affected lower extremity. One study noted that children with medial femoral condyle OCD walked with external tibial rota-

tion and that their pain was reproduced during knee extension with internal tibial rotation.[70] Tenderness may be present over the medial femoral condyle, as the knee is slowly brought into full flexion.

IMAGING

Various imaging modalities are helpful for diagnostic purposes (Fig. 18-20). Routine plain films often show a well-circumscribed fragment of subchondral bone separated from the femoral condyle. In addition to routine radiographic views of the knee, a tunnel view should be ordered on all active youngsters who have knee pain of unexplained etiology. The tunnel view provides the best view of the posterior aspect of the femoral condyles, where OCD lesions are most commonly located. MRI can often identify lesions that are missed on plain films. MRI with intra-articular gadolinium may be more helpful to differentiate a stable versus unstable lesion.[71]

A classification scheme for OCD lesions has been developed based on MRI findings.[72]

Type I   Intact articular surface with subchondral bony changes

Type II   Fracture or fissure of the articular surface

Type III Partial detachment (osteochondral flap)

Type IV   Detached osteochondral loose body with open crater on the articular surface

TREATMENT

Immobilization and non-weight-bearing may be adequate treatment for the young athlete with *open physes and a stable fragment* (type I and some type II lesions). Unloading of the joint provides the optimal environment for healing of such injuries and it may protect against progression of an OCD lesion. Symptoms, not radiographic healing, determine the time frame, as the healing changes on x-ray may take 3 months

Figure 18-20

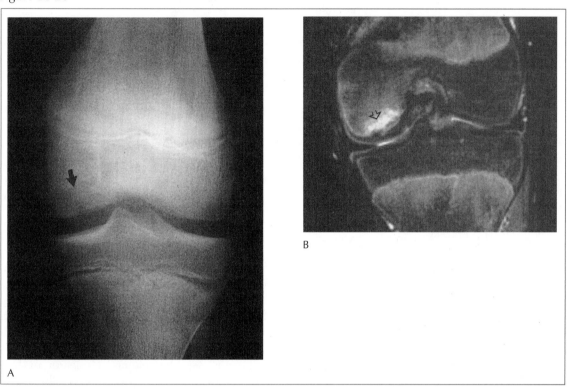

Osteochondritis dissecans of the knee. (**A**) Notice the subtle subchondral bony lesion on the lateral aspect of the medial femoral condyle (*solid arrow*). (**B**) MRI shows a similar lesion with white signal change suggestive of an active lesion on the T-2 weighted image (*open arrow*). (*Radiographs courtesy of James C. Puffer, MD, University of California at Los Angeles.*)

to appear. A gradual return to mobility is crucial with graded weight bearing, progressing to quadriceps, hamstring, and calf strengthening, and, later, functional rehabilitation focusing on sports-specific skills. If the symptoms do not subside within 8 to 10 weeks and bone scan or MRI does not show adequate healing, then arthroscopy is indicated.[67] For a skeletally immature patient with locking, catching, or severe swelling, the fragment must be considered unstable and more aggressive measures taken.

Indications for surgery in skeletally immature patients include: (1) unstable lesions (type III,

type IV, and some type II lesions) on plain films or MRI, (2) symptom recurrence, or (3) failure to heal as skeletal maturity approaches. Skeletally mature patients generally will not benefit from conservative management, with surgery offering the best possibility of obtaining union of the osteochondritic fragment.[69]

Decisions regarding surgical treatment are complex and vary widely among surgeons, due to lack of prospective data. Arthroscopy with debridement or abrasion followed by drilling is the most common procedure. Depending on fragment morphology and tissue damage, ORIF with pins, screws, and bone pegs with and without bone grafting are also potential procedures. Osteoarticular transplant technique (OATS) is now being studied, as well as autologous chondrocyte transplantation.[69,73]

PROGNOSIS AND COMPLICATIONS

Certain prognostic factors help to determine the overall risk for development of premature arthritis, which is the main complication of OCD. The primary factor is age of onset, but lesion size, progression, location, and stability must also be considered. The ultimate goal is a flat and smooth joint surface with as much articular cartilage, and as little fibrocartilage, as possible. Most investigators agree that children with open physes are more likely to heal spontaneously without major sequelae, as compared to patients who have reached skeletal maturity.[69,74,75] Pappas suggested that girls and boys less than 11 and 13 years old, respectively, have the best prognosis. Girls aged 12 to 20 and boys aged 14 to 20 years have a less certain prognosis, and anyone over 20 years old has a poorer prognosis and requires surgical intervention more frequently.[75]

If the articular cartilage mantle breaks down and the subchondral bone is exposed to synovial fluid, this lesion is considered open and the stability of the fragment is compromised; therefore, spontaneous resolution is unlikely. Radiographic evidence of sclerosis at the base of the fragment margin is generally considered a poor prognostic sign.[66]

RETURN-TO-PLAY GUIDELINES

Return to play criteria is based on the child's ability to perform necessary sports activities at full capacity, without symptoms. Average return to full activity is 3 to 4 months for low-grade OCD lesions. Up to 6 months may be necessary for more advanced lesions which require operative treatment.[67]

Distal Tibial Physeal Fractures

This discussion is limited to SH type I and II distal tibial fractures, because SH type III and IV fractures should be referred to an orthopedic surgeon for management.

HISTORY AND PHYSICAL EXAMINATION

The mechanism usually involves either external rotation or an eversion force applied to a pronated foot. These fractures are commonly seen in football and soccer players. Swelling and tenderness along the anterolateral portion of the ankle are seen on physical examination.

IMAGING

X-rays in nondisplaced SH type I distal tibial fractures may reveal growth plate widening or may be normal except for soft tissue swelling. Radiographs of the uninjured side may detect subtle growth plate widening. SH type II fractures show the typical metaphyseal flag, which is frequently displaced either laterally or posteriorly. X-rays should be reviewed carefully to look for associated fibular fractures.

TREATMENT

Displaced SH I and II fractures should be reduced using longitudinal traction and internal rotation of the ankle. If a satisfactory reduction cannot be achieved using closed techniques, then ORIF is necessary.

SH type I fractures can be treated in a long-leg non-weight-bearing cast for the first 3 weeks and then a weight-bearing short-leg cast or walking boot for 3 weeks. SH type II fractures are treated the same as SH type I fractures for the first 3 weeks. The final 3 weeks of treatment are spent non-weight-bearing in a short-leg cast.[76]

COMPLICATIONS

Growth arrest and/or angular deformity may result. The distal tibial growth plate contributes approximately 45 percent of the total tibial length but a leg-length discrepancy of less than 2 cm is generally well-tolerated.[2]

RETURN-TO-PLAY GUIDELINES

Distal tibial SH type I and II fractures require approximately 6 weeks for complete healing. Once the fracture is healed, the athlete may gradually return to practice and competition. Impact activities should be increased in a step-wise fashion and supplemented with nonimpact cross-training activities. Physical therapy is generally not needed unless there is a significant amount of atrophy or loss of ROM.

Tillaux Fracture

A juvenile Tillaux fracture is an SH type III fracture of the anterolateral portion of the distal tibial epiphysis (Fig. 18-21). To understand this fracture, the clinician must appreciate the normal asymmetrical pattern of physeal closure in the distal tibia. Closure of this physis starts between 12 to 15 years of age, beginning earlier in girls and later in boys. It takes about 1.5 years to completely close the distal tibial physis and it is during this time-period that a Tillaux fracture can occur. The central portion of the distal tibial physis closes first, followed by the medial portion, then the posterolateral portion, and, finally, the anterolateral portion.

A Tillaux fracture occurs when an excessive external rotation force places traction on the anterior inferior tibiofibular ligament. This ligament attaches distally to the tibial physis on the anterolateral portion of the distal tibia. Instead of the ligament failing, the forces are translated to the weak link in the chain, the anterolateral portion of the distal tibial physis.[1,4,77,78]

HISTORY AND PHYSICAL EXAMINATION

The patient will usually be between 12 to 15 years old and describe an external rotation

Figure 18-21

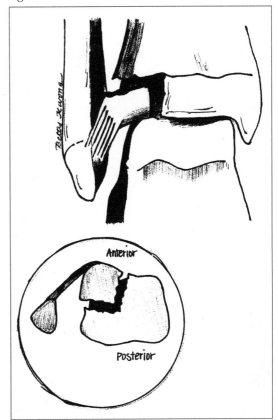

Diagram of a Tillaux fracture.

mechanism as the cause of the injury. Tenderness and swelling will be located over the anterior and lateral distal tibia. An ankle effusion will likely be present due to violation of the articular cartilage. External rotation of the ankle produces pain.

IMAGING

Standard ankle radiographs reveal this SH type III fracture and should carefully evaluated for displacement (Fig. 18-22). Further imaging with a CT scan is necessary; plain films do not always reveal the amount of displacement accurately.[79]

Figure 18-22

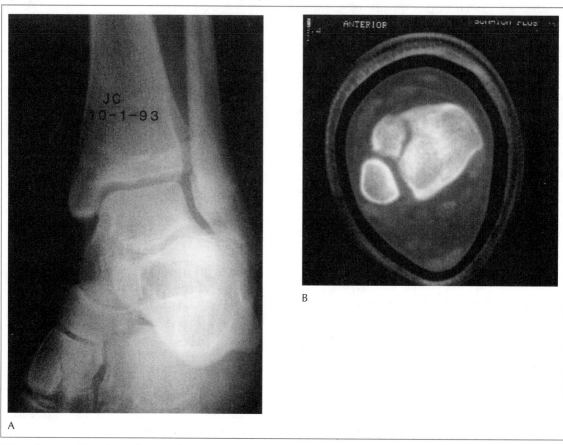

Tillaux fracture. (**A**) Radiograph of a Salter–Harris type III fracture of the distal tibia. (**B**) CT scan (axial section) more accurately reveals the degree of fracture displacement. *(Radiographs courtesy of James C. Puffer, MD, University of California at Los Angeles.)*

TREATMENT

Treatment of Tillaux fractures with no displacement and anatomic alignment of the tibial plafond consists of immobilization in a long-leg, non-weight-bearing cast with the foot in internal rotation for 3 weeks. The patient is then placed into a short-leg walking cast for the final 3 weeks of treatment.[76,79]

Consultation with an orthopedic surgeon is necessary for Tillaux fractures with displacement or malalignment of the tibial palfond. Closed reduction involves gentle internal rotation of the ankle with axial traction. Repeated attempts at closed reduction should be avoided. ORIF is indicated if the fragment is displaced greater than 2 mm, the alignment of the tibial palfond is disrupted, or attempts at closed reduction have failed.[4,79]

COMPLICATIONS

Failure to restore anatomic alignment of the articular cartilage can lead to chronic pain and degenerative arthritis.[77] Growth arrest may be a complication of this fracture, but is usually of little consequence because the physis is almost closed at the age when this injury is likely to occur.

Triplane Fracture

Orthopedic consultation is necessary for this fracture and, thus, a detailed discussion is beyond the scope of this chapter. Briefly, a triplane fracture is a fracture of the distal tibial physis in which the fracture line extends in 3 planes: transverse, sagittal, and coronal (Fig. 18-23). It is also described as a Tillaux fracture with a metaphyseal fragment.[1] In one study of 36 triplane fractures, approximately 50 percent occurred during sports activities.

Radiographs may not reveal the extent of the fracture and a CT scan is often required to detail the full extent of the fracture and to assess adequacy of closed reduction.[80] CT with three-dimensional reconstruction is recommended by some researchers.[81]

ORIF is indicated for displacement greater than 2 mm. The outcome of triplane fractures is surprisingly good with prognosis related to the restoration of joint congruency. Complications include growth plate arrest, loss of ankle mobility, degenerative arthritis, and chronic pain.

Fractures of the Lateral Process of the Talus

This fracture is commonly referred to as "snowboarder's ankle." This previously uncommon

Figure 18-23

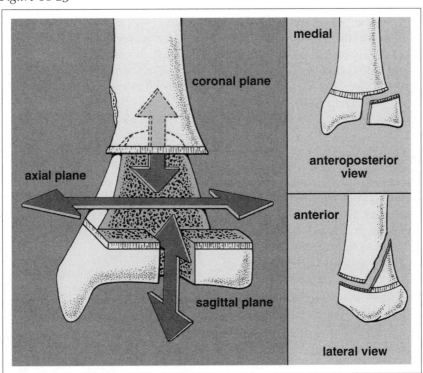

Diagram of a triplane fracture. A triplane fracture consists of three fracture components: axial, coronal, and sagittal. *(Reproduced with permission from Greenspan A. (ed): Orthopedic Radiology. Philadelphia: Lippincott, Williams & Wilkins, 2000.)*

Figure 18-24

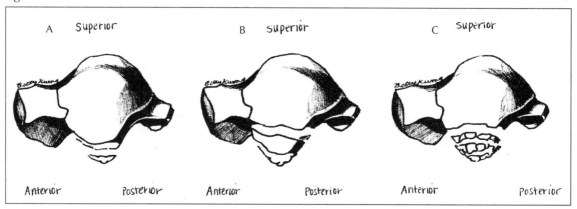

Classification of fractures of the lateral process of the talus. (**A**) Type 1. (**B**) Type 2. (**C**) Type 3.

fracture has increased dramatically since the inception of snowboarding.[82] This fracture is associated with more advanced levels of snowboarding and is estimated to account for 34 percent of all ankle fractures in snowboarders.[83] The lateral process of the talus has both an articular and a nonarticular surface. The lateral process is closely associated with the anterior talofibular ligament (ATFL).

HISTORY AND PHYSICAL EXAMINATION

Usually the patient will be a snowboarder. The mechanism of injury appears to involve forced dorsiflexion and inversion of the ankle.[82] Examination reveals tenderness and swelling over the lateral aspect of the ankle, particularly over the lateral process. The lateral process can be palpated 1 cm inferior to the tip of the lateral malleolus. This fracture is often misdiagnosed as a severe sprain due to the close proximity of the anterior talofibular ligament.

IMAGING

Fractures of the lateral process of the talus can be classified into 3 types (Fig. 18-24). Type 1 is

a chip fracture of the anterior inferior portion of the lateral process and probably represents an avulsion fracture of the ATFL. Type 1 fractures are best seen on lateral x-rays taken in 0° of dorsiflexion as well as with 10° to 20° of inversion. Type 2 is a fracture of a single large fragment, which involves both the talofibular and talocalcaneal articular surfaces. Anteroposterior x-ray views provide the best look at this fracture type. Type 3 fractures are comminuted and often involve the entire lateral process. Type 3 fractures involve the articular surfaces of the talofibular and talocalcaneal joints. This fracture is easily missed on plain films.[83] CT or MRI scanning may be necessary if the diagnosis is in question or to further define the extent of the fracture.[83,84]

TREATMENT

Nondisplaced (less than 2 mm) type 1 and 2 fractures can be treated with partial weight-bearing in a short-leg cast for 6 weeks. Displaced type 2 fractures and type 3 fractures should be treated with ORIF. Type 3 fractures may require excision of the entire lateral process if anatomic alignment is not achievable.

COMPLICATIONS

Data are lacking on the long-term outcome of these fractures. Two retrospective studies reported that 2 to 3 patients out of 13 developed subtalar degenerative changes that required subtalar fusion.[85,86] Other complications may include non-union, malalignment, and osseous overgrowth.[82]

RETURN-TO-PLAY GUIDELINES

For nondisplaced type 1 and 2 fractures, it is necessary to demonstrate healing of the fracture, resolution of pain, and full ROM and strength of the ankle prior to return to sports. For most patients, this represents a 6- to 10-week time frame.

Distal Fibular Physeal Fractures

Salter–Harris type I or II fractures are the most common fractures of the distal fibula seen in young athletes.[87]

HISTORY AND PHYSICAL EXAMINATION

The mechanism involves supination and inversion of the ankle. Athletes that wear cleats, such as football and soccer players, may be more prone to this injury, although it is important to consider this fracture in the differential diagnosis of any inversion ankle injury in athletes with open growth plates.

The patient will be tender at the distal fibular physis on palpation.[78] To palpate this physis, the examiner should palpate the tibiotalar joint line anteriorly and then move laterally to the distal fibula. The distal fibular physis lies approximately at the level of the tibiotalar joint. There may be swelling and ecchymosis along the distal fibula. The lateral ligaments will be nontender, unless there is an associated ankle sprain. External rotation of the ankle joint causes pain at the distal fibula. Neurovascular status of the foot should be normal.

IMAGING

Standard ankle radiographs (3 views) should be ordered to evaluate the physis. Most distal fibular physeal fractures are nondisplaced. Radiographs of a nondisplaced distal fibular SH type I fracture will typically show lateral soft-tissue swelling without evidence of fracture.[78] Remember, tenderness of the distal fibular physis alone is sufficient to make the diagnosis of a SH type I fracture. If there is doubt about growth-plate widening, radiographs of the opposite side should be obtained for comparison (Fig. 18-25). As with any SH type II fracture, those of the distal fibula will demonstrate the Thurston–Holland sign described earlier (metaphyseal flag).

TREATMENT

Nondisplaced SH type I or II fractures can be treated with a short-leg walking cast or boot for 3 to 4 weeks. If there is too much swelling present initially, such that casting would not be appropriate, use either a plaster or fiberglass splint or walking boot. If after 3 to 4 weeks of immobilization, the patient remains tender at the distal fibular physis, then further immobilization (2 to 3 weeks) in a short-leg walking cast or walking boot is necessary.[87]

Displaced SH type I or II fractures can usually be treated with closed reduction. After performing a hematoma block, the reduction is attempted by inverting and internally rotating the ankle. Post-reduction radiographs are necessary to document adequate reduction. If the clinician is uncomfortable attempting a closed reduction, then the athlete should be referred to a specialist for definitive treatment. Following an adequate reduction, the patient should be treated in a non-weight-bearing short-leg cast for 3 to 4 weeks. If tenderness is still present, further immobilization is required as outlined for nondisplaced SH type I or II fractures.[87]

Distal fibular SH fractures other than types I and II should be referred for orthopedic management.

Figure 18-25

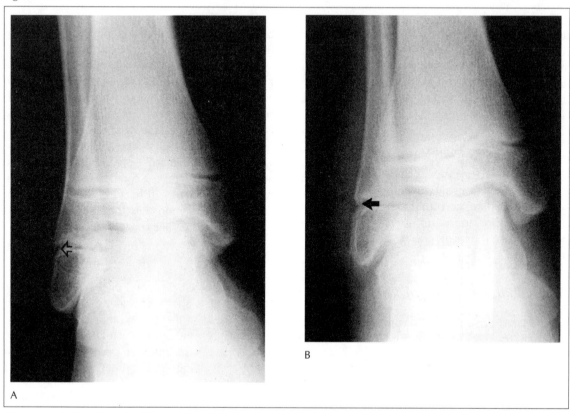

(**A**) A normal AP radiograph of the right distal fibular physis. (**B**) Salter–Harris type I distal fibular physis fracture. Abnormal widening (*solid arrow*) of the left distal fibular physis (3 mm) could easily be overlooked unless compared to the measurement of 2 mm on the uninjured side (*open arrow*). *(Radiographs courtesy of Michael Zucker, MD, University of California at Los Angeles.)*

COMPLICATIONS

Growth arrest is a possible complication, but is exceedingly rare in this location with SH I or II fractures.

RETURN-TO-PLAY GUIDELINES

Return to play is allowed after adequate healing of the fracture (typically 3 to 4 weeks), return of full ankle ROM and strength, and demonstration of the ability to perform sports-specific skills without pain.

Avulsion Fracture of the Proximal Fifth Metatarsal Apophysis

The apophysis of the proximal fifth metatarsal generally begins to ossify and appears visible on x-rays in girls between 9 to 11 years of age and in boys between 11 to 14 years old.[35] This apophysis is sometimes mistakenly identified as a fracture (Fig. 18-26). The normal apophysis lies parallel to the long axis of the metatarsal shaft. Other fractures of the proximal fifth metatarsal, including Jones fractures, are covered in Chap. 11.

Figure 18-26

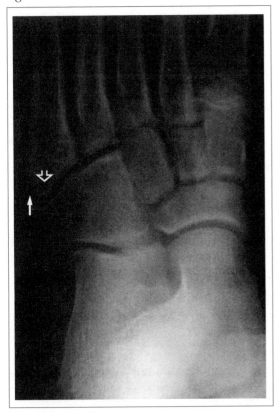

Note the normal apophysis of the base of the fifth metatarsal (*solid arrow*), which is oriented parallel to the long axis of the fifth metatarsal. The fracture in this radiograph is oriented in a horizontal position in the base of the fifth metatarsal (*open arrow*). (*Radiograph courtesy of James C. Puffer, MD, University of California at Los Angeles.*)

HISTORY AND PHYSICAL EXAMINATION

Avulsion of the apophysis occurs with a typical ankle sprain/inversion mechanism. This mechanism places traction on the apophysis via the attachment of the peroneus brevis tendon. The athlete will complain of pain and swelling at the base of the fifth metatarsal and may also complain of lateral ankle pain as well. Examination reveals tenderness to palpation and swelling at the base of the fifth metatarsal.

IMAGING

Foot x-rays, rather than ankle x-rays, are necessary for adequate visualization of this area. X-rays reveal widening of the apophysis. It may be necessary to x-ray the opposite foot to accurately assess for widening on the injured side.

TREATMENT

Treatment consists of full weight bearing as tolerated in a short-leg walking cast or walking boot for 2 to 3 weeks. Markedly displaced apophyseal avulsion fractures require orthopedic consultation.

COMPLICATIONS

Chronic pain secondary to nonunion is a possible complication.

RETURN-TO-PLAY GUIDELINES

Most athletes will be able to return to sports participation 3 weeks following this injury.

References

1. Maffulli N, Baxter-Jones A: Common skeletal injuries in young athletes. *Sports Med* 19:137, 1995.
2. Wascher DC, Finerman GA: Physeal injuries in young athletes. In: Stanitski CL, DeLee JC, Drez D (eds): *Pediatric and Adolescent Sports Medicine.* Philadelphia: WB Saunders; 1994;144.
3. Eiff MP, Hatch RL, Calmbach WL: *Fracture Management for Primary Care.* Philadelphia: WB Saunders; 1998.
4. England SP, Sundberg S: Management of common pediatric fractures. *Pediatr Clin North Am* 43:991, 1996.
5. Salter RB, Harris WR: Injuries involving the epiphyseal plate. *J Bone Joint Surg Am* 45:587, 1963.
6. Borsa JJ, Peterson HA, Ehman RL: MR imaging of physeal bars. *Radiology* 199:683, 1996.
7. Rogers LF, Poznanski AK: Imaging of epiphyseal injuries. *Radiology* 191:297, 1994.

8. Smith BG, Rand F, Jaramillo D, et al: Early MR imaging of lower extremity physeal fracture-separations: A preliminary report. *J Ped Orthop* 14: 526, 1994.

9. Carey J, Spence L, Blickman H, et al: MRI of pediatric growth plate injury: correlation with plain film radiographs and clinical outcome. *Skeletal Radiol* 27:250, 1998.

10. Naranja RJ, Gregg JR, Dormans JP, et al: Pediatric fracture without radiographic abnormality. Description and significance. *Clin Orthop* 342:141, 1997.

11. White PG, Mah JY, Friedman L: Magnetic resonance imaging in acute physeal injuries. *Skeletal Radiol* 23:627, 1994.

12. Post M: Current concepts in the treatment of fractures of the clavicle. *Clin Orthop* 245:89,1989.

13. Simon RR, Koehigsknecht SJ: *Emergency Orthopedics, the Extremities*, 3rd ed. Norwalk, CT: Appleton & Lange, 1995; 201.

14. Stanley D, Towbridge EA, Norris SH: The mechanism of clavicular fractures: A clinical and biomechanical analysis. *J Bone Joint Surg Br* 70:461, 1988.

15. Fu FH, Salyers S: Injuries involving the clavicle. In: Reider B (ed): *Sports Medicine, the School Aged Athlete*. Philadelphia: WB Saunders; 1991;190.

16. Arciero RA, Warme WJ: Traumatic shoulder injuries in athletes. In: Arendt EA (ed): *Orthopedic Knowledge Update, Sports Medicine 2*. Rosemont, IL. American Academy of Orthopedic Surgeons; 1999;165.

17. Ebraheim NA, Mekhail AO, Darwich M: Open reduction and internal fixation with bone grafting of clavicular nonunion. *J Trauma* 42:701, 1997.

18. Curtis RJ: Skeletal injuries. In: Stanitski CL, DeLee JC, Drez D (eds): *Pediatric and Adolescent Sports Medicine*. Philadelphia: WB Saunders; 1994;191.

19. Eiff MP: Management of clavicle fractures. *Am Fam Phys* 55:121, 1997.

20. Blasier RD, Aronson J: Injuries of the shoulder girdle. In: MacEwen GD, Kasses JR, Heinrich SD (eds): *Pediatric Fractures—A Practical Approach to Assessment and Treatment*. Baltimore: Williams & Wilkins; 1993;91.

21. Curtis RJ, Dameron TB, Rockwood CA: Fractures and dislocations of the shoulder in children. In: Rockwood CA, Wilkins KE, King RE (eds): *Fractures in Children*, 3rd ed. Philadelphia: JB Lippincott; 1996;878.

22. Saperstein AL, Nicholas SJ: Pediatric and adolescent sports medicine. *Pediatr Clin North Am* 43: 1013, 1996.

23. Gross ML, Flynn M, Sanzagni JJ: Overworked shoulders—Managing injury of the proximal humeral physis. *Phys Sports Med* 22:81, 1994.

24. Carson WG, Gasser SI: Little Leaguer's shoulder—a report of 23 cases. *Am J Sports Med* 26:575, 1995.

25. Axe MJ, Synder-Mackler L, Kanin JG, et al: Development of a distance-based interval throwing program for little league aged athletes. *J Sports Med* 24:594, 1996.

26. Andrews JR, Fleisig GS: How many pitches should I allow my child to throw? *USA Baseball News* April 5, 1996.

27. Hennigan SP, Bush-Joseph CA, Kuo KN, et al: Throwing-induced humeral shaft fractures in skeletally immature adolescents. *Orthopedics* 22: 621, 1999.

28. Branch T, Pantin C, Chamberland P, et al: Spontaneous fractures of the humerus during pitching—a series of 12 cases. *Am J Sports Med* 20:468, 1992.

29. Wilkins RE: Fractures of the humeral shaft. In: Stanitski CL, DeLee JC, Drez D (eds): *Pediatric and Adolescent Sports Medicine*. Philadelphia: WB Saunders; 1994;227.

30. Farnsworth CL, Silva PD, Mubarak SJ: Etiology of supracondylar humerus fractures. *J Ped Orthop* 18:38, 1998.

31. Sponseller PD: Problem elbow fractures in children. *Hand Clin* 10:495, 1994.

32. Bradley JP: Upper extremity elbow injuries in children and adolescents: In: Stanitski CL, DeLee JC, Drez D (eds): *Pediatric and Adolescent Sports Medicine*. Philadelphia: WB Saunders; 1994;243.

33. Higgins DL: Fractures about the elbow. In: Baker CL (ed): *The Hughston Clinic, Sports Medicine Book*. Baltimore: Williams & Wilkins; 1995;312.

34. Bryan W: Baseball injuries. In: Reider B (ed): *Sports Medicine, the School Aged Athlete*. Philadelphia: WB Saunders; 1991;447.

35. Dameron TB: Fractures and anatomic variations of the proximal portion of the fifth metatarsal. *J Bone Joint Surg Am* 57:788, 1975.

36. Irelano ML, Andrew JR: Shoulder and elbow injuries in the young athlete. *Clin Sports Med* 7: 473, 1988.

37. Radomisli TE, Rosen AL: Controversies regarding radial neck fractures in children. *Clin Orthop* 353: 30, 1998.

38. Irashad F, Shaw NS, Wegaz RJH: Reliability of fat-pad sign in radial head/neck fractures of the elbow. *Injury* 28:433, 1997.

39. McCoy RL, Dec KL, McKeag DB: Common injuries in the child or adolescent athlete. *Prim Care* 22:117, 1995.

40. Noonan KJ, Price CT: Forearm and distal radius fractures in children. *J Am Acad Orthop Surg* 6:146, 1998.

41. Kasser JR: Forearm fractures. In: MacEwen GD, Kasser JR, Heinrich SD (eds): *Pediatric Fractures: a Practical Approach to Assessment and Treatment.* Baltimore: Williams & Wilkens; 1993;165.

42. Lovallo JL, Simmons BP: Hand and wrist injuries. In: Stanitski CL, DeLee JC, Drez D (eds): *Pediatric and Adolescent Sports Medicine.* Philadelphia: WB Saunders; 1994;262.

43. Caine D, Roy S, Singer KM, et al: Stress changes of the distal radial growth plate: A radiographic survey and review of the literature. *Am J Sports Med* 20:290, 1992.

44. DiFiori JP, Puffer JC, Mandelbaum BR: Factors associated with wrist pain in the young gymnast. *Am J Sports Med* 24:9, 1996.

45. Mandelbaum BR, Bartolozzi AR, Davis CA, et al: Wrist pain syndrome in the gymnast: Pathogenetic, diagnostic, and therapeutic considerations. *Am J Sports Med* 17:305, 1989.

46. Roy S, Caine D, Singer KM: Stress changes of the distal radial epiphysis in young gymnasts: A report of twenty-one cases and a review of the literature. *Am J Sports Med* 13:301, 1985.

47. DiFiori JP, Mandelbaum BR: Wrist pain in a young gymnast: unusual radiographic findings and MRI evidence of growth plate injury. *Med Sci Sports Exerc* 28:1453, 1996.

48. DiFiori JP, Puffer JC, Mandelbaum BR: Distal radial growth plate injury and positive ulnar variance in nonelite gymnasts. *Am J Sports Med* 25:763, 1997.

49. Ruggles DH, Peterson HA, Scott SG: Radial growth injury in a female gymnast. *Med Sci Sports Exerc* 23:393, 1991.

50. Albanese SA, Palmer AK, Kerr DR, et al: Wrist pain and distal growth plate closure of the radius in gymnasts. *J Pediatr Orthop* 9:23, 1989.

51. De Smet L, Claessens A, Lefevere J, et al: Gymnast wrist: an epidemiologic survey of ulnar variance and stress changes of the radial physis in elite female gymnasts. *Am J Sports Med* 22:846, 1994.

52. Tolat AR, Sanderson PL, DeSmet L, et al: The gymnast's wrist: acquired positive ulnar variance following chronic epiphyseal injury. *J Hand Surg Br* 17:678, 1992.

53. Jobe MT: Fractures and dislocations of the hand and wrist. In: MacEwen GD, Kasser JR, Heinrich SD (eds): *Pediatric Fractures: A Practical Approach to Assessment and Treatment.* Baltimore: Williams & Wilkens; 1993;191.

54. Markiewitz AD, Andrish JT: Hand and wrist injuries in the preadolescent and adolescent athlete. *Clin Sports Med* 11:203, 1992.

55. Beaty JH, Kumar A: Fractures about the knee in children. *J Bone Joint Surg Am* 76:1870, 1994.

56. Thomson JD, Stricker SJ, Williams MM: Fractures of the distal femoral epiphyseal plate. *J Pediatr Orthop* 15:474, 1995.

57. Heinrich SD, Finney T, D'ambrosia RD: Bony injuries about the knee—Fractures. In: MacEwen GD, Kasses JR, Heinrich SD (eds): *Pediatric Fractures—A Practical Approach to Assessment and Treatment.* Baltimore: Williams & Wilkins; 1993;296.

58. Lombardo SJ, Harvey JP: Fractures of distal femoral epiphysis. Factors influencing prognosis—a series of 34 cases. *J Bone Joint Surg Am* 59:742, 1977.

59. Strizak AM. Knee injuries. In: Nicholas JA, Hershman EB (eds): *The Lower Extremity and Spine in Sports Medicine.* St. Louis: Mosby; 1995;1251.

60. Stanitski CL: Epiphyseal injury in a junior high school football player. In: Smith NJ (ed): *Common Problems in Pediatric Sports Medicine.* Chicago: Year Book Medical Publishers; 1989;313.

61. Stanitski CL: Acute tibial tubercle avulsion fracture. In: Stanitski CL, DeLee JC, Drez D (eds): *Pediatric and Adolescent Sports Medicine.* Philadelphia: WB Saunders; 1994;294.

62. Balmat P, Vichard P, Penn R: The treatment of avulsion fractures of the tibial tuberosity in adolescent athletes. *Sports Med* 9:311, 1990.

63. DeLee JC: Ligamentous injury of the knee. In: Stanitski CL, DeLee JC, Drez D (eds): *Pediatric and Adolescent Sports Medicine.* Philadelphia: WB Saunders; 1994;406.

64. Beaty JH: Fracture of the tibial spine. In: Rockwood CA, Wilkins KE, King RE (eds): *Fractures in Children,* 3rd ed. Philadelphia: JB Lippincott; 1996;1237.

65. Grankvist H, Hirsch G, Johansson L: Fractures of

the anterior tibial spine in children. *J Ped Orthop* 4:465, 1984.

66. Stanitski CL: Osteochondritis dissecans of the knee. In: Stanitski CL, DeLee JC, Drez D (eds): *Pediatric and Adolescent Sports Medicine.* Philadelphia: WB Saunders; 1994;387.

67. Harris JR: Chondral lesions. In: Baker CL (ed): *The Hughston Clinic, Sports Medicine Book.* Baltimore: Williams & Wilkins; 1995;473.

68. Beaty JH: Osteochondral fractures. In: Rockwood CA, Wilkins KE, King RE (eds): *Fractures in Children,* 3rd ed. Philadelphia: JB Lippincott; 1996; 1233.

69. Graf SK, Ilahi OA: Osteochondritis dissecans. In: Reider B (ed): *Sports Medicine, the School Aged Athlete.* Philadelphia: WB Saunders; 1996;273.

70. Wilson JN: A diagnostic sign in osteochondriitis dissecans of the knee. *J Bone Joint Surg Am* 49: 477, 1967.

71. Kramer J, Stiglbauer R, Engel A, et al: MR contrast arthrography (MRA) in osteochondritis dissecans. *J Comput Assist Tomogr* 16:254, 1992.

72. Obedian RS, Grelsomer RP: Osteochondritis dissecans of the distal femur and patella. *Clin Sports Med* 16:157, 1997.

73. Browne JE, Brach TP: Surgical alternatives for treatment of articular cartilage lesions. *J Am Acad Orthop Surg* 8:180, 2000.

74. Linden B: Osteochondritis dissecans of the femoral condyles. *J Bone Joint Surg Am* 59:769, 1977.

75. Pappas A: Osteochondritis dissecans. *Clin Orthop* 158:59, 1981.

76. Sullivan JA: Ankle and foot injuries in the pediatric athlete. In: Stanitski CL, DeLee JC, Drez D (eds): *Pediatric and Adolescent Sports Medicine.* Philadelphia: WB Saunders; 1994;441.

77. Duchesneau S, Fallat LM: The Tillaux fracture. *J Foot Ankle Surg* 35:127, 1996.

78. Griffin LY: Common sports injuries of the foot and ankle seen in children and adolescents. *Orthop Clin North Am* 25:83, 1994.

79. Koury SI, Stone CK, Harrell G, et al: Recognition and management of Tillaux fractures in adolescents. *Pediatr Emerg Care* 15:37, 1999.

80. Rapariz JM, Ocete G, Gonzalez-Herranz P, et al: Distal tibial triplane fractures: Long-term follow-up. *J Pediatr Orthop* 16:113, 1996.

81. Shin AY, Moran ME, Wenger DR: Intramalleolar triplane fractures of the distal tibial epiphysis. *J Pediatr Orthop* 17:352, 1997.

82. McCrory P, Bladin C: Fractures of the lateral process of the talus: A clinical review. "Snowboarder's ankle." *Clin J Sport Med* 6:124, 1996.

83. Kirkpatrick DP, Hunter RE, Janes PC, et al: The snowboarder's foot and ankle. *Am J Sports Med* 26:271, 1998.

84. Bladin C, McCrory P: Snowboarding injuries. *Sports Med* 19:358, 1995.

85. Hawkins LG: Fractures of the lateral process of the talus. *J Bone Joint Surg Am* 47:1170, 1965.

86. Mukherjee SM, Pringle RM, Baxter AD: Fracture of the lateral process of the talus. *J Bone Joint Surg Br* 56:263, 1974.

87. Dias L: Fractures of the tibia and fibula. In: Rockwood C, Wilken K, King R (eds): *Fractures in Children,* 3rd ed. Philadelphia: JB Lippincott; 1991;1271.

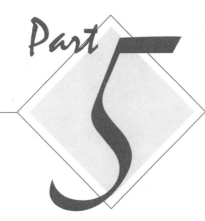

Part 5

Miscellaneous Problems

David J. Shaskey

Low Back Pain

Introduction

Low back pain is one of the most ubiquitous medical problems in primary care as it is the fourth most common complaint in ambulatory medicine. It is also the third most expensive medical problem to treat, following cancer and heart disease.[1] For better or for worse, the athlete and the physically active population are not immune to low back pain, and in certain circumstances, they are even predisposed to conditions that manifest as low back pain. Therefore, sports medicine practitioners and any primary care provider who treats physically active patients need some degree of expertise in diagnosing and treating low back pain. This task is made no less difficult by the fact that low back pain can be a frustrating and difficult problem to treat because a high percentage of patients are poorly responsive to therapy and continue to experience recurrent or persistent low back pain despite aggressive treatment. Low back pain is certainly a challenging problem for health practitioners everywhere—particularly sports medicine physicians.

Anatomy

The anatomy of the lumbar spine is complex and multifaceted and directly relates to function. The three functions of the lumbar spine are to: (1) provide support for upright posture, (2) protect the spinal cord and neural structures, and (3) allow motion. Anatomically, there are three major components of the lumbar spine: (1) the vertebral column, (2) the investing musculature, and (3) the spinal cord and associated neural structures.

Vertebral Column

The vertebral column consists of an alternating "sandwich" of vertebral bodies alternating with intervertebral discs (Fig. 19-1). The lumbar vertebrae are the largest, heaviest, and widest vertebrae of the spinal column, which relate to their location at the base of the spine. They act as a base of support for the more cranial vertebral elements. The lumbar vertebrae have short, heavy pedicles to protect the spinal cord and long transverse processes and broad strong spinous processes to act as origins and insertions for the numerous, large, and powerful investing musculature that encases the entire region in a myofascial envelope. The facet joints are sagittally aligned by ligaments to allow the motions of flexion and extension.[2]

The overall bony anatomy results in a three-joint complex of two facet joints and an intervertebral apophyseal joint. These function together to resist forces and allow motion, as well as protect the vital neural structures. The predominant motion of the lumbar spine occurs in the sagittal plane resulting in flexion and extension. However, a lesser degree of motion is also possible such as lateral flexion, and even lesser motion such as rotation. Most spinal rotation occurs in the thoracic and especially cervical spine.

The intervertebral discs are unique structures that provide not only a strong union between the adjoining levels of the vertebral column, but also intervertebral motion, especially rotation. They also function as "shock absorbers," particularly in relationship to axially loaded forces.

The anatomy of the disc lends itself to the aforementioned functions. Specifically, it is a bilayer of a strong outer laminar layer, the annulus fibrosis, which invests an inner compressible semi-fluid core, the nucleus pulposus. The annulus fibrosis is composed of a series of concentric lamellae with alternating fiber orientations that give the disc its torsional strength. Microscopi-

Figure 19-1

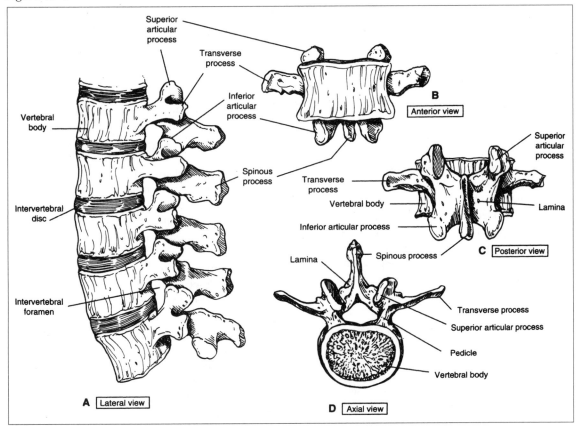

Views of the lumbar spine. (**A**) Lateral view (saggital plane). (**B**) Anterior view (frontal plane). (**C**) Posterior view (frontal plane). (**D**) Horizontal (axial plane). *(Courtesy of Nancy Shaskey, illustrator).*

cally, it is composed of collagen fibrils that give it its tensile strength, and 60 to 70 percent water. The nucleus pulposus is also predominantly water, approximately 80 percent in early age, which declines with advancing age. The predominant dry-weight component is proteoglycans. Proteoglycans are large negatively charged molecules that make them hydrophilic and, therefore, strongly attract water and give the nucleus its strength in compression. The proteoglycan and high water content of the nucleus pulposus decreases with age and, therefore, the

ability of the disc to withstand compressive force declines with age.

Investing Musculature

Surrounding the vertebral column is an incredibly strong myofascial envelope. The innermost layer of this myofascial envelope is the numerous ligaments that support the vertebral column. Two strong vertically oriented ligaments lie just anterior and posterior to the vertebral bodies:

the anterior longitudinal ligament and the posterior longitudinal ligament. More posteriorly located is the ligamentum flavum, which vertically unites the adjoining laminae. The most posterior ligamentous structure is the complex of interspinous ligaments that invests and connects each level from spinous process to spinous process. The entire ligamentous complex is thickest and strongest in the lumbar spine as it carries and distributes the greatest forces. The next layer toward the exterior is actually a multilayer, less defined investment of extensive musculature. The deep muscles of the spine fall into five groups including the splenius, the erector spinae, the transversospinalis, the interspinalis, and the intertransversarial. These muscles are quite large and strong, especially in the lumbar spine and together act to invest, protect, and initiate motion of the lumbar spine.

Spinal Cord and Neural Structures

The last anatomic component is the most important and therefore the deepest and most protected—the spinal cord and associated neural structures. Briefly, the cord tapers to a conus medullaris at approximately L1-L2 and below this level, the collection of nerve roots is known as the cauda equina. Each corresponding spinal nerve root then exits through the neuroforaminae, which are bordered above and below by the respective pedicles, posteriorly by the facet joints, and anteriorly by the posterolateral aspect of the intervertebral discs. The neuroforaminae and the accompanying nerve roots are at risk from derangements to the proximate discs and facet joints.

Clearly, the lumbar spine is a complex and amazing structure that when functioning normally protects the spinal structures, allows motion mainly as flexion and extension, and resists forces to allow and support upright posture.

Evaluation

History

The importance of a careful history and physical examination cannot be over-emphasized. This is actually truer in today's age of high tech imaging. As we all know, radiologic evaluation, particularly of the LS spine, can uncover a multitude of pathology that in many circumstances is simply incidental and unrelated to the problem at hand. Therefore, as radiologists frequently say, "clinical correlation is required" and this clearly hinges on a careful history and physical examination.[5]

The clinical evaluation of a patient or athlete with low back pain must follow a systematic approach. This approach includes the history, an appropriate physical examination, and specialized diagnostic testing based on the history and examination, if indicated.

Frequently, the history is the key to understanding the underlying cause of low back pain. The first historical feature of low back pain that points toward diagnosis is the timing and temporal relationships. For example, a direct blow with the immediate onset of pain directs the practitioner toward contusion or even fracture of the spinal elements. In contrast, the onset of pain gradually over hours after an inciting activity clearly directs the diagnosis toward a muscular etiology. Finally, the insidious onset of pain over days to weeks points toward inflammation or overuse problems of the muscles or spinal elements, such as spondylolysis.

Most cases of low back pain have their onset in a subacute or chronic fashion and, therefore, other historic features are also helpful. The PQRST mnemonic helps the practitioner further clarify and classify pain. P stands for precipitants or relieving factors. Q relates to the quality of the pain. R stands for radiation of the pain. S for associated symptoms, such as hematuria, numbness, etc.; and T relates to the temporal aspects of the pain (i.e., night pain such as osteoid osteomas or tumors). The specific activities and frequency and duration of activities in relationship to pain are also important aspects of the history, particularly in athletes.

The location of pain is also a key feature because that will narrow the diagnostic possibilities. For example, unilateral, focal pain in the lower lumbar region clearly suggests spondylolysis whereas diffuse bilateral perilumbar pain in contrast clearly suggests a muscular etiology.

The differentiation of localized low back pain from radicular pain is one of the most important elements of the evaluation. Radiation of the pain distally down the leg strongly suggests nerve root or cord irritation.

Physical Examination

The physical examination of an athlete is directed by the clinical setting. On the field, management of acute post-traumatic back pain clearly hinges on the question of spinal stability and neurologic status. In short, any acute back injury that has resulted from significant force or any injury with neurologic abnormalities must be treated as if there is an unstable spine, and the patient immobilized and transported for emergent radiologic evaluation. Adherence to these principles cannot be over-emphasized and the principle of "when in doubt overtreat" should be strictly followed, lest a permanent and severe neurologic compromise be the resultant outcome of a cavalier approach to acute traumatic low back pain.

In the absence of severe, acute traumatic injury, the evaluation of the athlete with low back pain should follow the basic principles for evaluation of any joint: (1) inspection, (2) palpation, (3) range of motion, (4) provocative maneuvers, and (5) neurovascular status.

Inspection should routinely be undertaken with the patient disrobed and standing. The patient should be viewed from behind as well as from the side, looking for asymmetry, masses, scoliosis, and the presence and degree of normal lumbar lordosis. The clinician needs to also take notice of associated skin lesions such as café-au-lait spots that may herald neurofibromatosis with its accompanying spinal abnormalities.

Palpation of the lumbar spine should include palpation of each spinous process, the paraspinal muscles, the SI joints, and the sciatic notches. The examiner is palpating for tenderness, muscular spasm, or any underlying masses or defects.

The range of motion of the lumbar spine is helpful not only in determining the severity of injury/problem, but may also direct the evaluation toward specific etiologies. The "normal" range of motion for the lumbar spine is quite variable but in general, normal flexion entails 40 to 60°, extension 20 to 35°, lateral flexion 20° to each side, respectively, and 90° of rotation to each side. Lateral flexion and rotation primarily occur in the thoracic spine, whereas flexion and extension occur in the lumbar spine.

In addition to the absolute range of motion, the effect of motion on the pain should be explicitly noted. The exacerbation of pain with flexion is nonspecific but suggests anterior column problems such as disc pathology. Pain with extension is less common and suggests posterior element pathology. In the young athlete, pain on extension is suspicious for spondylolysis whereas in an older athlete, facet joint pathology or even spinal stenosis is the more likely cause of extension pain.[3]

Special Maneuvers

Provocative maneuvers are clearly helpful and one of the mainstays of evaluation of the lumbar spine. The classic nerve root tension sign is the straight leg raise.[4] The objective of this test is to determine if the nerve roots are irritated. The patient is placed supine and the straight leg is slowly raised upward. A positive straight leg raise test is one that elicits pain down the leg. Clearly, more severe pain that radiates below the knee with less hip flexion is more suspicious for nerve root irritation, but hamstring "tightness" must be differentiated from radicular pain. One maneuver that can help distinguish these two clearly different entities is comparison to the contralateral side if it is not involved in the pathologic process.

A few other maneuvers warrant mention. Specifically, the exacerbation of the pain with popliteal compression or ankle dorsiflexion complements the positive straight leg raise and conversely, relief of leg pain with knee flexion also complements the positive straight leg raise.

In addition to the straight leg raise as a provocative maneuver to diagnose a radiculopathy, there are also various intrathecal pressure tests. These tests are designed to increase nerve root irritation by increasing intrathecal pressure. The Valsalva maneuver exacerbates or elicits radicular symptoms and radiculopathies. The milligram test is another intrathecal pressure test. It is performed by having the patient hold both legs 3 inches off the examining table for 30 sec while supine. An inability to hold the leg up with reproduction of the radicular pain is a positive test suggesting nerve root irritation.

The Patrick or FABER (Flexion, Abduction, External Rotation) test is one designed to exacerbate ipsilateral SI joint pain, but it is nonspecific and care must be used in localizing the pain that results from the test. The patient is supine and the ipsilateral hip is flexed, abducted, and externally rotated so that the foot rests on the opposite knee. Downward pressure is then applied to the knee and contralateral anterior superior iliac spine. A positive Patrick test is elicitation or exacerbation of ipsilateral SI pain.

The one-legged hyperextension test is the classic test to screen for spondylolysis, although it is also non-specific. It is performed by having

the patient stand on one leg while extending the back maximally (Fig. 19-2). A positive test elicits focal ipsilateral pain in the back just lateral to the midline.

Neurovascular Examination

The last, but certainly not the least important, part of the physical examination is evaluation of neurovascular status. The sensation of both lower extremities should be evaluated, at least to light touch, to include all the dermatomes. Particularly in the setting of high-velocity acute trauma, the sacral or perianal sensation should be specifically tested lest the examiner miss a sacral fracture with neurologic compromise. Manual muscle testing should be performed on all muscle groups to complement functional testing. The clinician may have the patient perform

Figure 19-2

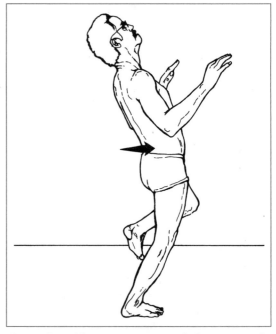

The one-legged hyperextension test, which is positive if it causes/exacerbates focal ipsilateral pain in the back just to the lateral of midline. *(Courtesy of Nancy Shaskey, illustrator).*

heel or toe walking as well as deep knee bends to more functionally assess the strength of the lower extremities. Finally, the reflexes should be tested with particular attention focused on symmetry.

Specific Conditions

Lumbar Strain

EPIDEMIOLOGY

Lumbar strains or paraspinal muscular injuries are the most common back injuries encountered, not only in athletes but also in the general population. An estimated 80 percent of the entire population suffers from at least one episode of low back pain during their lifetime[6] and in as many as 50 percent it will be recurrent.[7] Athletes are clearly not immune to this problem, although some studies suggest a lower incidence in athletes.

Between 5 to 8 percent of all sports injuries have been found to involve the low back by Harvey et al.[8] Nonetheless, certain sports do seem to predispose to low back problems including gymnastics, diving, swimming, skiing, and American football. Keene et al examined retrospectively the medical records of athletes participating in 17 varsity sports over a 10-year period and found the low back injury rate to be 7 per 100 participants. Football and gymnastics both had a significantly high rate of low back injury. Most of the injuries occurred during practice, 80 percent according to Keene, and only 6 percent occurred during competition.[9]

CLINICAL EVALUATION

The typical lumbar strain results in pain that begins insidiously after the inciting activity and is poorly localized and diffuse. The typical strain develops minutes to hours following activity and is worse in the ensuing days due to secondary muscular spasm. A key feature in the history, however, is a history of previous low back pain. This piece of information is common in simple lumbar strains but should be a "red flag" for considering other pathologies. The exacerbating factors should also be elicited. Typically with lumbar strain, standing and especially twisting exacerbate the pain. The pain is usually relieved with rest, particularly in the supine position or on the side.

The physical examination of a patient with a lumbar strain involves the various maneuvers described earlier. It is very nonspecific, yet the key to an adequate physical examination is ruling out other more serious pathology. Typically the range of motion, particularly to flexion, is reduced because of pain that is poorly localized along with perilumbar tenderness and spasm. Important aspects of the physical examination include nerve root tension signs, the neurologic examination of the lower extremities, and the one-legged hyperextension test. All of these tests should be negative to make the diagnosis of a lumbar strain based on clinical grounds.

The role of radiographic testing in lumbar injury in general, and suspected lumbar strain specifically, is controversial. Clearly, the overuse of radiologic testing has been demonstrated repeatedly in the medical literature with an apparent bias toward radiologic overuse.[10] Most clinicians would agree that plain films have little value in the setting of acute low back pain with the history and physical examination pointing toward lumbar strain. The vast majority of lumbar strains will resolve within 3 weeks, with a high percentage resolving in 1 week. Persistent pain should be a clear indication for obtaining plain films and possibly additional diagnostic imaging.[11]

TREATMENT

Treatment of simple lumbar strain is also controversial and the optimal regimen remains uncertain. A myriad of studies exists that examine the role and effectiveness of numerous treatment regimens and most have some proven efficacy. Nonetheless, the modern treatment recommendations have changed and have shifted toward a "conservative but active" approach. The 1995 Agency for Health Care Policy Research (AHCPR) guidelines for low back pain reflect this change.[12] Clearly, the effectiveness of prolonged bed rest has been disproved as patients assigned to prolonged (greater than 2 days) strict bed rest recovered no faster, and in one study even slower, than those who remained active.[13,14]

The details however, become cloudy when the specifics of "active treatment" are more carefully examined. Controversy exists about the specifics of which exercises and activities are most effective, when they should be conducted, and how much exercise should be conducted. Nonetheless, data exist to support, at least in part, numerous different regimens ranging from McKenzie extension exercises to Williams flexion exercises, and most recently in vogue, the "Back Stabilization Program," with exercises predominantly in the neutral position and consisting of both flexion and extension exercises.

In addition to exercise, other treatment modalities have merit. Specifically, chiropractic manipulation, TENS, NSAIDs, muscle relaxants, and analgesics all have some proven efficacy and have been specifically recommended by the AHCPR guidelines.[12]

One common approach to the treatment of acute lumbar strain is to stratify treatment based on severity of injury. For mild injuries, relative rest, icing, and gentle range-of-motion exercises may be enough. More severe cases, however, warrant some degree of activity restriction, plus nonsteroidals and possibly analgesics, and either a physical therapy or chiropractic referral. Plain films prior to chiropractic or physical therapy referral are obtained to rule out contraindications to manipulation.

The precise guidelines for activity restrictions and return to play guidelines are empiric at best and there is no substitute for common sense and clinical judgment. Nonetheless, in the acute and simple lumbar strain there are no absolute contraindications to allowing an athlete to continue to participate in sports. Depending on the severity of pain and the mechanism of the injury, it is sometimes important to obtain objective testing to more clearly rule out serious underlying pathology such as disc disease, bony pathology, or otherwise. As stated, there is no substitute for common sense and clinical judgment.

Spondylolysis/Isthmic Spondylolisthesis

EPIDEMIOLOGY

Spondylolysis and isthmic spondylolisthesis are common and certainly clinically relevant low back disorders to sports medicine because their prevalences are significantly higher in athletes who participate in certain sporting activities such as football, gymnastics, and diving. Some studies have suggested that 25 to 39 percent of low back pain in the athletic population arise from this entity.[15–17]

The etiology of spondylolysis is somewhat enigmatic, but it is certainly an acquired disorder. It has never been reported in stillborns or fetuses and it is exceedingly rare under the age of 5 years.[18] There is certainly a genetic predisposition to spondylolysis. Prevalence has been shown to be as high as 33 percent among those with a family history of spondylolysis,[11] and prevalence may be as high as 50 percent in certain subpopulations.[19]

The generally accepted theory is that spondylolysis represents a stress reaction or stress fracture of the pars interarticularis.[5,20–22] However, this stress reaction/stress fracture differs from other stress fractures in three ways. First, it develops at an earlier age. Second, it heals with less callus formation. Third, it forms fibrous nonunions much more frequently than other stress fractures.[22,23]

The risk for spondylolysis hinges on two factors: genetic predisposition as detailed previously, and predisposing activity. Clearly, there is a higher prevalence in athletes who participate in certain sports. In general, those activities that require repetitive axial loading of the spine, especially in extension, are more prone to spondylolysis. Rossi et al. showed that there was a marked association with particular sports, especially diving, weightlifting, gymnastics, and track and field.[24] The prevalence in these sub-populations ranges from 22 to 63 percent compared to less than a 5 percent prevalence in the general population. The frequency of hyperextension activities also seems to correlate with the risk, as young gymnasts that restricted gymnastics to less than 24 h per week had a significantly lower prevalence.[23] The age of greatest prevalence also seemed to vary with activities yet overall the greatest age prevalence is from 10 to 15 years.

In summary, spondylolysis seems to be an acquired stress reaction/stress fracture that occurs in adolescent athletes who perform axially loaded spine activities, particularly hyperextension activities. There is a genetic predisposition yet high volume hyperextension activities greatly increase the risk.

CLINICAL EVALUATION

The typical symptomatic patient with spondylolysis has well-localized unilateral paraspinal pain that is worse with extension or twisting activities. Unfortunately, there is a high percentage of patients with spondylolysis that are minimally symptomatic or even asymptomatic. This contributes to the difficulty in diagnosing and treating spondylolysis, because radiographic abnormalities do not necessarily indicate symptomatic spondylolysis. There is, however, a well-documented association with hamstring tightness although the cause of this association is unclear.[21–23] It is not certain if hamstring tightness is a primary problem that predisposes to spondylolysis or whether this is simply a result of the spondylolysis and a manifestation of the disease itself.

Typically, in symptomatic patients the pain has an insidious onset and there are usually no radicular or neurologic components. The patient typically notes exacerbation of the pain with hyperextension activities that gradually becomes worse.

On examination, the patient usually has localized, unilateral, paraspinal pain, along with tenderness and exacerbation of that localized pain with the one-legged hyperextension test. The combination of these findings is classic for spondylolysis. As above, hamstring tightness should also alert the clinician to the possibility of spondylolysis.

The diagnosis of spondylolysis rests mainly on the radiographic demonstration of a defect in the pars interarticularis seen on plain radiographs (although early lesions may be normal on plain films). Typically, oblique films demonstrate the defect best with the classic "collar on the Scottie dog" (Figs. 19-3 and 19-4) but the defect can also be seen on the anterior-posterior (AP) or lateral films as well. In 85 percent of cases, spondylolysis is seen at L5, with the remaining 15 percent at L4. Occasionally, case reports have documented its occurrence at nearly any spinal level, including even the thoracic and cervical spines.[25] Most of these unusual anatomic locations have been associated with congenital abnormalities of the spine that presumably result in excessive biomechanical force being placed on the posterior elements of the vertebral column.

Spondylolysis is more treatable when detected before plain x-rays become abnormal. Such cases can be detected with either a bone scan or SPECT scan. Therefore, in athletes with persistent, suspicious symptoms, and normal plain x-rays, the radiologic evaluation should be continued and the examiner should either obtain a bone scan or SPECT scan. Nevertheless, a high index of suspicion is needed to identify these "early spondylitic lesions." An athlete, especially one at higher risk from a predisposing activity, with low back pain lasting for greater than 2 weeks should be evaluated with plain films and either a bone scan or SPECT scan if the plain

Figure 19-3

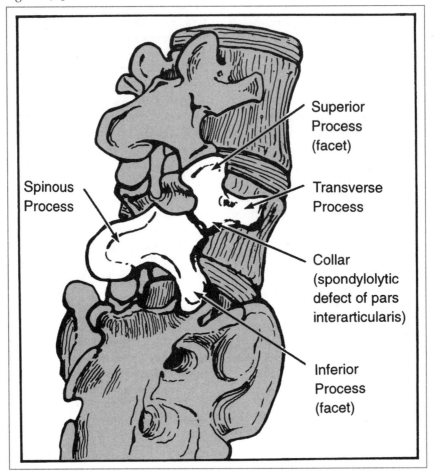

Spondylolytic defect of the pars interarticularis is evident as a collar on the "scottie dog" on oblique plain films. *(Reproduced with permission from Micheli L: How I manage low-back pain in athletes. Phys Sportsmed 21(3): 1993).*

films are normal. SPECT scans, however, are not universally available at this time.[21–22, 26]

Long-standing bilateral spondylolysis that has resulted in a non-union can cause isthmic spondylolisthesis. Spondylolisthesis is the anterior-posterior motion of one spinal segment in relation to the adjoining segment. It is graded from 1 to 4 depending on the degree of slippage. Grade 1 is an overlap of 0 to 25 percent of the vertebral body AP diameter, as seen on lateral films. Slippage of 25 to 50 percent is grade 2 and 50 to 100 percent is grade 3, with greater than 100 percent slippage being graded as grade 4.

TREATMENT

SPONDYLOLYSIS WITH NORMAL X-RAYS The treatment of spondylolysis is controversial. The degree, duration, and indications for activity restrictions and bracing are unclear; the exact role of surgery is poorly delineated.[27–28]

There is general agreement that spondylolysis

Figure 19-4

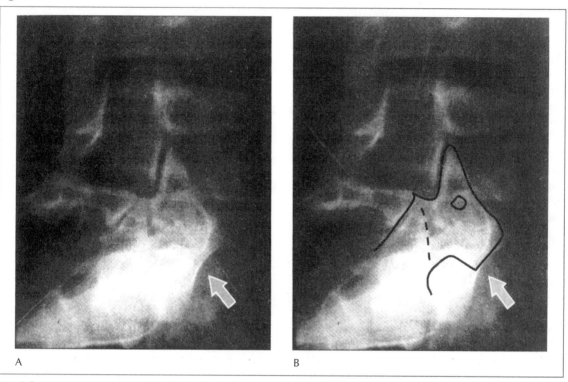

Pars defect is shown on oblique plain films without the "scottie dog" outlined in (**A**) and with the "scottie dog" outlined in (**B**). *(Reproduced with permission from Micheli L: How I manage low-back pain in athletes. Phys Sportsmed 21(3): 1993).*

with normal plain films and either a positive bone scan or SPECT scan has a greater chance for complete healing, and treatment in this situation should be directed toward cure. For treatment, most experts agree that the offending (i.e., hyperextension) activities should cease, and some argue for antilordotic bracing. The duration of activity restriction is unclear, however, and recommendations vary from 6 weeks to 6 months. Some investigators argue for continued treatment until the bone scan/SPECT scan becomes normal. Most clinicians will restrict activities until the patient is asymptomatic, and then proceed with a slow graduated return to full activities using symptoms as a guide.[20–22]

The role of surgery with debridement and bone grafting directed at healing is very controversial. Some clinicians will consider surgery for those that remain symptomatic with a positive bone scan/SPECT scan after 6 months. Return to athletics and full activities is unlikely after surgery and the overall benefit of this course of action is questionable.[28]

SPONDYLOLYSIS WITH ABNORMAL X-RAYS Once spondylolysis is evident on plain films, the "chance for healing" is lower and, therefore, treatment recommendations vary widely. Some practitioners will use bone scans to guide treatment recommendations with the idea that "hot" lesions have a greater propensity for healing and, therefore, activity restrictions and possible bracing should be used more often and for longer periods of time when bone scan abnormalities are present. Others will treat with activity restrictions and a spine-stabilization physical therapy program based on symptoms, and allow return to full activities using symptoms as the sole guide.

SPONDYLOLYSIS WITH SPONDYLOLISTHESIS The treatment recommendations for spondylolysis with resultant spondylolisthesis is clearer. Because there is essentially no chance for healing of the lesion, all treatment recommendations are based solely on relief of symptoms. Symptomatic treatment for limited periods is most widely recommended.

The role of surgery for advanced or progressive spondylolisthesis is controversial. Most experts recommend surgical stabilization with in situ fusion for spondylolisthesis greater than grade II, progressive spondylolisthesis, or spondylolisthesis with neurologic compromise due to either neuroforaminal encroachment or an associated herniated nucleus pulposus, which seems to increase in frequency with progressive degrees of spondylolisthesis.[28]

RETURN TO PLAY

The question of return to play depends not only on the stage of spondylolysis but also on the treatment protocol the clinician follows. One common approach is as follows.

A lesion that is only evident on bone scans with normal plain films has the greatest propensity to heal. Therefore, patients with such lesions should restrict extension activities for at least 6 weeks, but do not routinely require antilordotic bracing. After 6 weeks, there can be a slow, step-wise return to full activities using symptoms as a guide. Follow-up bone scans are not needed if symptoms resolve.

A lesion that is evident on plain films and on bone scan is treated as above. However, if the bone scan is negative or if spondylolisthesis is

evident, there is very little propensity for healing of the lesion. Therefore, patients are treated symptomatically with a spine stabilization program and activities modestly limited based on symptoms. These patients need to be monitored for radicular symptoms or neurologic compromise, and need serial plain films to rule out severe or progressive spondylolisthesis that would warrant surgical referral and severe activity restrictions. Unfortunately, most athletes who require spinal surgery will not be able to return to their sports, although this is not a hard-and-fast rule and individual determination needs to be made depending on the sport and extent of the lesion and symptoms.

Disc Herniation

EPIDEMIOLOGY

Acute lumbar disc herniation/herniated nucleus pulposus (HNP) with associated lumbar radiculopathy or sciatica needs to be considered in patients with low back pain. It is common, and may lead to neurologic compromise, and needs specific treatment and definite activity restrictions. Acute disc herniation is most common in the third and fourth decades of life but it may occur at any age, even in adolescents, especially in athletes performing high-force axial loading activities such as weightlifting.[29]

CLINICAL EVALUATION

There is a spectrum of symptoms and findings in acute herniated discs. The classic symptom complex is the acute sensation of a popping or tearing sensation with a lifting or axially loaded event followed by the acute or insidious onset of radicular pain. Tingling/numbness or focal weakness in the lower extremities may accompany the pain. The pain is typically exacerbated by coughing or sneezing. Not all herniated discs present with classic symptoms and a significant minority of patients have no back pain at all or only leg pain or neurologic complaints. This seems to be especially true of adolescents, in whom hamstring tightness may be the only presenting complaint.[30]

Physical examination demonstrates variable findings as well. Depending on the severity of HNP, patients may be relatively asymptomatic at rest or may list toward or away from the side of herniation to "unload" the herniation depending on the exact location. Typically, they are more comfortable supine or standing compared to sitting, as sitting results in greater flexion and load on the anteriorly located disc.

The hallmark finding is a positive nerve root tension sign induced by a provocative maneuver. Straight-leg raise is the classic provocative maneuver, but there is a host of similar nerve root tension signs including the sitting straight-leg raise, as well as the milligram test, which increases intrathecal pressure and aggravates an HNP.

Another key point in the physical examination is the neurologic evaluation to localize the lesion. Mapping out sensory or motor deficits to determine the level of nerve root involvement and, more importantly, to rule out cauda equina syndrome is imperative. About 90 percent of HNPs occur posterolaterally at L5/S1 (S1 nerve root) and 5 percent at L4/L5 (L5 nerve root), and both usually manifest as unilateral nerve root compression. When there are bilateral deficits or involvement of lower sacral nerve roots, cauda equina syndrome or central HNP needs to be considered.

Plain films are not usually helpful, although most clinicians perform them to rule out discitis, tumor, or masses that could result in neurologic compromise. The diagnostic test of choice is an MRI. However, there may be poor correlation between radiologic findings and clinical symptoms. Numerous studies have documented frequent, mild, disc abnormalities in MRI studies of asymptomatic individuals. Therefore, clinical correlation between MRI findings and clinical symptoms is very important.[31–32]

TREATMENT

The treatment of acute HNP hinges mainly on activity restriction, rest, and time. Most radicular symptoms and mild neurologic deficits will resolve with time and restriction of axial loading.[33] Nonetheless, numerous other adjuvant therapies are used frequently. These include nonsteroidal, anti-inflammatory drugs, physical therapy for modalities, as well as a gentle back stabilization program once radicular symptoms subside. Some practitioners advocate the use of pulse oral steroids to accelerate the resolution of radicular symptoms. Others advocate either nerve root or epidural steroid injections to hasten the recovery of neurologic symptoms, although studies have shown no long-term benefit with injectable steroids.[34–35]

Surgical therapy is indicated for cauda equina syndrome or severe or progressive neurologic deficits, although the definition of severe is not always clear in a given patient. Unfortunately, however, the most common situation in which surgery is contemplated is not severe neurologic symptoms, but rather persistent radicular pain with or without subtle neurologic deficits. The role of surgery in such cases is unclear, although most patients' symptoms will resolve with the nonsurgical therapies that have been outlined previously.

Most sports medicine physicians will severely restrict activities in patients with HNP, particularly axial loading, until the radicular symptoms are completely resolved. Some clinicians will restrict activities for a minimum of 6 weeks. Most clinicians will restrict activities for at least 8 weeks after a discectomy without fusion. A more extensive discectomy with laminectomy and fusion requires a more prolonged restriction from activities and usually would preclude contact activities in persons undergoing multiple level fusion.[20] As with many other issues in medicine, the optimal time period for activity restrictions is not clarified and clinical judgment remains the moniker of reason.

Fractures

Fractures of the osseus elements of the lumbar spine, fortunately, occur infrequently in athletics. They are most common in high-velocity, high-impact sports. Therefore, the index of suspicion needs to be higher in activities such as football, skiing, biking, and so forth. Obviously, severe fractures resulting in neurologic compromise are a medical emergency and the role of the primary care physician is to stabilize the spine and transport the patient to an appropriate medical facility for further evaluation in a timely fashion. Less severe, stable fractures also occur. These include compression fractures and nondisplaced transverse and spinous process fractures. Most of these injuries can be treated conservatively, yet rest and activity restriction, especially with compression fractures, is very important. Compression fractures usually necessitate 8 to 12 weeks of protection from contact and axial loading lest a stable, neurologically intact lesion be converted to a burst fracture with neurologic compromise.

Other Conditions

The aforementioned specific problems account for the majority of low back pain in younger athletes but other entities exist that can result in low back pain in physically active patients. Obviously, not all the specific entities that can cause low back pain can be detailed in this chapter but the more common conditions include inflammatory spondylitis (e.g., ankylosing spondylitis), degenerative disc disease, osteoarthritis, infection, and neoplasm. Although not specific to athletes, all may occur in athletically active individuals. These conditions are not discussed here, but clinicians should keep them in mind when evaluating patients whose sports-related back pain does not fit the disorders described earlier.

References

1. Hockberger RS: Meeting the challenge of low back pain. *Emerg Med* 22:99,1990.
2. Panjabi MM, White III AA: *Clinical Biomechanics of the Spine*, 2nd ed. Philadelphia: JB Lippincott; 1990.
3. Hoppenfeld S: *Physical Examination of the Spine and Extremities.* New York: Appleton-Century-Crofts; 1976.
4. Schamm S, Taylor T: Tension signs in lumbar disc prolapse. *Clin Orthop* 75:195, 1971.
5. Deckey JE, Weidenbaum M: The thoracic and lumbar spine. In: Scuderi GR, McCann PD, Bruno PJ (eds): *Sports Medicine. Principles of Primary Care.* St. Louis: Mosby; 1997;202.
6. Bigos SJ, Deyo RA, Romanowski TS, et al: The new thinking on low-back pain. *Patient Care* 29: 140, 1995.
7. Jenkins EM, Borenstein DG: Exercise for the low back pain patient. *Ballieres Clin Rheumatol* 8:191, 1994.
8. Harvey J, Tanner S: Low back pain in young athletes. A practical approach. *Sports Med* 12:394, 1991.
9. Keene JS, Albert MJ, Springer SL, et al: Back injuries in college athletes. *J Spinal Disord* 2:190, 1989.
10. Hart LGH, Deyo RA, Cherkin DC: Physician office visits for low back pain: frequency, clinical evaluation, and treatment patterns from a U.S. national survey. *Spine* 20:11, 1995.
11. Brigham CD, Schafer MF: Low back pain in athletes. *Adv Sports Med Fitness* 1:145, 1988.
12. Bigos SJ, Bowyer OR, Braen GR, et al: *Acute Low Back Problems in Adults: Clinical Practice Guideline, Number 14.* Agency for Health Care Policy and Research publication No. 953. Rockville, MD: Public Health Service, U.S. Dept of Health and Human Services, Dec 1994.
13. Deyo RA, Diehl AK, Rosenthal M: How many days of bed rest for acute low back pain? A randomized clinical trial. *N Engl J Med* 315:10640, 1986.
14. Malmivaara A, Hakkinen U, Aro T, et al: The treatment of acute low back pain: Bed rest, exercises, or ordinary activity? *N Engl J Med* 332:351, 1995.

15. Flemming JE: Spondylolysis and spondylolisthesis in the athlete. In: Hochschuler SH (ed): *The Spine in Sports*. Philadelphia; Hanley & Belfus; 1990; 101.

16. Alexander MJ: Biomechanical aspects of lumbar spine injuries in athletes: A review. *Can J Appl Sport Sci* 10:1, 1985.

17. Thomas, JC Jr: Plain roentgenograms of the spine in the injured athlete. *Clin Sports Med* 5:353, 1986.

18. Dubousset J: Treatment of spondylolysis and spondylolisthesis in children and adolescents. *Clin Orthop Rel Res* 337:77, 1997.

19. Stewart TD: The age incidence of neural arch defects in Alaskan native considered from the standpoint of etiology. *J Bone Joint Surg (Am)* 35: 937, 1953.

20. Eismont FJ, Kitchel SH: Thoracolumbar Spine. In: DeLee JC, Drez D (eds): *Orthopaedic Sports Medicine: Principles and Practice*. Philadelphia: WB Saunders; 1994;1018.

21. Micheli LJ, Couzens GS: How I manage low-back pain in athletes. *Phys Sportsmed* 21:183, 1993.

22. Johnson RJ: Low-back pain in sports: Managing spondylolysis in young patients. *Phys Sportsmed* 21:3, 1993.

23. Letts M, Smallman T, Afanasiev R, et al: Fracture of the pars interarticularis in adolescent athletes: A clinical-biomechanical analysis. *J Pediatr Orthop* 6:40, 1986.

24. Rossi F: Spondylolysis, spondylolisthesis, and sports. *J Sports Med Phys Fitness* 18:317, 1988.

25. Steiner ME, Micheli LJ: Treatment of symptomatic spondylolysis and spondylolisthesis with the modified Boston brace. *Spine* 10:932, 1985.

26. Garry JP, McShane J. Lumbar spondylolysis and adolescent athletes. *J Fam Pract* 47 (2):145, 1998.

27. Blanda J, Bethem D, Moats W, et al: Defects of pars interarticularis in athletes: A protocal for nonoperative treatment. *J Spinal Disord* 6:406, 1993.

28. Bradford DS, Iza J: Repair of the defect in spondylolysis or minimal degrees of spondylolisthesis by segmental wire fixation and bone grafting. *Spine* 10:673, 1985.

29. Saal JA: Natural history and nonoperative treatment of lunbar disc herniation. *Spine* 21(suppl24): 2S, 1996.

30. Yancey RA, Micheli LJ: Thoracolumbar spine injuries in pediatric sports. In: Stanitski CL, DeLee JC, Drez D (eds): *Pediatric and Adolescent Sports Medicine*. Philadelphia: WB Saunders; 1994;162.

31. Boden SD, Wiesel SW: Lumbar spine imaging: Role in clinical decision making. *J Am Acad Orthop Surg* 4:238, 1996.

32. Haughton VM: MR imaging of the spine. *Radiology* 166:297, 1988.

33. Weber H. Lumbar disc herniation: A controlled, prospective study with ten years of observation. *Spine* 8:131, 1983.

34. White AH, Derby R, Wynne G: Epidural injections for the diagnosis and treatment of low-back pain. *Spine* 5:78, 1980.

35. Snoek W, Weber H, Jorgensen B: Double blind evaluation of extradural methyl prednisolone for herniated lumbar discs. *Acta Orthop Scand* 48:635, 1977.

Thomas D. Armsey, Jr.

Chapter
20

Stress Fractures

Overview

A "stress fracture" is a common overuse injury that occurs to a bone when subjected to repetitive, submaximal stress at a rate beyond the bone's ability to accommodate. Numerous factors, which are discussed later in this chapter, have been reported to significantly lower this pathologic threshold of bone and are considered predisposing factors for injury. Stress fractures are common in competitive and recreationally active athletes and can lead to significant morbidity if inadequately treated.

Despite the frequency with which stress fractures are diagnosed today, the true incidence of this injury is still relatively unclear in the athletic population. This is due, in part, to the fact that a stress fracture is not a discretely defined entity, but develops over an injury continuum, making it difficult to objectively categorize disease.

In general, the management of stress fractures consists of rest, as the cornerstone of treatment. By reducing activity, the mechanical stress applied to a bone is decreased to a level below the pathologic threshold, which allows the bone to undergo the process of healing. Although most stress fractures improve with rest and time, some are resistant to conservative means and should be treated aggressively.

As with all overuse injuries, stress fractures are preventable. By individualizing training regimens, addressing biomechanic abnormalities, and altering an athlete's hormonal and nutritional milieu, stress fractures can be avoided.

Historical Perspective

The first diagnosis of stress fracture is credited to a Prussian surgeon, Breithraupt, in 1855.[1] He diagnosed the fracture in the painful, swollen foot of a young military recruit forced to endure repetitive, submaximal stresses. Although the term "march fracture" was used, this was clearly the first diagnosed metatarsal stress fracture. Over the next 100 years, stress fractures were predominantly studied in the military population. It was not until 1958 that the first stress fracture was reported in an athlete.[2] Since that time, stress fractures have become well recognized and widely reported.

Epidemiology

Although descriptions of stress fractures in the athletic population have been widely published, insufficient data are available to compare the incidence of stress fractures in different sports. It is not possible to identify sports with the greatest risk of stress fractures because of the lack of sound epidemiologic data.

Currently, there are only two published studies that allow direct comparisons of annual stress fracture rates in collegiate sports.[3,4] These studies suggest that track athletes are at the highest risk of stress fractures, but, because neither study reported incidence in terms of exposure, frequency, duration, and intensity of activity, these results may not be valid. To date, only one study has prospectively reported stress fracture injury rates in terms of exposure, with an overall rate of 0.70 stress fractures per 1000 training hours among track and field athletes.[5] More research is necessary before true comparisons can be made about the incidence of stress fractures in different sports.

The sites of stress fractures, on the other hand, have been well studied. Clanton reported that up to 95 percent of stress fractures occurred in the lower extremity, with tibial stress fractures the most common.[6] Several other locations are

Table 20-1

Summary of the Anatomic Location of Stress Fractures (percent) in Athletes

REFERENCE	SPORT	TIBIA	FIBULA	METATARSAL	FEMUR	NAVICULAR
Goldberg, 1994	Multiple	18.9	12.1	25.9	10.0	NA
Johnson, 1994	Multiple	38.2	0	20.6	23.5	11.8
Bennell, 1996	Track	45.0	12.0	8.0	8.0	15.0
Brukner, 1996	Multiple	20.0	16.7	23.3	3.3	20.0

also common sites of stress fractures in athletes including the metatarsals, fibula, tarsal navicular, and femur. Results of the anatomic location of stress fractures as a percentage of the total number of stress fractures in athletes is summarized in Table 20–1.

Stress fractures comprise a large proportion of injuries in the athletic population and may lead to significant morbidity. Although most are reported as case series, it seems that stress fractures account for up to 15.6 percent of all injuries sustained by athletes.[7] Hulkko and Orava found that 77 percent of athletes with stress fractures reported symptoms only during training, 13 percent complained of symptoms with activities of daily living and only 10 percent required "sick leave."[8] A direct correlation seems to exist between time delay in diagnosis and time to recovery, meaning that early diagnosis and treatment may be important in decreasing morbidity.[9] Anatomic location of injury may also be useful in predicting morbidity. In a review of 320 stress fractures in athletes, Matheson found that the mean time to recovery was 12.8 weeks, with tarsal stress fractures taking the longest time to recover and femoral stress fractures the least.[10]

Although most reviews suggest that females have a disproportionately higher number of stress fractures than males, a gender difference has not been proven in athletes. Studies either show no difference between male and female athletes or a slightly increased risk for women. When incidence rates are expressed in terms of exposure, women sustain 0.86 stress fractures per 1000 training hours compared with 0.54 in men, which is not a statistically significant difference. These results show that gender may not inherently affect the risk of developing a stress fracture in athletes, but further research in this area is necessary.

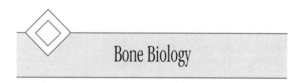

Bone Biology

Being a dynamic tissue, bone is in a constant state of change. Cycles of bone resorption and bone formation are continuously altering the mechanical properties of bone. This "remodeling" of bone is regulated intrinsically by local and systemic factors, as well as extrinsically by mechanical forces that combine to create a complex interplay between the regulatory factors and mechanical forces that determine the strength of bone.

During normal bone formation, osteoblasts synthesize a protein matrix of type I collagen and osteocalcin as a response to local mediators (namely, TGF-B, bone morphogenic protein, IGF I and II, PDGF, heparin-binding fibroblast growth factor).[11] This protein matrix is mineralized to form new bone, under strict control of 1,25 dihydroxyvitamin D. Bone resorption occurs with the same intricacies of bone formation. Osteoclasts demineralize bone and degrade the matrix through proton and proteolytic enzyme release. This process is controlled by many systemic hormones (PTH, calcitonin, 1,25 dihydroxyvitamin D, thyroid hormone, sex hormones) as well as numerous local factors (IL-1, TNF, lymphotoxin).[12] It is known that the resorptive phase takes only 7 to 10 days to complete, whereas new bone formation may take up to 3 months, thereby creating a window of vulnerability during which bone is susceptible to injury from lesser mechanical forces.

Although there are numerous intrinsic activities controlling the balance of bone resorption and formation, the mechanical forces imparted on bone may also alter this balance. First described in a series of articles by Julius Wolf in 1869, it was noted that stressed bone adapts by becoming more resistant to the stress. Carter and Caler later described the piezoelectric phenomena, which further defined stress as a compression or tension force.[13] In the piezoelectric model, compressive forces stimulate bone formation and tension forces stimulate bone resorption. Therefore, the effect that mechanical force has on a bone may lead to different outcomes dependent on the nature of the stress. More recently, Frost proposed the mechanostat theory of bone adaptation, which describes bone health on a continuum and accounts for both intrinsic and extrinsic factors.[14] This model may be used to explain the differences in stress fracture incidence among individuals subjected to similar training regimens. By taking into account an athlete's predisposing factors for injury, this model categorizes each athlete's unique physiologic loading zone, overload zone, and pathologic overload zone. When properly training, the athlete will remain in the overload zone, where adaptation by the musculoskeletal system will occur. If the athlete proceeds into the pathologic overload zone, the stress exceeds the body's ability to adapt and a stress injury occurs.

Clinical Considerations

History

Athletes with stress fractures complain of pain. This pain has an insidious onset and progressively worsens if the inciting stress is continued. The classical pain of overuse injuries can be categorized into stages, which may assist in treatment and prognosis. Initially, the pain of a stress fracture is apparent only after performing the inciting action, and it is relieved with rest (stage 1). The pain progresses so that at the initiation of the inciting action the pain begins, but does not affect performance (stage 2). The pain then continues to progress so that the pain compromises performance (stage 3). Finally, the pain is constant and even may occur during rest (stage 4). As previously mentioned, there is a direct correlation between when athletes are diagnosed and treated and when they return to pain-free activities.

Characteristically, athletes who sustain stress fractures will report a change in their training regimen in the 2 or 3 weeks prior to the onset of symptoms. So, a careful review of the athletes routine is essential, with special inquiry about any changes in duration, frequency, or intensity of activities. Theoretically, any increase in mechanical stress may surpass the athlete's overload zone, resulting in an inability to adapt, and a subsequent stress fracture.

When considering a stress fracture in females, it is imperative that a menstrual history be included. Delayed menarche has been associated with higher risk of stress fractures in ballet dancers and track athletes.[15] Secondary amenorrhea and oligomenorrhea also significantly increase an athlete's risk of stress injury (see Chap. 12).[16] Although the exact hormonal imbalance responsible for this increase in stress fracture rates is unknown, it is apparent that menstrual irregularities are correlated with a decrease in the pathologic overload threshold of bone.

The nutritional status of athletes must also be included in a focused history. Dietary calcium intake has a positive linear correlation with bone mineral density in athletes.[17] It has been reported that athletes who sustain stress fractures have lower intakes of calcium than those athletes without stress fractures, but the amount of dietary calcium necessary to significantly decrease the rate of stress fractures is still unknown. Currently, the National Institutes of Health (NIH) recommend 1500 mg/day for athletes with a history of menstrual irregularities, to maximize bone mineral density and potentially decrease the risk of stress fractures. Vitamin D intake may also prove noteworthy in regard to stress fractures in athletes, but there is little scientific evidence to elucidate its role in this process. Patterns of disordered eating and inadequate caloric intake are common in athletes and need to be addressed to avoid potentially profound bone loss. Retrospective studies have shown athletes with a history of stress fracture have significantly higher incidence of restrictive eating patterns and dieting.[18] But, the question still remains whether this is due to decreased "energy" necessary for bone repair or if it is due to an inadequate intake of a vital nutrient, or possibly a combination of both.

Physical Examination

The hallmark of stress fractures on physical examination is point tenderness on palpation of the affected bone. There may be localized swelling and erythema overlying the area of insult, but this is often apparent only late in the course of disease. Matheson reported that in athletes with bone scan-positive stress fractures, 66 percent had localized point tenderness and only 25 percent had any distinguishable swelling. With such a paucity of physical find-

ings, some pertinent negatives must also be included. In particular, if an athlete has atrophy, limited range of motion, or weakness, an alternative diagnosis should be considered.

Several provocative tests for stress fractures have been reported. The "hop test" has been described as a means to diagnose a femoral neck stress fracture. The "fulcrum test," in which a long bone is stressed over the examiner's bent knee, is used to diagnose femoral or tibial shaft stress fractures. Pain with hyperextension of the spine may indicate a stress fracture at the pars interarticularis. The "flamingo sign" is an extension of this test whereby the athlete hyperextends the spine while supporting body weight on only one leg; this may differentiate unilateral from bilateral spondylolysis. Although these maneuvers may assist in the diagnosis of stress fractures, adjunctive diagnostic studies are useful to clearly define the injury.

Ancillary Tests

When considering the diagnosis of a stress fracture, many advanced imaging techniques are available that provide insight into the spectrum of stress-related changes to bone. A logical initial assessment should include plain radiographs, which may show the stress fracture.

It has become increasingly recognized, however, that many significant injuries to bone may be initially, and in some cases, forever radiographically occult.[19] Previous studies in this regard have reported that stress fractures are not consistently visualized until 2 to 3 weeks after the initial pain onset.[20] At that point in the disease process, the stress fracture is evident as a periosteal reaction (Fig. 20-1). If no periostitis is visualized on plain films, either due to the time interval between injury and radiographic evaluation or location of the stress fracture, diagnostic studies with greater sensitivity are available.

Currently, the gold-standard for diagnosis of a

Figure 20-1

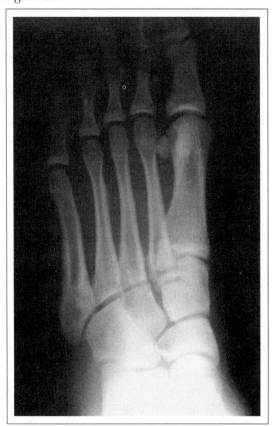

Periosteal reaction and callus formation at fourth metatarsal consistent with healing stress fracture.

stress fracture is a triple-phase bone scan (Fig. 20-2). It has been found that 95 percent of stress fractures in patients under 65 years of age can be demonstrated in the first day after injury and in 100 percent of patients by 3 days.[21] In addition to the diagnostic value of bone scans, these scans can also determine the approximate age of the stress injury and fracture healing can be monitored.[22] It has been noted that the radionuclide angiogram phase is only positive for the first 4 to 8 weeks with the blood pool phase being the next to revert to normal. The intensity of activity on delayed images decreases over 3 to 6 months, although minor abnormalities may persist up to 18 months. Due to the exceptional sensitivity that this study provides, it has been found that athletes will often demonstrate bone scan abnormalities without developing stress fractures. The most common condition being "shin splints," in which the radionuclide angiogram and blood pool phases are normal, but the delayed images demonstrate abnormalities involving the posterior cortex of the tibia. Therefore, the bone scan results must be correlated with the athlete's symptoms and physical findings to accurately assist in diagnosis.

An alternative diagnostic tool is magnetic res-

Figure 20-2

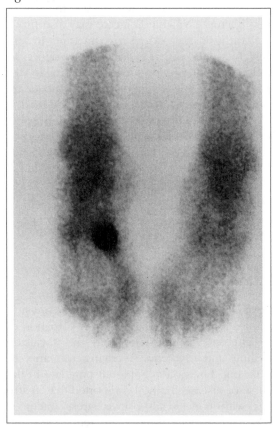

First metatarsal stress fracture in a 20-year-old runner. This bone scan was taken 3 days after the onset of pain and shows increased tracer uptake at the proximal first metatarsal. This injury was not visualized on plain radiographs.

onance imaging (MRI), which has become the primary technique for evaluating musculoskeletal injuries in athletes. It has comparative sensitivity to radionuclide techniques for detection of bone abnormalities, as well as, greater specificity.[23] In addition to visualizing stress response or fracture in bone, MRI demonstrates soft-tissue injury that is not otherwise detectable. With continued advances in technology and decreased cost of MRI, this technique could possibly challenge conventional radiography and radionuclide bone scans as the primary diagnostic tool for detection of stress injury to bone.

It is important to remember that standard x-rays in conjunction with a focused history and physical examination will be adequate to diagnose most stress fractures in athletes. Clinically, the high sensitivity of bone scan and MRI is necessary only when the diagnosis of stress fracture is in question or the exact location of the injury must be known to determine the treatment.

Site-Specific Stress Fractures

Tibia

The tibia is the most common location for a stress fracture in athletes. In a review of the literature, McBryde revealed that running was the most common activity associated with tibial stress fractures.[24] It has been shown that up to 25 percent of tibial stress fractures are due to training errors. The most common location of injury in "runners" is the posterior medial border at the junction of the middle and distal third of the tibia, whereas "jumpers" tend to injure the proximal and anterior areas of the tibia (Fig. 20-3). The vast majority of these fractures are visible on x-ray as a periosteal reaction.

Tibial stress fractures can be safely and effectively treated in a pneumatic leg brace (i.e., air cast).[25] The athlete may continue exercising, but

modifications of the training routine must be made to maintain pain-free activities. Partial weight-bearing with crutches is sometimes necessary in athletes who continue to complain of pain in the air cast, but this is the exception rather than the rule.

Figure 20-3

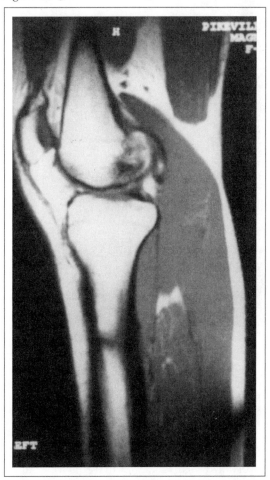

17-year-old female basketball player who complained of left knee pain with increasing intensity over the last 6 days. Physical examination revealed point tenderness at the proximal medial tibia with a positive "fulcrum test." Plain x-rays were negative, MRI revealed increased signal of the proximal tibia medullary cavity consistent with a compression-sided proximal tibial stress fracture. She was treated conservatively with pneumatic bracing and modification of activities and returned to pain-free activity in 4 weeks.

Figure 20-4

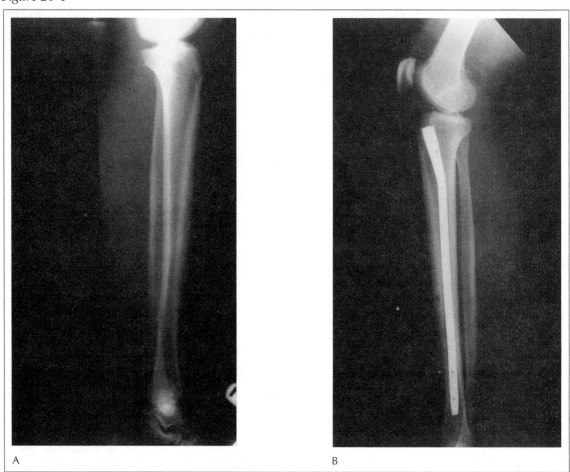

A   B

(**A**) A 17-year-old female collegiate cheerleader complained of intermittent shin pain and swelling for several months. The pain finally progressed to the point that the athlete was unable to ambulate without a limp. Point tenderness and swelling was noted overlying the anterior tibia. The "dreaded black line" was noted on radiographs. (**B**) An intramedullary nail was placed and the athlete returned to activities within 4 weeks.

Although most of these injuries do well with conservative management, there is one tibial stress fracture that needs much more aggressive management. Described radiographically as "the dreaded black line" (Fig. 20-4A), the anterior tibial cortex stress fracture has proven very difficult to manage without surgical intervention.[26] This is a result of extreme tension forces that occur across the anterior tibial cortex, which prevents adequate healing and may progress to non-

union. Currently, treatment with intramedullary rodding of the tibia (Fig. 20-4B) has proven to return athletes to activity faster and with more consistent results than any conservative management.[27,28]

Metatarsal

Stress fractures in the metatarsals are very common in athletes and usually are associated with running and dancing. The pain progresses along the stages previously described. Described as dull and achy, this pain is located in the midfoot or forefoot. The most usual location is the second metatarsal shaft, which is subjected to 3 to 4 times body weight during loading and push-off phases of gait.[29] These forces are even more extreme in a Morton's foot, in which the second metatarsal is the longest shaft.[30] Another structural variant found to increase the incidence of metatarsal stress fractures is the flexible, flat foot. Kinetically, the "flat foot" absorbs stress in the muskuloskeletal structures of the foot, versus the "cavus foot," which is rigid and passes the stress onto the tibia and femur.

Clinically, these injuries present as areas of point tenderness overlying the metatarsal shaft. An x-ray is usually adequate to document a metatarsal stress fracture, which is visualized as a periosteal reaction of the affected bone (Fig. 20-5). Bone scan and MRI have improved sensitivity and specificity if the diagnosis is in question.

These injuries may be treated symptomatically, allowing the athlete to continue activities that are not painful. Usually, immobilization is necessary for a limited time, which can be accomplished via a steel shank insole or a stiff, wooden-soled type shoe. Occasionally, a below-the-knee walking cast or removable walking boot is needed if the forefoot is severely painful. Although 4 weeks of rest is usually sufficient for healing, athletes may be allowed to continue modified conditioning with non-weight-bearing exercises (i.e., swimming and pool running), followed by cycling and stair-climbing. The athlete's training schedule should be scrutinized and adapted to prevent another overuse injury.

Although most metatarsal stress fractures respond well to conservative management, stress injuries to the proximal fifth metatarsal have a significant incidence of delayed and nonunion.[31] Due to potential morbidity of this injury in athletes, surgical treatment with percutaneous screw fixation is currently recommended.[32]

Figure 20-5

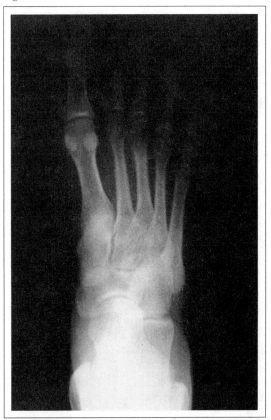

A 33-year-old recreational runner complained of forefoot pain for 6 weeks. She was training for a marathon and had increased her training program 2 weeks prior to the onset of pain. Physical examination revealed a thin, white female with a flexible, flat foot. Point tenderness was present overlying the distal shaft of the third metatarsal. X-ray shows a periosteal reaction at the distal shaft of the third metatarsal.

Femur

Stress fractures that occur in the femur may present in various locations, most notably in the femoral shaft or the femoral neck. This injury is mainly found in distance runners, jumpers, and ballet dancers. To diagnose this injury, the clinician must consider femoral shaft stress fracture in the differential diagnosis of pain in the thigh region or pain referred to the hip or groin (Fig. 20-6).

Figure 20-6

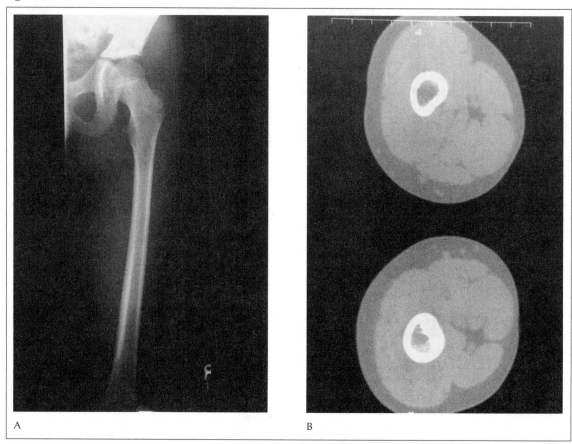

(**A**) X-ray findings of posterior cortical thickening in a 10-year-old soccer player with thigh pain. Although these findings are consistent with a femoral shaft stress fracture, the athlete required further testing due to his age and his intolerance to weight-bearing. (**B**) A CT scan was performed to further assess the femur of this 10-year-old child. It shows obvious cortical thickening of the posterior femur with a linear lucency, consistent with a healing stress fracture. The young athlete was placed on crutches with toe-touch weight-bearing progressing to full weight-bearing over 2 weeks. He modified his activities to pain for the next 2 weeks and returned to athletics in 4 weeks.

If the diagnosis is considered, an x-ray may reveal the injury as a periosteal elevation, usually at the junction of the proximal and middle thirds of the femur. This anatomic location is the origin of the vastus medialis and the insertion of the adductor brevis, implicating traction from these muscles as a causative factor in femoral shaft stress fractures. Due to the location and radiographic appearance, it may be mistaken for a malignant tumor, in which case, a CT scan or MRI is necessary to elucidate the nature of the lesion.[33] The fulcrum test has been reported to assist the early diagnosis of this fracture.[34]

Most femoral shaft stress fractures are successfully treated with a period of rest followed by gradual return to activities. More specifically, a rest period of 1 to 4 weeks (partial-weight-bearing progressing to full-weight-bearing as tolerated), followed by low-impact activities (swimming and cycling), and finally, resumption of high-impact exercise allows return to competitive athletics in 8 to 16 weeks.

Unlike most overuse injuries, stress fractures of the femoral neck have a high complication rate if untreated. Presenting as pain in the groin, anterior thigh, or knee, this stress fracture can be missed if not considered in the differential diagnosis. The pain is exacerbated with weight-bearing (i.e., hop test) as well as internal rotation at the hip. Due to the potential complications that may result from this injury, imaging studies are necessary to assure the correct diagnosis. Plain radiographs will often detect the periosteal reaction, but currently, MRI and bone scans are the tests of choice for early diagnosis of femoral neck stress fractures.

As described by Devas, femoral neck stress fractures can occur as two distinct entities based on the anatomic location of injury (Fig. 20-7).[35] The compression fractures are more common in young athletes, with the injury limited to the inferior part of the femoral neck. If nondisplaced, these are treated with rest until the athlete is free of pain and the hip regains full motion. Non-weight-bearing is maintained until radiographic evidence of healing is complete. If these fractures progress or fail to heal with conservative management, then internal fixation may be necessary. In striking contrast, tension-sided femoral neck stress fractures should be acutely treated with internal fixation due to the high likelihood of progression to displacement and the subsequent risk of avascular necrosis of the femoral head.

Tarsal Navicular

Stress fractures involving the tarsal navicular are uncommon in athletes but are also probably under diagnosed. Torg reported a mean interval of 7 months between onset of pain and diagnosis.[36] Due to this significant delay in diagnosis, it has been difficult to determine an accurate incidence of injury.

Figure 20-7

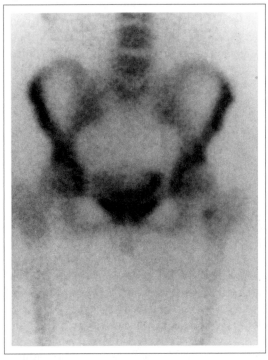

Bone scan of a 25-year-old collegiate runner with left groin pain. Pain was exacerbated with one-legged hopping and passive internal rotation. X-rays were negative. The bone scan shows abnormal uptake at the compression side of the femoral neck. The athlete modified her activities and was cleared to return to collegiate athletics in 6 weeks.

Athletes who participate in basketball, football, and track seem to sustain the most tarsal navicular stress fractures. The presenting complaints usually include an insidious onset of vague midfoot pain. Tenderness on palpation of the dorsum of the midfoot or the medial longitudinal arch, should prompt further evaluation. Radiographs plus bone scan or MRI, are usually necessary to diagnose this stress fracture.

Uncomplicated, partial fractures and complete nondisplaced fractures of the tarsal navicular should be treated by immobilization in a non-weight-bearing cast for 6 to 8 weeks. Return to weight-bearing activities is guided by radiographic evidence of healing and the athlete's clinical picture. Complete, displaced fractures are treated with open reduction and internal fixation followed by cast immobilization and non-weight bearing for 6 weeks. Although these treatment plans may seem extreme for an athlete with stress fracture, the data is clear that without non-weight-bearing cast immobilization, these injuries do not consistently heal.[37]

Conclusion

Whenever a young healthy-appearing athlete is diagnosed with a stress fracture, a thorough history must be obtained, including a detailed nutritional and menstrual assessment. Is the athlete restricting calories? Avoiding dairy products and protein due to fat content? Using laxatives or diet pills? These questions may reveal an underlying eating disorder that if recognized and treated early, may significantly benefit the athlete throughout his or her entire lifetime. Simple modifications, such as calcium or estrogen supplementation, may decrease the rate of recurrence of stress fractures, as well as improve overall bone health in the athlete.

In addition to dietary and hormonal factors, an athlete's training routine must be evaluated. Is the athlete increasing activities in a cyclical progression? Is there adequate time available for physiologic adaptation to the increasing stress? Does the athlete participate in cross training? Individualizing each athlete's conditioning program is essential because no two athletes adapt in exactly the same manner.

Finally, education of athletes, parents, coaches, and trainers is necessary for effective management and prevention of these injuries. As previously noted, when a stress fracture is diagnosed early in the course of the disease, the athlete returns to play sooner. Therefore, recognizing the signs and symptoms of these injuries

can assist in early intervention and decreased morbidity.

References

1. Breithraupt MD: Zur pathologie des menschlichen fusses. *Med Zeitung* 24:169, 1855.
2. Devas MB: Stress fractures of the tibia in athletes or "shin soreness." *J Bone Joint Surg* 40B:227, 1958.
3. Goldberg B, Pecora C: Stress fractures: A risk of increased training in freshmen. *Physician Sportsmed* 22:68, 1994.
4. Johnson AW, Weiss CB, Wheeler DL: Stress fractures of the femoral shaft in athletes—More common than expected: A new clinical test. *Am J Sports Med* 22:248, 1994.
5. Bennell KL, Malcolm SA, Thomas SA, et al: The incidence and distribution of stress fractures in competitive track and field athletes. *Am J Sports Med* 24:211, 1996.
6. Clanton T, Solcher B: Chronic leg pain in the athlete. *Clin Sports Med* 13:743, 1994.
7. James SL, Bates BT, Osternig LR: Injuries to runners. *Am J Sports Med* 6:40, 1978.
8. Hulkko A, Orava S: Stress fractures in athletes. *Int J Sports Med* 8:221, 1987.
9. Benazzo F, Barnabei G, Ferrario A, et al: Stress fractures in track and field athletes. *J Sports Traumatol Rel Res* 14:51, 1992.
10. Matheson GO, Clement DB, McKenzie DC, et al: Stress fractures in athletes: A study of 320 cases. *Am J Sports Med* 15:46, 1987.
11. Hauschka PV, Maurakos AE, Iafrati MD, et al: Growth factors in bone matrix, isolation of multiple types by affinity chromatography on heparin-sepharose. *J Biol Chem* 261:12665, 1986.
12. Mundy GR: Cytokines and local factors which affect osteoclast function. *Int J Cell Cloning* 10:215, 1992.
13. Carter DR, Caler WE: A cumulative damage model for bone fracture. *J Ortho Res* 3:84, 1985.
14. Frost HM: A new direction for osteoporosis research: A review and proposal. *Bone* 12:429, 1991.
15. Bennell KL, Malcolm SA, Thomas SA, et al: Risk factors for stress fractures in female track and field

athletes: A retrospective analysis. *Clin J Sports Med* 5:229, 1995.

16. Barrow GW, Saha S: Menstrual irregularity and stress fractures in collegiate female distance runners. *Am J Sports Med* 16:209, 1988.

17. Wolman RL, Clark P, McNally E, et al: Menstrual state and exercise as determinants of spinal trabecular bone density in female athletes. *Br Med J* 301:518, 1990.

18. Frusztajer NT, Dhupar S, Warren MP, et al: Nutrition and the incidence of stress fractures in ballet dancers. *Am J Clin Nutr* 51:779, 1990.

19. Anderson MW, Greenspan A: Stress fractures. *Radiology* 199:1, 1996.

20. Meyer SA, Saltzman CL, Albright JP: Stress fractures of the foot and leg. *Clin Sports Med* 12:395, 1993.

21. Matin P: The appearance of bone scans following fractures including immediate and long term studies. *J Nucl Med* 20:1227, 1979.

22. Roub LW, Gumerman LW, Hanley EN, et al: Bone stress: A radionuclide imaging perspective. *Radiology* 132:431, 1979.

23. Martin SD, Healey JH, Horowitz S: Stress fracture: MRI. *Orthopedics* 16:75, 1993.

24. McBryde, AM: Stress fractures in athletes. *J Sports Med* 3:212, 1975.

25. Swenson EJ, Dehaven KE, Sebastianelli WJ, et al: The effect of pneumatic leg brace on return to play in athletes with tibial stress fractures. *Am J Sports Med* 25:322, 1997.

26. Reddick AC, Shelbourne KD, McCarrol JR, et al: The natural history and treatment of delayed union stress fractures of the anterior cortex of the tibia. *Am J Sports Med* 16:250, 1988.

27. Barrick EF, Jackson CV: Prophylactic intramedullary fixation of the tibia for stress fractures in the professional athlete. *J Orthop Trauma* 6:241, 1992.

28. Knapp TP, Mandelbaum BR: Stress fractures. In: Garret WE (ed): *The U.S. Soccer Sports Medicine Book*. Baltimore: Williams & Wilkins; 1996.

29. Eisele S, Sammarco GJ: Fatigue fractures of the foot and ankle in the athlete. *J Bone Joint Surg* 75A:290, 1993.

30. Rodgers MM: Dynamic biomechanics of the normal foot and ankle during walking and running. *Phys Ther* 68:1822, 1988.

31. Stewart IM: Jones' fracture: Fracture at the base of the fifth metatarsal. *Clin Orthop* 16:190, 1960.

32. Kavanaugh JH, Brower TD, Mann RV: The Jones fracture revisited. *J Bone Joint Surg* 60A:776, 1978.

33. Burks RT, Sutherland DH: Stress fracture of the femoral shaft in children: Report of two cases and discussion. *J Pediatr Orthop* 4:614, 1984.

34. Johnson AW, Weiss CB, Wheeler DL: Stress fractures of the femoral shaft in athletes more common than expected: A new clinical test. *Am J Sports Med* 22:248, 1994.

35. Devas MB: Stress fractures of the femoral neck. *J Bone Joint Surg* 47B:728, 1965.

36. Torg JS, Pavlov H, Cooley LH, et al: Stress fractures of the tarsal navicular. *J Bone Joint Surg* 64A(5):700, 1982.

37. Khan KM, Fuller PJ, Brukner PD, et al: Outcome of conservative and surgical management of navicular stress fractures in athletes. *Am J Sports Med* 20:657, 1992).

Index

Page numbers followed by "t" indicate tables; page numbers in italics indicate figures.

441

NOTES

NOTES

NOTES

NOTES

NOTES

NOTES

NOTES

NOTES

NOTES

DATE DUE